Medical Ethics

Raimondo G. Russo

Medical Ethics

Springer

Raimondo G. Russo
Milano, Italy

ISBN 978-3-031-42443-4 ISBN 978-3-031-42444-1 (eBook)
https://doi.org/10.1007/978-3-031-42444-1

Translation from the Italian language edition: "Etica Medica" by Raimondo G. Russo, © Nuova Editrice Medica e Scientifica 2020. Published by Nuova Editrice Medica e Scientifica. All Rights Reserved.

This Springer imprint is published by the registered company Springer Nature Switzerland AG
The registered company address is: Gewerbestrasse 11, 6330 Cham, Switzerland

To Aunt Anna and Uncle Giorgio

Foreword I

Ethics is a "big word" that spans millennia. It comes from *éthos*, which in the language of Hippocrates means "behavior" and which, according to Aristotle, defines *tà ethikà*, "moral things" (in Latin *mores*). It is linked to a high value concept of human action since the origins of ancient Greek thought, where philosophy was tripartite in the knowledge of *physis*, *logos*, and *ethikos*.

Physiology had, as its object, the natural world (including the nature of man); logic had as its object the discourse on the ideas of metaphysics (in Plato) and on the concepts of gnoseology (in Aristotle); ethics, finally, dealt with the forms, ways, and means of human actions. Among these, in the first place, there were the civil and political ones (with Pericles), educational and dialogic ones (with Socrates), and the curative ones of Hippocratic medicine. From then on, the "art of healing"—*techne iatriké*—is inscribed, as well as in a methodology and epistemology of its own, in an area of values that include virtues, duties, utilities, and rights.

Aristotle (384–322 B.C.) consolidates a tradition centered on *arete*, in Latin *virtus*, which arrives at the tetralogy of the "cardinal virtues"—fortitude, prudence, temperance, justice—considered cornerstones of the "good life and good death," that is, of living and dying in the ways most suited to the rational nature of the human being. Reflecting on "what is good" and "what is right," Epicurus (241–271 B.C.), in line with his ideal of wisdom, interprets the virtues as attitudes and habits aimed at an "*ataraxic*" life, devoid of turmoil, freed from fear of gods and death.

In the Middle Ages, the theory of virtues is filtered by the sancta doctrina of Thomas Aquinas (1224–1270) who fixes Aristotelian ethics and the moral philosophy of Seneca (4–65 A.D.) and Galen in the role of *ancilla fidei* (130–200 A.D.): *salus* is not only corporal "health," but also and above all spiritual "salvation." A different way of dealing with ethical problems has historically established itself on the basis of the idea of duty.

In the late eighteenth-century Age of Enlightenment, "enlightened" reason makes clear the duties that, having brought "reason within the limits of pure" reason—as Immanuel Kant (1724–1804) wrote in 1793—man finds conscience: "Act as if the maxim of your action should be elevated by your will to universal law." The theory and practice of duties come to constitute deontology, as dating back to the work of the English jurist Jeremy Bentham (1748–1832) entitled "Deontology, or the Science of Morality." With Bentham, the "ethics of principles," founded on virtues, is replaced by the "ethics of consequences," based on results. He is the philosopher of "utilitarianism": the criterion of utility, which is the foundation of moral judgments and the rules of civil coexistence, implies that in seeking the greatest possible good or well-being, the quantity of pleasure is maximized and the quantity reduced to a minimum pain, taking into account the harmful consequences of selfishness and those instead useful for the renunciation of one's own pleasures, compensated by the benefits deriving from the same renunciation by others.

Ethical thought is on the threshold of an era in which "moral" is also assuming the meaning of "social": 30 years after Bentham, the English economist John Stuart Mill (1806–1873), in his work *Utilitarianism*, expresses the golden rule of associated living, which makes good coincide with the greatest possible happiness for the greatest number of people.

Alongside duty, there is another word that resounds in the nineteenth century echoing the "Declaration of the rights of man and citizen," promulgated in 1789 by the French Revolution: the word "law."

In 1990 Norberto Bobbio, a master of ethics and ideas, periodized the age of rights in four successive generations, articulated over the last two centuries: the first three are attributable to the revolutionary message of 1989, the fourth to today's thought. The first generation contemplated individual rights under the banner of liberty, the second the social rights under the banner of egality, the third the rights to solidarity under the banner of fraternity.

Fourth is the current generation that contemplates political and ecological rights, such as the right to peace and protection of the environment and the rights deriving from the problems due to the impact of today's science and technology with human life and which constitute the field of "bioethics." Bioethics is a word that makes its appearance in 1970, coined by Van Resselaer Potter as a "bridge to the future" to define the disciplinary area where the moral and normative problems of the life sciences are drawn and to indicate that every present and future scientific-technical achievement in the fields of biology and medicine must be used to improve the quality of life and nothing else. It broadens the area of deontology applied to medicine, as the French physician Maximilien-Isidor Simon had done in 1845 in his work Déontologie Médicale, which contemplated, with duties, "the rights of doctors in the current state of our [nineteenth century] civilization." As is well known, in the area of bioethics various "questions of life" can be distinguished: first of all, questions of the beginning and end of life, ranging from the status of the human embryo and the modalities of assisted procreation and fertilization to therapeutic persistence and to active and passive euthanasia.

Follow the questions of ethics of everyday life, ranging from the "dual" relationship between the caregiver and the cure to the "plural" relationship between doctor and community, then the ethics of biological and clinical experimentation and finally the questions of economic, bio-juridical, and biopolitical ethics, concerning inter alia the just distribution and allocation of available resources.

These presentation pages are intended to provide a historical frame to the large picture that Raimondo G. Russo offers to the readers of this book entitled *Medical*

Ethics which he crosses with meticulous precision and critical rigor the bases and the development of Medical Ethics in centuries' for better clarity.

The author, doctor, with multiple experiences in scientific research and pharmacovigilance, in Italy and abroad, undertakes a challenging and important historiographical itinerary that starts from before Hippocrates to zigzag between Greeks, Romans, Byzantines, and Barbarians, to then take us to the extreme, medium, and the Near East, going back from the charitable contribution of the Christian Middle Ages to the contemporary contribution of Arabs and Jews, and then leading us into the centuries of modernity, confronting opposing ethical-political ideologies and finally arriving at the life issues that all of us, men and women today, experience in the full and residual life that is reserved for us.

The book keeps what it promises, and for this recognition and praise must be given to its Author.

Historian of Medical Thought and Biosciences
Vita-Salute San Raffaele University,
Milan, Italy

Giorgio Cosmacini

Foreword II

Raimondo Russo's book is an outstanding achievement with its combination of extraordinarily wide coverage of his topic combined with fascinating detail and commentaries. Ethics in medicine, with more than 2000 years of history, still arouses debate, even though its recommendations are not only accepted throughout most of the modern world, but most doctors take an oath to observe them, using terms that Hippocrates himself would recognize. The book compares attitudes dictated by laws, religions, and centuries of common usage, in countries and regions widely differing in their climates, levels of development and education, and health services, from the earliest centuries before Christ, in China and Egypt, to modern discoveries that have themselves posed, and are posing—ethical questions. Bioethics, that "bridge to the future," has been tackled by various committees and organizations—including an Italian Bioethical Committee—and it is astounding to see how little the basic opinions on ethics in medicine differ. This book provides admirable coverage of all these questions, and the author is to be congratulated for his research and this informative result.

Mario Negri Institute
Milan, Italy

Silvio Garattini,

Foreword III

This book, which focuses on ethical questions, always prevalent in the medical profession, finds some answers and underlines not only the deontology expressing its values and tasks. Ethics in medicine is viewed here from various angles, almost always founded on respect for the dignity of the person. Today's scientific and ethical approaches tend to converge in what is called bioethics. Raimondo Russo cites the most commonly accepted definition, that of Warren T. Reich, 1978: "The systematic study of human conduct in the area of life sciences and health the light of moral values and principles." In these pages one senses the culture and the desire to have the doctor return to his function and role "at times to cure, often to relieve, always to comfort." Doctors, sociologists, and ordinary citizens often ask: "What is a doctor, what is special about medical ethics?" The book closely looks at medical ethics over the centuries and in various parts of the world. The first principle was set down by Hippocrates: "I will make use of the regimen (of medicine) to help the sick according to my strength and my judgment, but I will refrain from causing harm and injustice." Since those distant times, doctors virtually everywhere still take this Oath at graduation. The book highlights the modernity of what Hippocrates did for the medical profession. The medical profession is closely intertwined with the right to life and the protection of health, now universally recognized in Western countries, and reflected in Article 32 of the Italian Constitution. The author deals systematically with the ethics of the doctor-patient relationship, and the careful choice of topics gives both historical and descriptive information. Some statements in the book are still very topical today. In medical times ethics was initially a matter of classical medical etiquette together with Christian ethics. The attitudes of other religions and in other epochs cast interesting light on this age-old question, and the similarities are striking. Common features are belief in the figure of a God, and Fate. The art of healing has always been part of man's development, and the chapters dedicated to various institutions are very informative, listing Ethics Committees such as the Nuffield Council on Bioethics, and many others. Regrettably, during the Covid-19 pandemic ethics sometimes got lost under the pressure on doctors and medical staff and facilities. Raimondo Russo points to some of the main tasks of medical ethics in the third millennium: (1) to define ethical issues arising from recent advances in biological and medical research and to foresee, and address, public concerns; (2) to investigate and report on these issues in a form that facilitates public understanding and informed debate; (3) always to seek expert analysis and ensure transparency and reliable publication. The author's analysis of all the medical ethical implications from prehistory to the present day offers the doctor unprecedented cultural enrichment, his ethics, and his profession.

Raimondo's fine and learned book illustrates that life is Man's highest good, and requires the Doctor's ethical fidelity to respect all the natural stages of human existence. Someone like me who has done this job for many years can only recommend reading this enjoyable and fascinating book and reflecting on all the ethically sensitive topics: a better doctor and a better man will come out of it. After all, as the author stresses, the book wants to boost the knowledge of medical ethics and a doctor reading it will be stimulated to ensure better ethical behavior in daily medical practice.

Federation of Italian Medico-Scientific Societies Antonino Mazzone,
Milan, Italy

"Make sure that the principal of your actions becomes a universal law of human conduct"
—Immanuel Kant[1]

[1] "Handle so, daß die Maxime deines Willens jederzeit zugleich als Prinzip einer allgemeinen Gesetzgebung gelten könne." § 7 Grundgesetz der reinen praktischen Vernunft in der KpV, S. 54.

Acknowledgments

I am indebted to Prof. Giorgio Cosmacini, Prof. Silvio Garattini, and Prof. Nino Mazzone for the forewords they kindly prepared, and to other scholars who have provided me with valuable indications and suggestions to allow a drafting as faithful as possible to a moral and historical basis. For these reasons I thank my friend Mr. Diego Fiacchino who assisted me, step by step, in the revision of the text and the inevitable corrections to be made.

Last but not least, my thanks go to Dr. Judith Baggott, who assisted me with the translation of the text into proper English.

Contents

1 **Introduction** 1
References 4

2 **Medical Ethics Before Hippocrates** 5
Egypt 5
Mesopotamia 8
India 11
References 17

3 **Hippocrates and Greece** 21
Pre-Hippocratic Medicine 22
The Basics of Medical Ethics 22
Hippocrates 23
Hippocrates and Medicine 24
Hippocrates and Medical Conduct 26
Ethics in the Oath 26
Main Historical Stages of the Oath 27
White Coat Ceremony 28
Below Are a Few Versions of the Hippocratic Oath for Comparison . . 29
Hippocratic Oath and Code of Ethics 33
Comments and Considerations 34
Importance in Time 36
Some of His Aphorisms 36
Hippocrates in Recent Times 37
Hippocrates in Ecclesiastical Writings 37
Oppositions to the Oath 38
Other Comments 40
Review of the Hippocratic Oath ? 41
In Conclusion 43
References 43

4 **Rome, Barbarians, and Medieval Codes** 47
Morals and Medical Ethics 49
Romans: Public and Private Health 51
Barbarians 52

Medical-Assistential Codes in the Middle Ages 56
Fourth to Fifteenth Century A.D. 56
Doctors and Patients 57
The Beginnings of Medical Ethics 58
Salerno Medical School 61
Health and Disease 62
The Apothecaries 62
References 64

5 Far East: China 67
More Data on TCM 71
Confucianism 73
Influence of Confucianism in Chinese Medical Ethics 74
Moral Education 75
Ancient Chinese Medical Ethics (ACME) 75
Other Notes 76
Medical Writings and Medical Ethics 80
Teaching 80
The Purpose of Medical Practice 81
What Is Required to Be a Great Doctor 81
After Sun Simiao 81
Medical Ethics 82
Japan 85
The Seventeen Rules of Enjuin (Twenty-Fifth Century A.D.) and Notes of Medical Ethics 85
Seventeen Rules of Enjuin 86
Ethics 87
The Influence of Japanese Culture 88
References 88

6 Near and Middle East 91
Israel 91
Jewish Medicine and Ethics 91
Jewish Medical Ethics 95
Basic Principles 95
Sources of Medical Ethics 95
Distinctive Criteria 96
Halakhah 96
Law for Gentiles 99
In Conclusion 99
Oath of Asaph the Doctor and Yohanan Ben Zabda 100
Asaph's Oath 102
Abukrat (Hippocrates)'s Moral Precepts: Twelfth Century 104
The Moral Precepts Attributed to Hippocrates (Considered to Be the Right) 104
Comparison with the Original Hippocratic Text 105

Islam (2) 106
History and Ethics of Muslim Medicine, Eightieth to Twelfth Century 106
Moral Commandments of the Koran 108
Guiding Principles of Islamic Law 109
Medicine 109
Ethics. 110
Origin of Ethical Principles 110
Medical Ethics 111
In Conclusion 113
Muslim Doctors 114
The Doctor–Patient Relationship 115
Doctors' Ethics 116
List of (8) Major Muslim Doctors 117
The Chapters of Adab al-Tabib by al-Ruhawi 119
Other Islamic Doctors, Subsequently 123
Maimonides and Medicine 124
His Death 124
His Works 127
Medical Ethics in Maimonides 128
Marcus Herz 129
Arab Medicine, After Maimonides 130
The Islamic Perspective 132
More Critical Remarks 133
Islamic Code of Medical Ethics, 1981 136
The Doctor's Oath, 2005, Kuwait 136
Character of The Doctor 137
The Patient 138
The Islamic Oath. 139
Turkey (3) 141
Islamic Bioethics. 142
References. 144

7 Portugal, Italy, England 147
Amatus Lusitanus 147
Sixteenth Century (Portugal) 147
Jewish Doctors in Italy 150
Yaacov Zahalon Ben Isaac 151
The Doctor's Prayer 153
Medical Ethics: John Gregory (Scotland) and Thomas Percival (England). 153
Eighteenth to Nineteenth Century. 153
Historical Period 154
John Gregory. 155
The Profession of Medicine 156

Thomas Percival . . . 156
Extracts from Dr. Percival's "Medical Ethics" . . . 158
A Few More Points on Medical Ethics . . . 160
Code . . . 160
Profession . . . 160
Percival's Innovations . . . 161
Some Consequences of These Definitions . . . 162
After Percival's Death . . . 162
Other Contemporary English Authors . . . 163
Conclusion . . . 165
Florence Nightingale . . . 166
Nineteenth Century . . . 166
The Nightingale Commitment . . . 168
References . . . 169

8 Statement and Initial Development of Medical Ethics in the Nineteenth and Twentieth Centuries . . . 173
Historical Note and Updates to Recent Times . . . 173
First Activities on Medical Ethics in Various Countries . . . 175
British Medical Association, 1832 . . . 175
Confederation des Syndicats Médicaux Francais 1845 . . . 176
In USA . . . 176
Principles of Medical Ethics . . . 177
The Phisician's Pledge . . . 178
Historical Dates of the AMA'S Activities . . . 178
Development of the AMA Code . . . 179
Declaration of Professional Responsibility for Medicine and Social Contract with Humanity . . . 180
Preamble . . . 180
In Conclusion . . . 180
Sir William Osler . . . 182
In Conclusion . . . 184
References . . . 186

9 Italy . . . 187
Sassari (Island of Sardinia) . . . 187
Florence . . . 189
Law 10 July 1910, n. 455, (OJ no. 168 of July 19, 1910) Which Sets Rules for Healthcare Orders. (Published in the Official Gazette No. 168 of 19, 1910) . . . 189
Turin . . . 190
FNOMCEO . . . 190
After World War 2 . . . 191
Turin . . . 192
Como . . . 192
Bari . . . 193

Code of Conduct in Italy . . . 193
In Conclusion . . . 196
Positive Duties . . . 197
Negative Duties . . . 198
References . . . 198

10 Ethics and Professionalism . . . 199
More Declarations Followed . . . 199
More Notes on Profession and Professionalism . . . 200
Ethics in Professionalism . . . 202
Moreover (Added to Previous Declarations) . . . 203
Social Contract of Medicine with Humanity . . . 203
The Meaning of Medical Professionalism . . . 203
In Conclusion . . . 204
Principles of European Medical Ethics and Approval of the European Charter of Medical Ethics (Greece) . . . 204
Presentation . . . 211
Object and Scopes of Application . . . 213
General Duties of the Doctor . . . 213
Relations with the Citizen . . . 213
Relations with Colleagues . . . 214
Relations with Third Parties . . . 214
Relations with the National Health Service and with Public and Private Bodies . . . 214
Professional Oath . . . 214
References . . . 216

11 U.S.A. and U.R.S.S. . . . 219
ACP: American College of Physicians (U.S.A.) . . . 219
2021 ACP Resources for Internists Catalog . . . 219
Background . . . 219
Ethical Issues . . . 220
Physician's Charter on Professionalism . . . 221
About Internal Medicine . . . 221
Oaths in the U.S.A. (XX Sec.) . . . 222
The Healer's Oath . . . 222
Ethical Oath of the Christian Doctor . . . 222
Oath of the Loma Linda University (LLU) . . . 223
In U.S.S.R . . . 224
Supreme Soviet Oath . . . 224
Development of Medical Ethics in Russia . . . 225
Specific Areas of Ethical Debate and Decisions . . . 226
Human Rights in the Soviet Union . . . 226
Brief Notes on Medical Ethics in Recent Russia . . . 230
References . . . 231

12 Informed Consent . . . 233
Historical Premises . . . 233
Medical Experiments Permitted . . . 238
70 Years Later . . . 239
Informed Consent . . . 240
In Conclusion . . . 242
Italy . . . 242
In Conclusion . . . 249
References . . . 250

13 Medical Ethics in the World . . . 251
WMA . . . 251
The Handbook of WMA Policies . . . 253
Medical Ethics Manual . . . 253
WMA Oath: 1948 . . . 254
WMA: White Paper on Social Media and Medicine . . . 254
Geneva Declaration, 1948 . . . 254
Comments . . . 255
Proposed Changes . . . 256
International Code of Medical Ethics, 1949 . . . 256
To Summarize . . . 258
Universal Declaration of Human Rights, 1948 . . . 258
Preamble . . . 258
The General Assembly . . . 259
Helsinki + Taipei, 1964 . . . 260
Basic Principles of Clinical Research, According to the HD . . . 261
The Taipei Declaration (TD) . . . 262
Meetings Indicated and Sponsored by the WMA in the Twentieth and Twenty-First Centuries . . . 263
Sidney Declaration, Australia (1968) . . . 263
Oslo Declaration, Norway (1970) . . . 263
Tokyo Declaration, Japan (1975) . . . 264
Hawaii Statement (1977) . . . 264
Lisbon Declaration, Portugal (1981) . . . 265
Declaration of Venice, Italy (1983) . . . 265
Declaration of St. Julians, Malta (1991) . . . 266
Stockholm Declaration, Sweden (1994) . . . 266
Ottawa Declaration, Canada (1998) . . . 266
Tel Aviv Declaration, Israel (1999) . . . 267
Ferney-Voltaire Declaration, France (2001) . . . 267
Washington Declaration, U.S.A. 2002 . . . 267
Declaration of Divonne-les-Bains, France (2003) . . . 268
Manual of Medical Ethics, U.S.A. (2005) . . . 268
Resolution of Pilanesberg, South Africa (2006) . . . 268
Copenhagen Declaration, Denmark (2007) . . . 269

Seoul Declaration, South Korea (2008) 269
General Assembly, Montevideo, Uruguay (2011) 269
General Assembly, Moscow, Russia (2015) 270
General Assembly, Chicago, U.S.A. (2017) 270
General Assembly, Harpa, Reykjavik, Iceland (2018) 270
Adopted by the 70th WMA General Assembly, Tbilisi, Georgia (October 2019) 271
WMA General Assembly, Cordoba (Spain) (2020) 271
(October 26, 2021) 271
World Health Organization (WHO) 272
WHO: Ethical Principles. 273
Offenses 274
Exploitation and Prevention of Sexual Abuse. 274
Responsible Search Code of Conduct. 274
Conflicts of Interest. 275
Statements for Staff. 275
Declarations for Experts 275
References. 275

14 The Catholic Doctor's Prayers: Vatican City 277
Historical Background 277
The Doctor's Prayer (Saint John Paul II) 278
Another Doctor's Prayer. 279
The Sick Person's Prayer 279
More Prayers from the Doctor 280
Ethical Analysis and Conclusion 282
Religion and Medical Ethics. 283
Moreover, a Few Comments. 283
References. 285

15 Ethics in the Twentieth and Twenty-First Centuries 287
Belmont Report (U.S.A.) 287
Historical Notes 287
Ethical Principles and Guidelines for Research Involving Human Subjects. 289
Applications 289
Nuffield Council on Bioethics (London) 289
Nuffield and Medical Ethics. 291
Activities for Ethical Issues in Medicine 291
The Ethics of Animals. 291
CIOMS (Switzerland). 291
Historical Notes 291
Main Objectives 292
Ethics in CIOMS. 293
Fundamental Ethical Principles 294
A Few Extracts from the CIOMS Guidelines. 295

Good Clinical Practice (GCP): EU, U.S.A., Japan, etc. 297
Background 298
Italy: The National System of Guidelines [297] 298
References 299

16 Medical Ethics and Bioethics in the Twentieth Century 301
The American Revolution[2] 301
Preamble 303
Medical Deontology 304
"Ethics" and "Medical Ethics" 304
Causes of Problems in Medical Ethics 305
Medical Ethics in the World 306
WMA 306
EACME 307
Code of Medical Ethics of the Federal Council of Medicine of Brazil 308
Seychelles Medical and Dental Council (SMDC), 1994 308
Medical and Dental Council of Nigeria, (MDCN), 1995 309
India Ethics Committee: Notified, 6 April 2002 (Babu, India) 309
Association for Medical Ethics, 2008: Cambridge, Massachusetts, USA 309
Australian Medical Association (Aust MA) 310
Twenty-First Century: U.S.A., Europe 310
Technological Advances 311
Pluralism of Values 311
Patients' Rights 311
Concern for Faith 311
Other Important Topics 311
Forecasts for the Twenty-First Century 313
Other Aspects 314
In Conclusion 315
Moreover[16] 316
On Hold 316
References 316

17 Ethics Committees 319
Birth of Ethics Committees 319
What Are They? 320
Ethics Committees and Biomedical Research 326
Bioethics vs. Medical Ethics 327
What's New About Bioethics? 328
General Conclusions 328
Doctor-Patient Relationship 329
References 332

18 Update to Years 2020, 2021, and 2022, with Information on COVID-19 333
Introductory Notes 333
Infectious Diseases 334
Viruses. 334
RNA Viruses 336
Effects on the Host Cell 336
Epidemiology 336
Outbreaks 336
Epidemic 337
Pandemic. 337
Ethics in Infectious Diseases 338
Current Pandemic and Epidemic Risks Around the World. 340
Quarantine (See Footnote 13). 340
The Ethical Issues of Quarantine 341
Coronavirus. 342
Transmission of the Coronavirus 343
Incubation Period 343
Death Rate. 343
Cycle of Disease with the Coronavirus. 344
Risk Factors 344
Ethical Questions 344
COVID-19. 344
Symptoms 344
Worldwide, the WHO Stated on 11 March 2020 That the Disease Is a Pandemic. 345
Intensity and Severity 346
A Necessary Choice in the Absence of Adequate Health Resources 346
Predictions for the Next Treatment 347
A Few Further Notes. 348
Forecasts: COVID-19: Certain and Uncertain Aspects of the Pandemic 348
Vaccination Strategies: Serious Disease and Equity. 349
New Variants 349
COVID Vaccines. 350
How Many and What COVID Vaccines Are There Around the World?. 350
Medical Resources 351
COVID-19 and Medical Ethics. 352
In Conclusion: Ethical Priorities. 352
References. 354

1 Introduction

The ability to reason, shared by all human beings, may always have been the basis of our actions. Reasoning became moral when it specified how right or wrong the events in a particular situation were and suggested what people should (or might) do. With the invention of writing,[1] historically attributable to the end of the fourth millennium B.C., mankind documented the first attempts not only to remedy the suffering that has always plagued him, but also to restore the legitimacy or justification of the proposed remedies.

The lengthy and laborious interpretations, from Sumerian catalogs and the subsequent textual descriptions made by the scribes who worked in this field, bear witness to this. Their descriptions were based on the treatise "Mesopotamian Doctor," written on stones and tablets in large letters, but these have gradually deteriorated, leaving scholars with very little room for investigation.[2]

Some sentences and terms, appropriately interpreted and translated, remain as evidence by the many meticulous historical researchers who have alternated. These are some examples: "When an exorcist goes to the home of a sick person ..."—"The disease"—"Symptoms"—"The medicine man is an expert in finding the true cause"—"The Shaman is able to study the means of achieving trance, or other divination techniques"—"Diagnosis means to find out who possesses the ability—and why—that the patient seeks in those who treat him"—"Treatment of the cause appears to be of secondary importance ... " and so on.

[1] Cosmacini (2011), Cavalli (2013-2014) and Mark (2009).

[2] Some moral and ethical teachings derived from the Sumerians. In addition to the first analysis of the symptoms in the various clinical cases described in the "Diagnostic Manual" written by the *Ummânū* (chief scholar) Esagil-kin-apli (1067–1046 BC) the manual introduced, in the diagnosis, the methods of therapy, etiology, empiricism, logic and rationality. A patient's symptoms and illnesses were treated with therapeutic means, such as bandages, creams and pills. If a patient could not be physically cured, doctors resorted to exorcisms to cleanse him of any curse.

Rutz (2011).

R. G. Russo, *Medical Ethics*, https://doi.org/10.1007/978-3-031-42444-1_1

It was at that time that the two great river civilizations (Mesopotamia and Egypt), previously ruled by "shamanism,"[3] first introduced legal codes to define the conduct and the teaching formulations relating to what was acceptable or not. Similar conclusions were drawn almost simultaneously in India. It was around that period that the concept of "morality"[4] was defined, as the "science" of duty and human behavior, regardless of the professional or institutional roles covered.

Medical ethics was therefore still far from properly investigated.[5] It was in fact widely debated and often mentioned, as if to testify to its appropriateness and close relations with the professional activity of medicine.

From the original philosophical definition relating to "what is good and what is not good" over time it has come to be understood as a set of moral principles inherent in every activity. Over the millennia, the morality of human actions has been widely scrutinized, and has resulted in the deontology that subsequently accompanied and aimed to stimulate the "Noble Art" of medicine in the right direction.

This study is divided into 18 chapters, where some known paths and others, still unexplored, are retraced in order to analyze the terminology most appropriate to medical ethics and to compare what mankind has produced, in the various historical eras, as well as in parallel with growing medical and social culture.

Referring to the writings and prescriptions of ancient times, I wanted to leave their texts unchanged, without recomposing them to make the language easier to read and less obscure and repetitive. The relationships between the various pronouncements, such as "Oaths" and "Codes of Conduct," often had a religious basis[6] or else were purely practical, always respecting the principles of "respect for autonomy, equity, charity and justice."

---

[3] Traditions and myths could help recognize and accept the presence of external conditioning "forces". Some members were more willing than others to interpret such "mysterious events". These people (known as *Shamans*), were devoted to philosophy, religion or medicine. "Magic" was their reference tool: they were the first to formulate the primitive foundations of ethics itself, as they passed judgments and evaluated "values" and "roles" in some actions or in certain rituals. These shamans preceded today's doctors.

Loewy and Loewy (2005).

[4] "Ethics" comes from the Greek "ethos" (*ἔθος*), as attested by L. Rocci (in his Greek-Italian Dictionary, XIX ed. Dante Alighieri, 1966) and the term was coined by Aristotle in "Nicomachean Ethics" and understood as use, habit, "behavior", or the conduct to be followed in order to live a happy existence ("eudaimonistic" ethics). The term ethikos (*ἔθικός*)—the "theory of living"—refers to the concept of "morality". These terminologies can be traced to the fourth century B.C. so any attempt at assigning an "ethical connotation to works prior to that date" is pleonastic, if not actually anachronistic.

Bird (1989), Gabel (2010), Gert (2005a, b), Wear et al. (1993), II Ed. 2003 and Vegetti (1989).

[5] Bell (1847).

[6] For millennia, religion was considered the primary source of morality; alternatives were provided by science or tradition. Religious tradition, focused on rituals, sacrificial offerings or taboos designed to ward off bad luck and evil, contributed to the success of the gods, with a moral sense, as in Egyptian culture. Medical ethics was later to group the connotations of "morality" and "tradition" with their religious basis.

Gillon (1994), Radomysk (2011) and Sritharan et al. (2001).

The most recent codes of conduct are commented as indicating the moral and responsible professional conduct involve all health workers and communities dedicated to the care of sick people.

A few different visions are sometimes included, changing over the centuries, to illustrate how developments in medicine also lent themselves to interpretation and preconceptions based on questionable beliefs and superficial certainties.

The "instructions" for the correct application of medical ethics[7] have been gradually transformed from precise and unequivocal assertions (typical of oaths), to debated and questionable regulations, up to the most modern "deontological" codes of conduct.[8]

This is a story based on medical behavior, past, present, or future and its morals. There is no universally recognized and accepted *modus operandi*; some differences may be significant, depending on education, location, social class, to name just some influencing factors.

Additions to the chapter list the main bibliographic links, often with some comments for a fuller understanding of lesser known historical passages. I have generally used *italics* characters to indicate the citations of foreign Authors or topics reported in Italian or another foreign language. The words or phrases reported without changes in Italian or in the original language are indicated in quotation marks. Like for the bibliography, I have used a form that should make it easy to find the main references for the individual chapters. Bibliographic references are listed consecutively in the whole text. References or quotations that appear several times, some in different chapters, are listed as "Already cited." The search for the original texts was done using computerized surveys and databases, and consultation of bibliographic material in my possession or available in libraries.

---

[7] Ethics has a particular connotation when applied to medicine. Certainly the basic requirements must be respected, but there are some basic definitions (tentatively reported here) that can help us understand better.

Angeletti and Gazzaniga (2008), Amundsen (1980), Boyd (2013), Kottow (1999) and Percival (1849).

Nimesis Filosofie, 2015 (Italian Translation), Sugarman and Sulmasy (2010).

[8] Nearly 200 years ago, the science of morality was identified as a "deontology" in which the harmony and coincidence of duty and personal interest, virtue and happiness, prudence and benevolence, were explained and exemplified.

Bowring and Bentham (1834).

References

Amundsen DW. The development of medical ethics. Vancouver: The University of British Columbia; 1980.
Angeletti LR, Gazzaniga V. History, philosophy and general ethics of medicine. 3rd ed. Milano: Elsevier Masson; 2008.
Bell J. Introduction to the code of medical ethics. Chicago: American Medical Association; 1847. Original code of medical ethic. Chicago: AMA Press; 1891.
Bird LP. Medical ethics. In: Bird LP, Barlow J, editors. Oaths & prayers, an anthology. Richardson, TX: Christian Medical & Dental Society; 1989. p. 1–15.
Bowring J, Bentham J. Deontology, or, the science of morality, vol. 1. London: Longman; 1834.
Boyd K. The making of medical ethics. J Med Ethics. 2013;39:661.
Cavalli F. Breve storia della medicina. Antichità e Medioevo. (IT. A brief history of medicine. Antiquity and the middle ages). Anno Accademico; 2013-2014.
Cosmacini G. L'arte lunga – Storia della medicina dall'antichità a oggi. (IT. The long art—history of medicine from antiquity to today), II Mondo Classico. Bari: Laterza; 2011. p. 51–100.
Gabel S. Ethics and values in clinical practice: whom do they help? Mayo Clin Proc. 2010;86(5):421–4.
Gert B. The definition of morality. In: Zalta EN, editor. The Stanford encyclopedia of philosophy. Stanford: The Metaphysics Research Lab; 2005a.
Gert, B. Morality: its nature and justification. Revised ed. New York: Oxford University Press; 2005b.
Gillon R. Medical ethics: four principles plus attention to scope. BMJ. 1994;309(6948):184–8.
Kottow MH. In defense of medical ethics. J Med Ethics. 1999;25:340–3.
Loewy EH, Loewy RS. Textbook of healthcare ethics. Dordrecht: Kluwer Academic Publishers; 2005.
Mark JJ. Mesopotamia. Ancient history encyclopedia; 2009.
Percival T. Etica Medica, ovvero un Codice di istituzioni e precetti adattati alla condotta professionale dei medici e dei chirurghi (IT. Medical ethics, or a code of institutions and precepts, adapted to the professional conduct of physicians and surgeons). 3rd ed. Oxford/London: John Henry Parker/John Churchill; 1849.
Radomysk M. Medical oaths: when religion and ethics collide. Amsterdam Law Forum. 2011;3(1):68–80.
Rutz M. Threads for Esagil-kīn-apli. The medical diagnostic-prognostic series in middle Babylonian Nippur, Zeitschr. f. Assyriologie Bd., vol. 101S. Berlin: Walter de Gruyter; 2011. p. 294–308.
Sritharan K, Russell VG, et al. Medical oaths and declarations. BMJ. 2001;323(7327):1440–1.
Sugarman J, Sulmasy D, editors. Methods in medical ethics. 2nd ed. Washington, DC: Georgetown University Press; 2010.
Vegetti M. L'Etica degli Antichi. (IT. The ethics of the ancients). Bari: Laterza; 1989.
Wear A, Geyer-Korash J, French R. Doctors and ethics. The earlier historical setting of professional ethics, Clio Medica, vol. 24. Amsterdam: BRILL; 1993.

Medical Ethics Before Hippocrates 2

The first historical documents referring to medicine were those regarding the Egyptians and the peoples of Mesopotamia. They did not necessarily have medical ethics connotations *stricto sensu* but are equally reported as he early paths of a historical, philosophical, and medical journey.

Egypt

During the 3000 years of ancient Egypt's history, a great medical tradition developed.[1] The studies done up to now give us a broad picture of the extraordinary scope and enlightened acumen of this ancient culture. Even before the hieroglyphs were deciphered, Homer, Herodotus, Hippocrates, Pliny, and other writers mentioned Egyptian Medicine in positive terms.[2,3]

[1] Breasted (1908, 1935), Cavalli (2013–2014), pp. 8–10; 10–13; 14–31 and Shaw (2000).

[2] Egyptian medicine was aimed at non-invasive surgery, bone repair and pharmacopoeia. Homer (800 B.C.), wrote in the Odyssey: "In Egypt men are more skilled in medicine than any other people and more evolved in it of any other art they practice" and "whose fertile land produces many drugs" and where this could be practiced by anyone. "Herodotus (fifth century BC), defined the Egyptians as the people of the very healthy".

Pliny the Elder wrote favorably about it in a historical review. Hippocrates, Erofilo, Erasistrato and then Galen recognized the contribution of ancient Egyptian medicine which they studied at the temple of Amenhotep. Diodorus Siculus (first century A.D.) declared: "... he whole way of life of the Egyptians was so ordered that it appeared as if it had been predisposed to the rules of health by an enlightened physician rather than a legislator."

Homer (Odyssey, IV, 220–232).

Encyclopedia Italiana Treccani - Papirologia di Orsolina Montevecchi, v. App. (1994) (XXXVI, p. 257; App. I, p. 920; II p. 502; III, p. 361: IV.II).

Rossi (2010), Subbarayappa (2001) and University of Manchester (2007).

[3] The gods who watched over the exercise of medicine: Thot, Sekhmet and Horus. Nunn, John F. Ancient Egyptian medicine, London, British Museum Press, 1996.

Redford (2001) and Wilkinson (2003).

R. G. Russo, *Medical Ethics*, https://doi.org/10.1007/978-3-031-42444-1_2

Scientists from the KNH Center for Biomedical Egyptology in Manchester, with the guidance of Professor Rosalie David, spent almost 5 years meticulously studying the papyri written 1500/1000 years before Hippocrates was born (460 B.C. circa), and asserted that the origins of modern medicine should be ascribed to Egypt, not to Greece,

> *The Egyptians, not the Greeks, are the true fathers of medicine.*

The priests devoted to the "goddess *Sekhmet*", civilian doctors (*sun-nu*) and helpers (*ut*), with the use of natural herbs and holistic medicine, saved many lives and cured many diseases.[4] Treatments also included: (1) prayer, sacrifice and repentance; (2) the exorcism of demons; (3) the practices of combatting black magic; (4) the empirical application of medicines and drugs or surgery.

The documents also attested that "*Imhotep*" (defined by Sir William Osler as "*The first medical figure to rise from the fog of antiquity*") had diagnosed and treated over 200 diseases. Prayers and supplications were, in different historical eras, addressed to the gods for healing intercessions or magical practices. With this plethora of information, one can understand how initial "moral and ethical"[5] assumptions were formed.

Proper medical behavior was subjected to close scrutiny by the ancient Egyptians. The main exponent was the noble "*Ptah-hotep,*"[6] court physician in the 5th dynasty, who lived between 2420 and 2380 B.C. He was the author of some profound precepts: a "teaching" and 37 maxims were reported according to his view, and formed a complex system to foster tolerance and mental balance. This text (539 lines) is preserved in papyri and on a clay tablet. Basically it is a moral treatise on good manners, based on the clear distinctions between virtue and vice, law, and illegality. Ptah-hotep had emphasized the rules of behavior that all wise men had to pass on to their children. He said, among other things:

> *Respect the one who sent you. Spread his message as transmitted. Avoid any risk of harm in your speech. Keepto the truth. Do not malign anyone.*

In Egypt one had to have a basic knowledge of the divinity "*Ma'at,*"[7] who represented justice, balance, norms, order, truth and what is correct and just. The reasons for compliance with the rules were basically practical; ignoring them was reason

---

[4] Dunn J. as John Warren The Ethics and Morality of the Ancient Egyptians—www.touregypt.net. Ghalioungui (1983).

Westendorf and Leitz (2001, 2003).

[5] Lichtheim (2000), Redford (2002) and Walsh (2012).

[6] Ptah-hotep was also "Vizier" (among the highest officials and judges, head of the administration and high priest of Ma'at).

Chamblee (2005).

[7] Ma'at was the daughter of the divinity of the sun (Ra) and wife of the god of the moon (Thoth) and was in antagonism to "isfet"_ chaos. Justice consisted in circulating life in the microcosm and in the macrocosm. It seems that the Egyptians used the term "mtw" to refer to any long, thin structure that carried substances, such as intestines, blood vessels or nerves; the causes (unknown to

enough for punishment. Ma'at was a goddess to whom "cosmic balance" and at the same time obedience to the Pharaoh, were attributed; both helped sustain the Egyptian state.

The "Book of the Dead"[8] reported evidence that the deceased had led their lives with integrity and they could declaim their blamelessness, using "Negative Confessions," as follows:

I have not committed sins against men.

I have not opposed my family or my relatives. I have not acted fraudulently or sneakily.

I have never been friend with "useless" or dissolute persons and time wasters.

I have not indulged in evil.

I never allowed my first daily consideration to be aimed at useless work.

I have never put my name first to respect the dignity (of others).

I have not diminished the importance of the Gods.

I have not defrauded the humble man of his property. I have never done anything the gods loathe.

I have not defamed a slave in the presence of his master. I have inflicted no pain.

I have not starved anyone. I have made any man cry. I have not committed murder.

I have not given the order to carry out a murder.

I have not caused calamities to befall men and women.

I have not plundered the offerings in the temples.

I have not defrauded the gods of their offerings.

I have not stolen any offer made to the Spirits.

I have not masturbated in the sanctuaries of God.

I have not removed weight from the bushel.

I have not stolen my neighbor's land, I have not added it to mine.

I have not invaded the fields of others.

I have not altered the weights of the measuring scales. I have not changed the final balance.

I have never taken the milk out of the mouths of children. I have never led the cattle away from their pastures.

---

them) that blocked them, eliminating the natural balance, could be something different from the mechanics of human physiology.

David (2002), Mancini (2010) and Mark (2016).

[8] The Book of the Dead (found with the Papyrus of Ani, now in the British Museum) was a sacred text with some magical formulas used to serve the deceased in order to protect him and help him on his journey to the afterlife. During the "Ceremony of the Heart", the weight of the feather of Ma'at was compared with that of the heart of the deceased; if the heart was lighter or in balance, this meant that the deceased had passed the first test on the way to the afterlife or had no hope for an afterlife. (For the ancient Egyptians there was no hell; the worst fate after death was: "not having lived".)

De Rachewiltz (1992), Horne (1917), Karenga (2004), Shaw and Nicholson (1995), Wallis Budge (2007) and Zucconi (2007).

I have never caught the geese bearing the feathers of the Gods. I have not used bait made of the type of fish to be caught. I never stopped the water when it should have flowed out.

I never diverted the flow of running water in a canal.

I have never put out a fire or a lamp when they should have been burning.

I have not violated the time limits for offers.

I have not taken cattle away from the estates of the Gods. I have not opposed the Gods and their apparitions.

I am pure. I am pure. I am pure. I am pure.

Such statements were deemed correct conduct. According to Ma'at, balance, order, and justice had to govern relationships between people. The goddess personalized this harmony and the divine order of the universe; she governed not only natural phenomena but also social relationships. The ancient Egyptians did not see any great dichotomy between medicine and religion. Health and disease were manifestations of a person's relationship with the universe that included not only people and animals, but also spirits and gods. Although they perceived a distinction between the earthly/mortal human beings and the supernatural/divine worlds, they recognized and supported an interaction between them.

The need to be pure (*wab*) was particularly important for those who came into contact with the deities, i.e., the priests. The cleansing process was body-centered (washing, shaving, circumcising, and sexually abstaining when working in a temple). This purity ensured perfection in all the rituals.

Mesopotamia

The Sumerians, whose origin is uncertain, lived in Mesopotamia for over a thousand years between the fourth and the third millennium B.C. They drew up the first collections of laws. The most significant Codes were the following:

- Code of Ur-Nammu,[9] probably the oldest text of laws of mankind, created around the twenty-first century B.C. by a former general who started the third dynasty of Ur and reigned from 2113 to 2096 B.C. "Ur-Nammu established equity in his

[9] It is perhaps surprising that a uniform system of laws is relatively recent in about two million years of human history! It was written during the reign of Ur-Nammu, king of the city of Ur (now in Iraq), who founded the third Sumerian dynasty and ruled the Babylonian Assyrian Empire. The code, identified on clay tablets, precedes the code of Hammurabi by about three centuries and probably influenced its composition. It consists of a prologue and 32 laws. Only 40 of the 57 allegedly existing laws have been reconstructed and deciphered. It provided for penalties for various crimes and established standards of capacity and weights, defined the economic value of a person for the purposes of compensation for damage. It is considered as the first foundation of "Forensic Medicine".

Code of Ur-Nammu: http://en.wikipedia.org/w/index.p9hp?oldid=50481196.

Cavalli (2013–2014), pp. 8–10, Mark (2009, 2014), Pettinato (1994), Roth et al. (1995), Saporetti (1998) and Myer (1935).

Death penalty for murder and theft.

land; he outlawed the curse, violence and strife and set the temple's monthly expenses at 90 *gur* of barley, 30 sheep and 30 *sila* of butter. He modeled the size of a *sila* with bronze, standardized the weight of a *mine* and the stone weight of a silver *shekel* in relation to a coin" (A *mine* corresponded to 60 *shekels*).

- Epic of Gilgamesh, one of the first monarchs of the ancient Sumerians,[10]
- Code of Lipit-Ishtar, king of Isin, who ruled from 1934 to 1924 B.C.[11]
- Code of Hammurabi:[12] Hammurabi, who lived between 1792 and 1750 B.C., was king of Babylon and unified all of Mesopotamia under his rule; he was the sovereign who established above all the greatness of this city as the first metropolis in the world. His famous "Code" is one of the best preserved legal documents of antiquity; it was found in 1901 and had been engraved on a basalt stele about 2.5 m high so that its contents could be easily read by the people. It is currently on display in the Louvre Museum. Of the 282 laws that make it up, only 9 deal with "medicine." The old consideration of the medical profession is illustrated in the following sentences:[13]

Compensation for damages in money or other assets (value of man = 100 camels; value of woman = 50 camels) Five fragments can be indicative of sanctions in the medical field: For being the oldest existing law in history, it is considered incredibly advanced.

Five centuries before the Bible, which still provided for the "law of retaliation", monetary compensation was also recognized for bodily damage. For the cut of a foot the guilty party had to pay 10 "shekels" of silver and for the cut of the nose two thirds of a "mine" (350 g) of silver. However, murder, robbery, adultery and rape involved capital punishment.

[10]The Epic of Gilgamesh narrates the deeds of the king who, grappling with the problem of death and the impossibility of overcoming, instituted an ethical system to show that destiny was correlated with service and with loyalty to correct and responsible principles. The Sumerian king was known for his desire to "inform, examine, judge, perceive and do good" despite having a violent and irascible character. The poem was written approximately in 1870 B.C., and dates before the Homeric poems (eighth century B.C.) and the Indian Vedas (fifteenth century B.C.); the text has many similarities with them. Brandon (1961).

Kott (1997), Saporetti (1998, 2003) and Sandars (1986).

[11]The code of laws edited by the Semitic king Lipit-Ishtar was composed about 1860 B.C. and is 200 years older than the Code of Hammurabi. Discovered in 1899 near Nippur its decryption took 30 years. It mainly concerns the ethics of family work with the aim of "establishing justice on earth, to rectify complaints, eliminate hostilities and armed insurrection and to bring peace to the Sumerians and Akkadians". Social injustice is condemned by law and enmity, rebellion, weeping and lamentations are thus eliminated.

Duhaime (2011–2012), Robbins (1990), Steele (2005), vol 52(3): 425–450, 1948.

[12]The topics covered in the Hammurabi Code range from economic justice to property, from lawsuits and business practices to the conclusion of contracts.

Code of Hammurabi (eighteenth century B.C). www.agenzialebrariaeditrice.

Dadies (1905), Denison et al. (1997), Owen (2013), Pettinato (1994), Slanski (2012) and Souvay (1910), 30 Oct. 2016.

[13]The Code of Hammurabi explained the patient's rights according to the proclaimed Code of the King. The justice of the principle "an eye for an eye" and the practice of medicine were regulated by the state. "Malpractice" was recognized and punished by law. The Code can be considered the originator of modern health care concepts. The incapable doctor was punished: in case of loss of life or limbs, his hands were cut off. Surgical cure was practiced; there were opportunities for legal action to ensure justice and equity for each social class in the kingdom.

215. If a Doctor makes a large incision with an operative knife and treats it or if he opens a tumor (above the eye) with an operative knife and saves the eye, he receives ten *shekels* in money.
216. If the Patient is a free man, he receives five *shekels*.
217. If he is a slave, his owner must give the Doctor two *shekels*.
218. If a Doctor, with his bronze lancet (scalpel), causes a citizen a serious injury which leads to death or opens the eyebrow arch and causes him to lose his eye, his hands will be cut off.
219. If a Doctor makes a large incision on the slave of a free man and causes his death, he will have to replace the slave with another slave.
220. If a Doctor opens a tumor with the operative knife and causes the loss of an eye to extract it, he must pay back half of its value in money.
221. If a doctor heals a broken bone or other part of the body, the patient must pay the doctor five *shekels*.
222. If he was a free man, he must pay three *shekels*.
223. If he was a slave his owner must pay the Doctor two *shekels*.

The medical profession began to acquire importance and a few sanctions specified financial punishment for carelessness, negligence, and inexperience when causing therapeutic and surgical mistakes.

Positive outcomes received benefits. In both cases it was generally a question of establishing a "price" in money. The Code influenced subsequent medical practices in Babylon, Mesopotamia, and then in ancient Egypt.[14]

Here are some more examples:

Art.153: If a wife has her husband killed because of another man, this woman will be impaled
Art.196: if serious damage is caused to a man's eye, an eye will be extracted from the person responsible
Art.197: if another man's bone is broken, the bone of the person responsible will be broken
Art.198: if you damage the eye or break the bones of a freedman, you will pay a silver *mine* (350 g)
Art.199: if the eye is injured or the bone of a slave is broken, half of its value must be paid
Art.200: if someone breaks the tooth of a man equal, his tooth will be broken
Art.205: if the slave of a free man hits a free man, his ear must be cut off
Art.209: if a citizen strikes the daughter of another citizen and causes her to have an abortion, he will pay 10 *shekels* of silver (84 g).

Halwani and Takrouri (2006) and Larue (1988).

[14] F. Grotefend (1775–1853) deciphered the cuneiform writing in the years 1802–1803, thus allowing the systematic study of the thousands and thousands of clay tablets produced in over three millennia, that archaeological research (or clandestine excavations) brought to light.

US History.Org (2016) and Younan (1910).

From the situations listed it can be deduced that the so-called "Law of Retaliation" was also applied: "You will give life for life, an eye for an eye, a tooth for a tooth, a hand for a hand, a foot for a foot, a wound for a wound."

The laws concerning health, however, provided guidelines that emphasized the concept of "do no harm" in medicine and, at the same time, outlined the existence of new professionals. The code set clearly-defined terms, disciplining the organization of society and regulated procedural law based on social status.

The treatment of diseases attributed to divine, demonic, or magical causes fell within the purview of a different class of healers than those who treated disease attributed to natural causes. Ethical principles were not (yet) of primary importance in the ancient Middle East, but similar concepts were present in commercial documents, codes of law, stories of heroes, and myths.

At that time it was not always possible to distinguish exorcism from medicine; all evil was caused by impiety or the action of a god, a demon, a ghost or a witch. The words that opened the legislative and deontological code of Hammurabi are indicative, as if to guard against the evils that are wished on "enemies":

> May Nin-Karak, the daughter of Anu, who dispenses grace for me, cause her members in E-kur to have a high fever, wounds that cannot be understood, healed or removed by the doctor, so as to compromise their future lives.

India

Indian ethics was philosophical from its inception.

In the fifteenth century B.C. approximately the religion and culture of the Indo-European peoples, called "*Arii,*" developed and migrated to North-western India, giving rise to "Vedism." The first records concerning medical practice in India date back to that historical period, together with the ethical regulations that were announced and adopted. In the Vedas ethics was an integral aspect of philosophical and religious speculation on the nature of reality, and indicated how people should live.

The word "Dharma"[15] had already been in use in the Vedic religion since the thirtieth century B.C. and its meaning and conceptual framework evolved over several millennia. Dharma is the reality that makes "one thing to be," or "the way things are" or as an equivalent to the Western term for "religion." In fact, Dharma is often understood as "religious law" since it involves the due observance of moral duties

[15] Dharma is a key concept with multiple meanings in Indian religions: Hinduism, Buddhism, Sikhism and Jainism, but there is no common translation among them. The word "Religion" literally means "that which leads to God". The word "Dharma" means "to hold together" and therefore has a different setting. Hinduism does not "lead to God", but rather seeks unity, the "holding together" of the human race and therefore is not a "true" religion. It is similar to the terms "Tao" in Chinese, "Maat" in ancient Egypt, "Me" in Sumerian.

Jonsen (2000), Keown (2002), Majumdar (2003), Rosen (2006), Guha (2007), Pandya (2000), Veatch (2000), pp. 240–258 and Veatch (2000), pp. 258–260.

and characterizes those actions that generate or maintain the cosmic order. The parallel with ethics (and therefore with medical ethics) is easily grasped. The antonym of the Dharma is "Adharma," which means that it is unnatural, immoral, incorrect or illegal. Besides disease, Adharma causes suffering, conflict, discord, and various imbalances.

Like other beliefs or religions, Hinduism had its own distinctive and philosophical derivation of ethics and morality too.[16] The teaching of Indian medical ethics focuses on principles and guidelines derived from rules and laws. Its practice is seen as a matter of social and professional etiquette, besides being a regulatory requirement.

Today most medical professionals enter careers with a commitment to morality and ethics; Dharma, in daily practice, can ensure this safety and can balance and temper a person's vital aspirations. The Dharma represents a way of life that awakens, promotes and supports an ethical attitude.

It can even influence decision-making in many aspects of health care; it has many areas in common with today's practice of medical ethics and enriches it further. The Dharmic perspective also attributes a more categorical force to ethics as a spiritual imperative.

Two of the main types of Dharma are worthy of mention here:

1. *Sanātana-Dharma* (thirtieth to sixth century B.C.) is the original name of what is today popularly called "Hinduism."

The two words indicate "what does not cease to be eternal." Dharma has an impact on the development and practice of health care, shared with other countries around the world.

Morals and ethics remain firmly attached to a spiritual and behavioral code for achieving "moksha" ("the good," enlightenment, liberation from the chains of being born/dying).[17]

A path of "Dharmic" life contemplates and respects ten fundamental rules: patients, forgiveness, mercy and/or self-control, honesty, holiness, control of the senses, reason, knowledge and/or learning, truthfulness, and absence of anger. Ethics and Medicine appear as two inseparable units. Ethics, or "*Shila*" in *Sanskrit*, concerns the correct way of life and the resulting mental attitude. Dharma and Medical Science have a common goal: to make humanity happier by reducing suffering.

Treat sometimes, relieve often and always give comfort

The cornerstones of Indian Medical Ethics are the well-known four principles: autonomy, charity, justice, and non-maleficence. Ethical issues related to health care have been discussed but very rarely published in India.

[16] Masui (1949), Prakash (1988) and Seetharam (2013).

[17] Huilgol (2012), Bellavite et al. (2000), Dash and Junius (2005).

The literature is very limited and the themes of ethics, closely related to the concept of "Dharma," are present in Ayurvedic treatises. This statement gives an indication of concern for the poor and justice: "The treatment given as charity, giving food to the hungry and water to the thirsty leads to paradise." However, this does not prevent the good doctor from making a profit. "The doctor must constantly observe the patient's condition and prescribe the appropriate treatment: with this method the patient is cured and the doctor obtains four benefits: virtue, wealth, serenity and emancipation."

Vaidya in Sanskrit means "doctor" and also "he who knows." Some royal families had a personal Vaidya called Raja Vaidya "the king's doctor." The oath of the Hindu doctor, adopted around the fifteenth century B.C., prescribed that the doctor should not conduct dishonest practices. It also pleaded with doctors not to harm their patients or to devote themselves exclusively to their care, even if this might endanger their ownlives (see Footnote 9).

It bears valid testimony to the high level of professional ethics in ancient India and the universal adoption of medicines. The one who held "the honorary rank of Vaidya was presumed to possess learning, specific knowledge, memory, devotion and the ability to instill happiness in living beings." Some texts also advised the Vaidyas to acquire knowledge of particular herbal remedies by living in the forest, with mountain people or shepherds.

(a) It is necessary to avoid anything that can generate desires, anger, greed, madness, pride, selfishness, jealousy, harshness, slander, lies, laziness, and wrongdoing.
(b) You must have short nails, be clean and ritually dressed in an orange robe.
(c) You must be committed to the cause of truth and have full respect for those who turn to you.
(d) If, on the other hand, you behave properly while professing false views, you will be guilty of sin and your knowledge will bear no fruit.
(e) When you have finished your studies, with your medicines you will assist the Brahmins, the venerable people, the poor, the women, the ascetics, the pious people who seek your help, the widows, the orphans and anyone you meet on your erratic path, as if it were your own relative. This will be your right course. Doctors were also required to refrain from eating meat, drinking alcohol and committing adultery.

The *Vimana Sthana* of the *Charaka Samhita*[18] provides an exposition of the deontological directives of the Vaidya, based on allopathic medicine. The Charaka Samhita sets out a seventh century B.C. discipline which invites the observance of certain rules of conduct.

Here are some excerpts:

[18] Crush et al. (2008), Gellhorn (1977) and Glucklich (2005). For L.A., Cinba (2010).

- The teacher must give instructions to the disciple in the presence of the sacred fire of the Brahmins and doctors.
- You will lead the life of a celibate, you will grow your hair and beard, you will only tell the truth, you will not eat meat, but only pure food, you will be free from envy, and you will not carry weapons.
- If you desire success, wealth, and fame as a doctor and heaven after death, you will pray for the welfare of all creatures starting with the cows and the Brahmins.
- Day and night, however, busy you will be, you will strive for the relief of patients with all your heart and soul.
- You will not commit adultery, not even with the mind. You will have no secret possessions.
- You will be modest in your clothing and appearance. You will not be a drunkard or a sinner or associate with accomplices in crimes.
- You will only use words that are sweet, pure, fair, pleasant, worthy, true, wholesome, and moderate.
- When entering a patient's home, you will be accompanied by a man known to the patient, and who has his permission to enter, and you will be well dressed, with bowed head, with mastery of yourself and your conduct.
- Once you have entered, your word, mind, intellect, and senses must be solely and entirely dedicated to the patient.
- In medicine there is no limit to knowledge, so you will have to apply yourself diligently.

This is the way you will need to act "*Acharya Charaka,*" recognized as the father of (Indian) medicine, composed the oath for students. This also reflects the concepts and beliefs of ancient Indian literature, not just medical. His famous work, "Charaka Samhita" (probably approximately from the seventeenth century B.C.), is considered to be the encyclopedia of Ayurveda.[19]

Ayurveda is the oldest known system of medicine. It originated in Vedic India and is still extensively practiced in the country of origin and in many other nations. The term "Ayurveda" literally means "The Science of Life" in Sanskrit and expresses the aim of taking care of human life in all its aspects, psychological, physical, behavioral, and environmental. Disease is an imbalance of the fundamental components of physiology. WHO has recognized the universal validity of Ayurveda, recommending its study and application.

According to the *Susshruta Samhita*, one of the oldest Ayurvedic texts: "Health is that condition in which the physiological principles of the body are in balance, digestion is efficient, the tissues are in a normal condition, the excretory functions are regular and mind, senses and spirit are fully satisfied." Its principles, together with the diagnoses and treatments, still hold true after a couple of millennia. Charaka provided data on anatomy, embryology, pharmacology, blood circulation, and some diseases including diabetes, tuberculosis, and cardiac dysfunctions. He described

[19] Bird (1989), pp. 23–24, Hassler (1893), Hilton (2007), Iannacone (2014), and Tavani et al. (2007).

the medicinal qualities and functions of as many as 100,000 plants and also how diet affects the activities of the mind and body.

He demonstrated how spirituality correlated with physical health and prescribed an ethics charter for doctors, two centuries before the Hippocratic oath.

In a medical conference of that time, not only were matters relating to life and health discussed, but also matters relating to morality and religion. A very interesting chapter deals with "Aggregation of the Four," that is: the doctor, the nurse, the drug, and the patient.

2. *Buddhadharma* (from the sixth century B.C.)

In this sense, the Dharma no longer has the original Hindu meaning, only as a religious duty, but denotes a series of behaviors to be observed in daily life that lead to Enlightenment (Nirvana). It is the teaching established by the Buddha about 2500 years ago and is symbolized by a wheel (*dharmacakra*): the universal law (see Footnote 7).[20]

The 84,000 teachings of the Buddhadharma can be summarized with what the Buddha himself concluded:

I teach about suffering and how to end it

Master Shantideva (eighth century A.D.) remembered and stressed the following:

- Medicine is the only source of happiness to counter suffering.
- May respect and practice accompany you and be the basis of your teaching.
- The definitive cure is that obtained within the individual.

Buddha emphasizes the value of justice, correct mediation, and an enduring state of peace and happiness.

All suffering is caused by the three basic "poisons": desire, hatred, and ignorance.

The ultimate cure is achieved by eliminating them all with the strength of compassion and wisdom. According to ethics, Buddhism and Medicine are two inseparable units.[21]

In the "Four Noble Truths" the Buddha stressed that one should: Know the disease; Eliminate the causes; Aim for healing; Rely on medical care.

The ethical code of Buddhism is essentially based on: Right Actions, Right Words, Adequate Livelihoods and lends itself to application in medicine. The ethical principles are known as "The Five Precepts" and consist in refraining from:

---

[20] Assuming that medicine is one of the most important fields of knowledge, each individual must respect the dharmic norms of his own social caste (varṇa) and of the various stages of life (āśrama).

Basham (1977), Creel (1975, 1977), Dhand (2002), Doniger (1996), Keown and Keown (1995), Keown (2002), Magi (2006), Mahony (2006) and Silvia (2013–2014).

[21] Hughes and Keown (1995), Keown (2002), Piantelli (2001), Veatch (2000), pp. 262–267 and Zysk (1991).

- killing or harming living beings;
- stealing;
- erroneous sexual behavior;
- using vulgar or offensive speech and lies;
- abusing intoxicating substances such as alcohol or drugs that cause neglect and loss of consciousness. The comparison is with the moral principles of non-maleficence, beneficence, autonomy and justice, can be found in the single verse 183 of the *Dhammapada*.[22]

This is the Buddha's teaching:

- **Do no harm,**
- **Indulge what is good**
- **Purify your mind**

Vejjavatapada, the Buddhist doctor's oath, is taken by Buddhist doctors and other professionals who work with the sick; it consists of a preamble followed by seven articles.

It is taken from the statements attributed to the Buddha between the fifth and third centuries B.C.

The Lord said: **health is the greatest resource**

(a) I will use my skills to promote health and to serve the sick with care, kindness and compassion.
(b) I will be able to prepare medicines
(c) I will know which medicine is suitable and which is not suitable: I will not give the unsuitable, but only the suitable
(d) I serve the sick with a loving heart, not out of desire for gain
(e) I will also deal with feces, urine, vomit or spit
(f) From time to time I will be able to instruct, inspire, excite and awaken the sick thanks to the teaching (received). Even if I fail to heal a patient with proper nutrition, proper medicine, and proper care, I will continue to serve him with compassion.

[22] The Dhammapada exposes, in the form of poetic stanzas, the fundamental concepts of ancient Buddhism. The work, probably composed around the third century B.C., means "words of Dharma" to indicate "support", something solid and stable: the law that governs the universe.

References

Basham AL. The practice of medicine in ancient and medieval India. In: Leslie C, editor. Asian medical Systems: a comparative study. Berkeley: University of California Press; 1977. p. 18–43.

Bellavite P, et al. Le Medicine Complementari, a cura di, O.M.C. Verona. Milano: Utet periodici; 2000.

Bird LP. Medical ethics. In: Bird LP, Barlow J, editors. Oaths & prayers, an anthology. Richardson: Christian Medical & Dental Society; 1989.

Brandon SGF. The epic of Gilgamesh: a Mesopotamian philosophy. History Today. 1961;11(1).

Breasted JH. A history of the ancient Egyptians. New York: Charles Scribner's Sons; 1908.

Breasted JH. Ancient times, a history of the early world. 2nd ed. Boston: Ginn; 1935.

Cavalli F. Breve storia della medicina. Antichità e Medioevo A. A.; 2013–2014.

Chamblee A. The ancient African wisdom commentary on the instruction of Ptahhotep. Bloomington: iUniverse Publications; 2005.

Cinba SJ. When doctors kill. Who, why and how. Berlin: Copernicus Books/Springer Science; 2010. p. 11.

Creel A. The reexamination of dharma in Hindu ethics. Philos East West. 1975;25(2):161–73.

Creel A. Dharma in Hindu ethics. Calcutta: South Asia Books; 1977.

Crush D, Robinson C, York M, editors. Encyclopedia of Hinduism. London: Routledge; 2008. p. 311.

Dadies WW. The Codes of Hammurabi and Moses with copious comments. Cincinnati/New York: Jennings & Graham/Eaton and Mains; 1905.

Dash VB, Junius MM. Manuale di Ayurveda. Roma: Ed. Mediterranee; 2005.

David R. Religion and magic in ancient Egypt. London: Penguin Books; 2002.

De Rachewiltz B. The book of the dead of the ancient Egyptians. Pentagramma series. Roma: Ed. Mediterranee; 1992.

Denison TS, et al. Hammurabi, King of Babylon. Ancient civilizations. Torrance: Mesopotamia: Frank Schaffer Publications; 1997. p. 26–8.

Dhand A. The dharma of ethics, the ethics of dharma: quizzing the ideals of Hinduism. J Relig Ethics. 2002;30(3):347–72.

Doniger W, editor. The laws of Manu. Milan: Adelphi; 1996.

Duhaime L. 1860 BC: the code of Lipit-Ishtar. Law Museum; 2011–2012.

Gellhorn A. Medical ethics—so what's the story? In Vitro. 1977;13(10):589.

Ghalioungui P. The physicians of Pharonic Egypt. Cairo: Al-Ahram Center for Scientific Translations; 1983. 115 pp.

Glucklich A. Dharma: Hindu dharma—encyclopedia of religion, vol. 4. New York: MacMillan; 2005.

Guha S. The Indus civilization. History Today. 2007;57(10):50–7.

Halwani T, Takrouri M. Medical laws and ethics of Babylon as read in Hammurabi's code. Internet J Law Healthcare Ethics. 2006;4(2).

Hassler FA. Charaka Samhita. Science. 1893;22(545):17–8.

Hilton C. Death and dying in the Upanishads Bhagavad-Gita and Caraka Samhita. Opticon1826. 2007;2(1):1–7.

Horne CF. The sacred books and early literature of the east, Egypt, vol. II. New York: Parke, Austin, & Lipscomb; 1917. p. 62–78.

Hughes JJ, Keown D. Buddhism and medical ethics: a bibliographic introduction. J Buddhist Ethics. 1995;2:105–24.

Huilgol NG. Medical ethics in Ayurveda. J Cancer Res Ther. 2012;8(4):661.
Iannacone E. Charaka Samhita and Vimasthana, ilmio libro, pubblicato in proprio. microbook; 2014.
Jonsen AR. Medical history in India and China (Chap. 3). In: A short history of medical ethics. Oxford: Oxford University Press; 2000. p. 27–41.
Karenga M. Maat, the moral ideal in ancient Egypt: a study in classical African ethics. Routledge: Taylor & Francis; 2004.
Keown D. Buddhism and medical ethics: principles and practice. In: Schmithausen L, Sobisch J, editors. Buddhismus in Geschichte und Gegenwart. Hamburg: Universität Hamburg; 2002. p. 39–70.
Keown D, Keown J. Killing, karma and caring: euthanasia in Buddhism and Christianity. J Med Ethics. 1995;21:265–7.
Kott L. Eros and Thanatos Ed. SE; 1997. p. 75–103.
Larue GA. Ancient myth and modern life. Long Beach, CA: Centerline Press; 1988. p. 29–40.
Lichtheim M. Moral values in ancient Egypt. J Near Eastern Stud. 2000;59(3):199–202.
Magi G. Dharma. In: Philosophical encyclopedia, vol. 3. Milan: Bompiani; 2006.
Mahony WK. Hinduism. In: Encyclopedia of religions, Hindu dharma, vol. 9. Milan: Jaca Book; 2006.
Majumdar SK. History of evolution of the concept of medical ethics. Bull Indian Inst Hist Med Hyderabad. 2003;33(1):17–31.
Mancini A. The goddess of justice of ancient Egypt. Buenos Books America LLC; 2010. 128 pp.
Mark JJ. Mesopotamia—ancient history encyclopedia; 2009.
Mark JJ. Ur-Nammu, ancient history encyclopedia; 2014.
Mark JJ. "Ma'at." Ancient history encyclopedia; 2016. Web.07 Dec 2017.
Masui J. How Hindu Dharma addresses, controversial medical issues frequently encountered by Approches de l'Inde (Les Cahiers du Sud); 1949.
Myer I. The oldest book in the world, Baltimore; 1935.
Owen J. Code of Hammurabi: Ancient Babylonian Laws. Live Science Contributor I September 3, 2013.
Pandya SK. History of medical ethics in India. Eubios J Asian Int Bioethics. 2000;10:40–4.
Pettinato G. Sumeri, Rusconi Ed., 1994. p. 283–9.
Piantelli M. Il Buddhismo Indiano. In: Filoramo G, editor. Buddhismo. Bari: Laterza; 2001.
Prakash ND. Medical ethics in India. J Med Philos. 1988;13(3):231–5.
Redford DB, editor. The Oxford encyclopedia of ancient Egypt. Cairo: The American University in Cairo Press; 2001.
Redford DB. The ancient gods speak: a guide to Egyptian religion. Oxford: Oxford University Press; 2002.
Robbins S. Law: a treasury of art and literature. New York: Hugh Lauter Levin Associates; 1990. p. 19–20.
Rosen SJ. Chapter 3: Dharma and the Hindu system. In: Essential Hinduism. Westport: Praeger; 2006. p. 35–6.
Rossi M. Homer and Herodotus to Egyptian medicine. Vesalius. 2010;Suppl: 3–5.
Roth MT, et al. In: Mochalowski P, editor. Law collections from Mesopotamia and Asia Minor, Code of Ur-Nammu. Atlanta: Scholars Press; 1995.
Sandars NK. Epopea di Gilgameš. Piccola Biblioteca Adelphi. Milano: Adelphi Ed; 1986.
Saporetti C. Antiche Leggi.I "Codici" del Vicino Oriente Antico. Milano: Rusconi Ed; 1998.
Saporetti C. Saggi su il Gilgameš per approfondire la conoscenza del più famoso poema della letteratura sumero-babilonese. Milano: Simonelli Ed; 2003.
Seetharam S. Dharma and medical ethics. Indian J Med Ethics. 2013;10(4):226–31.
Shaw I. The Oxford history of ancient Egypt. Oxford: Oxford University Press; 2000.
Shaw I, Nicholson P. The dictionary of ancient Egypt. London: The British Museum; 1995.
Silvia M. The medicine of the Dharma, degree thesis. Venice: Ca' Foscari University; 2013–2014.
Slanski KE. The law of Hammurabi and its audience. Yale J Law Human. 2012;24(1):Article 3.

Souvay C. Hammurabi. In: The Catholic encyclopedia, vol. 7. New York: Robert Appleton Company; 1910.
Steele FR. The code of Lipit-Ishtar. Am J Archeol. 2005;51(2):158–64.
Subbarayappa BV. The roots of ancient medicine: an historical outline. J Biosci. 2001;26(2):135–43.
Tavani M, Picozzi M, Salvati G, et al. Manuale di Deontologia Medica. Milano: Giuffré Editore; 2007. p. 524–5.
University of Manchester. Egyptians, not Greeks were true fathers of medicine. Science Daily, 9 May 2007.
US History.Org. Hammurabi's code: an eye for an eye-ancient civilization online; 2016.
Veatch RM, editor. Cross cultural perspectives in medical ethics. 2nd ed. Boston: Jones and Bartlett Publications; 2000.
Wallis Budge EA. The 42 negative confessions. Rosicrucian Digest. 2007;85(1):12–3.
Walsh J. Sexual morality in ancient Egyptian literature. Vexillum. 2012;2:178–87.
Westendorf W, Leitz C. Egyptian science. Medicine—history of science, 2001.
Westendorf W, Leitz C. Encyclopedia Treccani, Egyptian science, medicine, history of science; 2003.
Wilkinson RH. The complete gods and goddesses of ancient Egypt. London: Thames & Hudson Ltd; 2003.
Younan A. The code of Hammurabi. In: Rich, Hooker, editors. Political philosophy. Translated by L.W. King, 1910. p. 1–34.
Zucconi LM. Medicine and religion in ancient Egypt, Religion Compass, Wiley Online Library; 2007.
Zysk KG. Asceticism and healing in ancient India: medicine in the Buddhist Monasteries. Delhi: Motilal Banarsidass Publishers; 1991.

Hippocrates and Greece

3

The waning of Egyptian civilization coincided with the early years of the Greek one, around the tenth century B.C. This lasted until 146 B.C., [1] with the arrival of the Romans. City states divided the territory and were governed by local authorities. In Athens there was a democracy, in Macedonia a dictatorship and in Sparta military rule.

The ancient Greeks initially regarded disease as divine punishment and healing as a gift (the cult of Asclepius, the god of healing in Roman mythology too: Aesculapius in Latin and English now). [2] Most diseases could be healed by prayers to the demigod; many people went to temples known as *Asclepions*, to pray for healing. The intervention of the daughters of Asclepius was also invoked: Hygieia (goddess of health, cleanliness, and hygiene), Iaso and Aceso (goddesses of healing), and Panacea (who healed all ills). The Greeks began to recognize the importance of the figure of the doctor. This can be seen in the classical works of the time where the necessary care was dispensed to wounded warriors. The medical knowledge of those who worked in this field was based on the practices adopted by the Egyptians.

Scientific medicine had its place in the philosophical schools and those who practiced it came closer to rational thought than many other populations, who were still linked to magic and spells. Over time, doctors acquired a basic knowledge of human anatomy following the observation of seriously wounded soldiers and the dissection of animals (fourth century B.C.).

[1] We have news of Hippocrates in the *Protagora* and in *Phaedrus*, 2 of the 34 "Dialogues" written by Plato; Aristotle also talks about it in "Politics". Sorano d'Efeso remembers him in his "Life" (first to second century AD); Claudio Galen of Pergamum often deals with it.

Boylan (2002), Ede and Cormack (2012), Fioranelli and Zullino (2008), Nordqvist (2012), and Veatch (2000). Chap. 1, The Hippocratic Tradition, pp. 1–24, Chap. 2 Modifying the Hippocratic Tradition, pp. 25–54.

[2] Cavalli (2013-2014), pp. 14–31, Cartwright (2013), Cosmacini (2011), Jonsen (2000), Hellenic, Hellenistic, and Roman Medicine (2000) and Sprengel (1814).

R. G. Russo, *Medical Ethics*, https://doi.org/10.1007/978-3-031-42444-1_3

Pre-Hippocratic Medicine[3]

What medicine aimed at was the good of mankind in general, in the perspective of "happiness":[4] treatments appeared to be the only possible way to solve many dilemmas. Doctors began to show interest in the human body and the symptomatic relationships of diseases, following the successes or failures of the various treatments.

Pre-hippocratic medicine tried to reconcile the different forms of "primitive ethics" (Babylonian, Persian, and Egyptian) with that highlighted in the *Corpus hippocraticum.* It became possible to identify a form of "etiquette" that respected adequate performance and could be used to distinguish experts from charlatans.

The oldest of the pre-hippocratic medical schools was the philosophical one of Miletus in the seventh century B.C. His masters (Thales, Anaxagoras, Anaximander, Archelaus, and Diogenes) tackled medical ethics not only as the study of Man but also from a naturalistic point of view and began to outline rules of conduct. A well-known phrase attributed to Hippocrates: "The doctor who is also a philosopher becomes equal to a god" expressed the first—main—properties (and also the aspirations) of those who took up the medical profession. Treating diseases unquestionably brought financial gain, and the patient had to place himself in a state of dependence on the person he was addressing.

At that time doctors were not subject to any regulations; they acquired scientific skills on their own initiative and presented themselves to patients as a "doctor-friend." Such conduct distinguished them professionally from the many charlatans who professed themselves to be "healers."

The Basics of Medical Ethics

Its foundation might be traced to Democritus, and it was taken up by Socrates, Plato, and above all by Aristotle; the latter explained the analogy between medicine and ethics in the three treatises that have come down to us: "Nicomachean Ethics" (written for his son Nicomacus), "Eudemia," and "Magna Moralia." Ethics became that branch of philosophy that studied behavior, right or wrong, moral concepts (such as justice, virtue, duty) and language.

Aristotle was born in Stageira (Macedonia) in 383/4 B.C. and was a philosopher, scientist, and biologist. Although he was not a doctor, he made an important contribution to the development of medicine by carrying out dissections on numerous animals. He was the founder of comparative anatomy. The introduction of the term "ethics" (*éthos*) can be attributed to him. He died in Euboea (an Aegean island) in 322 B.C.

---

[3] In the Iliad Homer reports that the doctors who assisted the warriors in the expeditions of the Achaeans were of the aristocratic class; in the Odyssey they were described as artisans.
Armocida and Zanobio (2002).

[4] Aristotle (2014), Carrick (2001), Jouanna (2012), Loewy (1989), Aristotle (2009), Koios et al. (2006) and Vegetti (2006).

When considering medical ethics in classical Greece and subsequently in Hellenistic and then Greco-Roman society, some points must be underlined:

1. Never in the classical world was there an explicit authorization for the practice of medicine. Anyone who undertook undertaken to treat patients could call themselves a physician.
2. There were no professional rules that involved sanctions against doctors who violated what were considered professional ethics.
3. It is in fact misleading to speak of professional ethics. At no time were physicians asked to take any oaths, nor were they obliged to follow any code of ethics, formal or informal.
4. The ethical standards referred to in the literature of the time were not always applied by most doctors.
5. Even when some ethical precepts were considered optimal, they never remained unchanged (at least from the ninth century B.C. to the second century A.D.)
6. Medicine was certainly practiced in the Hellenic world long before Hippocrates. From the fifth century B.C. ethics and the parallel development of medical practice, made it necessary to distinguish "doctors" (*iatroi* in Greek, *medici* in Latin) from magical-religious "healers."

Hippocrates

Hippocrates is a real historical figure, even if the myths surrounding him have sometimes undermined this fact. [5] At that time, Greece was enjoying military and cultural splendor. Hippocrates was born on Kos, a Greek island in the Dodecanese, around 460 B.C., in an aristocratic family. He was believed to be the 17th descendant of Asclepius, revered in Greece as a demigod. His contemporaries were Sophocles, Pericles, Herodotus, Euripides, Socrates, Aristophanes, and Plato.

He later met Pythagoras and became a follower. In one of Plato's works, the *Phaedrus*, we find news about the "Hippocratic system," involving knowledge of the body and of the balance of the four humors (blood, phlegm, yellow bile, and black bile) which govern the origin and the development and treatment of diseases.

Hippocrates was responsible for the eradication of an epidemic of plague that struck Athens in 429 B.C.; there he founded a real medical school. He lived for some years "in confinement" due to a restrictive measure imposed on him. However, he exercised his medical profession in Egypt, Libya, Macedonia, Chalcis, Thrace and on the island of Thasos, in the Propontis. Finally, he went to Thessaly (the mythical land of the Asclepiades family), near Larissa, where he died, between 375 and 355 B.C. Hippocrates' ethics and moral duties are reported in some of his works written before the famous Oath, which is described below.

[5] Boylan (2002), Fioranelli (2008), already cited, Gosić (2008), Jones and Withington (1868), Jori (1996), Jacques (1994), Lanata (1961) and Russo (2014).

"The doctor must lead a regular and reserved life, he must not speculate [financially] on the illnesses of patients who must, on the contrary, be treated free if in need. However, a bond of sincerity must be established with the sick." This oath specifies the fundamental principles that those who practice this profession must apply: responsible dissemination of knowledge, commitment to life, awareness of one's limits, integrity, and professional secrecy.

Hippocrates and Medicine[6]

Hippocrates was the first to introduce the concept that disease and health depend on the specific circumstances of the person himself and not on superior divine interventions. He was also the first to study anatomy and pathology, using the dissection of cadavers. He always kept his scientific interest and the ethical concept of medicine alive, together with questions of an ethical-moral order. He also dictated some general criteria for medical practice, always affirming the strict principles of deontology. Hippocrates and his school were the first to use the following medical terms for diseases: acute, chronic, endemic, epidemic, convalescence, crisis, exacerbation, paroxysm, peak, relapse, resolution.

He reported all these considerations in his Oath, which for millennia was taken as the true foundation of medical ethics. Since his time the oath has developed, including in its application multiple influences dictated by history, philosophy, theology, sociology, and anthropology. A fundamental concept of Hippocratic medicine derives from Babylonian and Egyptian medicine. The individual "gnosis" possessed the characteristics and functions of a vital energy, regulator of the harmony necessary for life. In the field of pathology, the Hippocratic school suffered from the doctrine according to which medical ethics may explain that the organism constitutes a unit and not a sum of organic entities. The fundamental doctrine of the school is what was called the "humoral pathology" mentioned above, according to which the four humors form the elements of the human body and of life. The health of a sick organism is brought back to a proportional relationship (*crasis*) between the humors. When this relationship is altered (*dyscrasia*), disease arises, classified as sanguine, phlegmatic, biliary or atrobiliary, depending on the organ concerned.

Finally, under the heading of therapy, the Hippocratic school attributed the greatest importance to the healing power of nature.

The organism has its own natural tendency to recover and disease is the alternation of successes and failures operated by the organism itself in attempts to achieve a remedy.

> Nature is the doctor of diseases and the doctor must only carry out his teachings

Hippocratic medicine is based only on reasoning and experience, completely detached from priestly and magical medicine. Hippocrates also hypothesized—well

[6] Reich (1995), Jones (1868), already cited, Jones (2003), Nutton (2013).

ahead of his time—that the doctor's hygiene benefitted the patient. The teachings of Hippocrates remained, almost unchanged, through to the end of the eighteenth century.

His works about 69 of them were collected in the *Corpus Hippocraticum*; they were mostly composed between the end of the fifth and the beginning of the fourth century B.C. Different topics were covered, dealing with legislative or more strictly medical or surgical aspects.

These were the most common diseases for the time, with medicaments, wounds for surgery, fractures, dentition, ulcers, fistulas, and hemorrhoids, but there were also topics related to nutrition or gestation. Specific attention was dedicated to epilepsy and to ecology.

Probably only a fraction of them were actually written by Hippocrates; the others date to his pupils or doctors from other schools. Ahead of the times by about 2000 years, human health was considered related to the influence exerted by the climate.[7]

The main aim of Greek medicine was a science free from superstition and philosophical hypotheses. The Hippocratic texts had a common characteristic: they denied that diseases were a divine punishment and did not attribute any therapeutic value to the prayers, spells, and mysterious healings that were said to take place at sanctuaries. A new rational medicine was opposed to the old, religious and magical, and everything was traced back to nature and its phenomena (even though they were still largely unknown).

Another recurring feature in Hippocratic medicine was the importance attached to the close observation of the sick and the systematic recording of all data concerning the course of the disease. This attention to detail led, for the first time in the history of medicine, to the compilation of clinical records of individual patients (a few dozen specimens have been retrieved and documented). Hippocrates introduced the use of medical records and theorized the need to observe patients rationally, taking account of their appearance and symptoms; he is also credited with having introduced the concepts of diagnosis and prognosis. The two surgical treatises "On fractures" and "On joints" can be traced back to Hippocrates, as well as the "Prognostic" and "The Epidemics."

As an example, in the second chapter of the Prognostic, there is a description of the signs that foretell death and are still called *Facies Hippocratica*[8] today in medical terminology :

[7] Little is known about the climate. Important studies have brought out this important variable that has accompanied and perhaps truly conditioned the development of mankind. The global situation is increasingly topical and seems to restrict even more the time to make the necessary and indispensable corrections. see: Behringer (2014).

[8] Similarly: The *risus sardonicus*, a continuous spasm of the face muscles, is also referred to as "Hippocratic smile". The "hippocratic succussion" (abrupt shaking of the chest) indicates the typical noises of "sprays" seen in cases of hydropneumothorax or pyopneumothorax. The "Hippocrates bench" (today referred to as inversion bench) is used for spinal traction to help reduce back pain, for physical well-being and to facilitate the correct position of the bones. Hippocrates observed and described numerous symptoms; he studied the dislocations, fractures, and head wounds. He prepared new surgical instruments and studied epidemiological elements in the air and water. He also

In diseases, the doctor must be useful or at least not do harm

The specification to "do no harm" expresses the awareness of the difficulties of the medical art and recommends a prudent and respectful attitude towards the patient. It is the disease, Hippocrates underlined, that is the real protagonist. The one who fights the disease—the doctor—is only the patient's ally, helping him in that dramatic struggle.

Hippocrates and Medical Conduct

Hippocrates also set down the rules of medical conduct in his famous oath. The doctor's task is to help the body by trying to restore the right conditions for its proper functioning, trying to make all the external factors that caused the disease harmless. From this point of view the disease is not to be considered a sudden or accidental event: it has a history that can be reconstructed by identifying its causes and predicting their course.

Ethics in the Oath

The oath reflects the ideas not only of doctors and caregivers in general. Certainly it was never imposed as a necessary qualification for the exercise of the profession. Hippocratic ethics honors the universal healing pact between a competent doctor and a sick person. Promoting life, alleviating suffering, being virtuous, protecting medical education and confidentiality are themes that are repeated over the centuries and in all cultures throughout the world. The broad ethical prohibition of murder, lying, and theft have their positive implications in medicine, considering certain elements as "essential" for "responsible medical activity":

1. respect for the patient;
2. the doctor and the relationship of trust and "alliance" between doctor and patient;
3. the intention not to harm (*primum non nocere*);
4. the confidentiality of the relationship;
5. professional decorum;
6. medical education to promote the advancement of the profession. These "virtues" are all reported and respected in the Oath.

dictated some general criteria for medical practice, always affirming the strict principles of deontology. Hippocrates seems to have been the first to describe the "drumstick fingers" characteristic of Pierre Marie's hypertrophic pneumatic osteopathy and of the "Eisenmenger" syndrome, labeled "hippocratic fingers" in semiotics.

Main Historical Stages of the Oath

Almost all classicists accept the idea that many Greek and Roman doctors did not follow the precepts of the Oath in their practice and in their ethics.

The authorities neither invoked it nor imposed it on future doctors. In fact, they practiced abortions and euthanasia, without being in any way condemned for this. Complex surgeries were performed, including lithotomy, with no remorse.

Although the Oath was widely known and shared, it was never imposed by law or custom in Greece, Rome, the Muslim world or in medieval Europe.

The Hippocratic oath, starting from the Middle Ages, has undergone several extensions and re-propositions over the centuries. It was first mentioned in 47 A.D. by *Scribonius* Largus. [9] From the eleventh century Western medical Ethics adopted the moral values of the Catholic religion; doctors therefore had to abide by the duties and principles of professional ethics. In the Middle Ages, more and more professional training and clinical skills were required to respond to the responsibility of caring, safeguarding the health of others and doing all possible to extend life even in severe or hopeless cases.

The first certain date on which the oath was taken in an academic context is 1508, in the Faculty of Medicine of Wittemberg (Germany). The "doctor's oath," composed by its Rector Von Scheurl and the first professor of medicine Von Mellerstadt, incorporates some phrases from the original Oath. Some time later, in 1558, the Dean had to recite the Oath at the Heidelberg Faculty of Medicine after taking office. Here it was the Headmaster who supervised, not the students or graduates. A similar procedure was adopted at the University of Basel where a version was adopted that replaced "Apollo doctor and Aesculapius" with the Trinity. This remained in force until 1868. At the University of Iena (1591) and at the University of Giessen (1607) the Statutes cite the Oath as a regulation to be observed.

From 1750 onwards more specific medical oaths were developed in Germany. These concerned what a doctor should do or think together with the loyalty to be given to the state and the university. In 1771 John Morgan, an Edinburgh graduate reported that the Hippocratic Oath was commonly adopted in universities and related medical schools in the USA. In Great Britain the Royal College of Physicians of London, founded by Henry VIII, applied it to ensure the lawfulness of the practice of medicine.

In the nineteenth century, words such as "holiness" and "purity," with their strongly religious connotations, disappeared from some translations of the oath. In the period following the French Revolution, from July 1804, those who graduated in medicine in Montpellier had to recite the Oath in Latin, facing a bust of Hippocrates donated by the French government. He then had to promise, in the

[9] Scribonius Largus wrote his Medical Recipes in 271 texts, with all kinds of "medical" curiosities of the time. He was a highly regarded author in the late imperial age, but was then misunderstood and little esteemed.

Mantovanelli (2012) and Sterpellone (2004).

name of God, to be faithful to the laws of man and honor in exercising his profession. The universities of Paris and Strasbourg followed suit—without the bust!

As early as 1806 Benjamin Rush (one of the founding fathers of the United States) called his students to treasure the Hippocratic heritage in their daily actions. In the United States, in the years 1840–1860, doctors were adapting medical ethics to the prescriptions of the Hippocratic oath. However, from 1880 at McGill University in Canada and at St. Thomas' Hospital in London, allegiance to the Oath was considered anachronistic and antiquated at a time when medical science was steadily, but despite this the Oath was still used at graduation ceremonies in many universities. Beginning in 1928, only in some American medical schools was the degree accompanied by the Hippocratic Oath ceremony, recognized as mandatory to this day. A modern English version, around 1930, takes up the original text, with the prohibition of deliberately causing the death of a person.

White Coat Ceremony[10]

From 1965, several US schools adopted the Hippocratic Oath, or parts of it. The White Coat Ceremony was instituted in American universities, taking place on the first day of the so-called Freshman Year. During the ceremony, each graduate student receives a white toga from the Dean, as a symbol of medicine. The Freshmen then have to stand up and recite an oath (Physician's Oath of Hippocrates) which, however, only re-proposes the name, having been revised to make it more "politically correct." In 1996 the Oath appeared in the "American Medical Association Code of Medical Ethics."

Finally, in this brief excursus on recent trends relating to the ethics of medicine, it is appropriate to recall what initiation ceremonies to start the school year for doctors are essentially a rite of passage to welcome the new students into the medical profession. They are scheduled at the very beginning of the course before the students have attended any lessons or do any laboratory work. Whole classes, families, and friends of students are welcome to attend. Students are congratulated on being selected and reaffirm the commitment they are making as future doctors to become and remain competent in the science and technology of medicine, together with the human obligations that go with it, the main obligation being to take proper care of their patients. Students are urged to make sure they put their patients' interests ahead of their own and conduct themselves honorably throughout their medical career, always striving to be worthy of the privilege of being doctors and never abusing it. The first "White Coat Ceremony," based on reading the Hippocratic Oath, seems to have taken place in 1993 at the College of Physicians in New York. It was sponsored by a grant from a foundation created by a neurologist/pediatrician,

[10] Berdine (2016), Published electronically: Jan. 2015. Wikipedia, White coat ceremony. Carrick (2001), Couch (1934), Guinan (2012), Hulkower (2010), Jones (1923), Littrè (1839-1841), Nutton (2013), Pellegrino (1990) and Trueman (2015), 4 Apr 2018.

"dedicated to promoting the human component in medicine." The ceremony is increasingly held in many American and European medical schools.[11]

Below Are a Few Versions of the Hippocratic Oath for Comparison

The Classic Hippocratic Oath (Fifth Century B.C.)

[From The Hippocratic Oath: Text, Translation, and Interpretation, by Ludwig Edelstein. Baltimore: Johns Hopkins Press, 1943.]

I swear by Apollo Physician and Asciepius and Hygieia and Panaceia and all the gods and goddesses, making them my witnesses, that I will fulfill according to my ability and judgment this oath and this covenant:

To hold him who has taught me this art as equal to my parents and to live my life in partnership with him, and if he is in need of money to give him a share of mine, and to regard his offspring as equal to my brothers in male lineage and to teach them this art, if they desire to learn it, without fee and covenant; to give a share of precepts and oral instruction and all the other learning to my sons and to the sons of him who has instructed me and to pupils who have signed the covenant and have taken an oath according to the medical law, but to no one else.

I will apply dietetic measures for the benefit of the sick according to my ability and judgment; I will keep them from harm and injustice.

I will neither give a deadly drug to anybody if asked for it, nor will I make a suggestion to this effect. Similarly I will not give to a woman an abortive remedy. In purity and holiness I will guard my life and my art.

I will not use the knife, not even on sufferers from stone, but will withdraw in favor of such men as are engaged in this work.

Whatever houses I may visit, I will come for the benefit of the sick, remaining free of all intentional injustice, of all mischief and in particular of sexual relations with both female and male persons, be they free or slaves.

What I may see or hear in the course of the treatment or even outside of the treatment in regard to the life of men, which on no account one must spread abroad, I will keep to myself holding such things shameful to be spoken about.

If I fulfill this oath and do not violate it, may it be granted to me to enjoy life and art, being honored with fame among all men for all time to come; if I transgress it and swear falsely, may the opposite of all this be my lot.

Primum non nocere.

Primum non nocere is a **Latin** phrase that means "first, do no harm."

The origin of the phrase is uncertain. The Hippocratic Oath includes the promise "to abstain from doing harm" but not the exact wording. That sentence was probably introduced into American and British medical culture in 1847.

[11] Kantarjian and Steensa (2014).

"Pagan Oath"

by Mr. W. H. S. Jones, in his book The Doctor's Oath (Cambridge University Press, 1924).

"I swear by Apollo Physician, by Asclepius, by Health, by Heal-all, and by all the gods and goddesses, making them witnesses, that I will carry out, according to my ability and judgment, this oath and this indenture:"

"To regard my teacher in this art as equal to my parents; to make him partner in my livelihood, and when he is in need of money to share mine with him; to consider his offspring equal to my brothers; to teach them this art, if they require to learn it, without fee or indenture; and to impart precept oral instruction, and all the other learning, to my sons, to the sons of my teacher, and to the pupils who have signed the indenture and sworn obedience to the physicians' Law, but to none other."

"I will use treatment to help the sick according to my ability and judgment, but I will never use it to injure or wrong them."

"I will not give poison to anyone though asked to do so, nor will I suggest such a plan. Similarly I will not give a pessary to a woman to cause abortion. But in purity and in holiness I will guard my life and my art."

"I will not use the knife either on sufferers from stone, but I will give place to such as are craftsmen therein."

"Into whatsoever houses I enter, I will do so to help the sick, keeping myself free from all intentional wrongdoing and harm, especially from fornication with woman or man, bond or free."

"Whatsoever in the course of practice I see or hear (or even outside my practice in social intercourse) that ought never to be published abroad, I will not divulge, but consider such things to be holy secrets."

"Now if I keep this oath and break it not, may I enjoy honor, in my life and art, among all men for all time; but if I transgress and forswear myself, may the opposite befall me."

(BMJ 1948;ii:616)

The Revised Hippocratic Oath

Modern Oath of Physicians: Written in 1964 by Louis Lasagna, Academic Dean of the School of Medicine at Tufts University, and used in many medical schools today. ... There is no promise by the physician that they will "do no harm" or never give a "lethal medicine" as is contained in the Hippocratic Oath.

> *I swear to fulfill, to the best of my ability and judgment, this covenant:*
>
> *I will respect the hard-won scientific gains of those physicians in whose steps I walk, and gladly share such knowledge as is mine with those who are to follow.*
>
> *I will apply, for the benefit of the sick, all measures [that] are required, avoiding those twin traps of over-treatment and therapeutic nihilism.*
>
> *I will remember that there is art to medicine as well as science, and that warmth, sympathy, and understanding may outweigh the surgeon's knife or the chemist's drug.*
>
> *I will not be ashamed to say "I know not," nor will I fail to call in my colleagues when the skills of another are needed for a patient's recovery.*
>
> *I will respect the privacy of my patients, for their problems are not disclosed to me that the world may know.*

Most especially must I tread with care in matters of life and death. If it is given me to save a life, all thanks.

But it may also be within my power to take a life; this awesome responsibility must be faced with great humbleness and awareness of my own frailty. Above all, I must not play God.

I will remember that I do not treat a fever chart, a cancerous growth, but a sick human being, whose illness may affect the person's family and economic stability. My responsibility includes these related problems, if I am to care adequately for the sick.

I will prevent disease whenever I can, for prevention is preferable to cure.

I will remember that I remain a member of society, with special obligations to all my fellow human beings, those sound of mind and body as well as the infirm.

If I do not violate this oath, may I enjoy life and art, respected while I live and remembered with affection thereafter.

May I always act so as to preserve the finest traditions of my calling and may I long experience the joy of healing those who seek my help.

The Physician's Oath

World Medical Association (Geneva, Switzerland) The Oath was amended by the 22nd World Medical Assembly, in August 1968. The Physician's Oath, to be sworn at the time a person enters the medical profession, was added to the Declaration of Geneva and adopted by the General Assembly of the World Medical Association in September 1948, 3 months before the General Assembly of the United Nations adopted the Universal Declaration of Human Rights, which upholds the right to security of person.

This oath was written as a direct response to the atrocities committed by the physicians in Nazi Germany.

The second last line reads, "I will maintain the utmost respect for human life; even under threat, I will not use my medical knowledge contrary to the laws of humanity."

The "Physician's Oath on Retirement" is being proposed "to address the moral, psychological, social, and cultural responsibilities that a physician assumes when voluntarily relinquishing the responsibilities of active medical practice."

I solemnly pledge myself to consecrate my life to the service of humanity;

I will give to my teachers the respect and gratitude which is their due;

I will practice my profession with conscience and dignity;

The health of my patient will be my first consideration;

I will respect the secrets which are confided in me;

I will maintain by all the means in my power, the honor and the noble traditions of the medical profession;

My colleagues will be my brothers and sisters;

I will not permit considerations of religion, nationality, race, gender, politics, socioeconomic standing, or sexual orientation to intervene between my duty and my patient;

I will maintain the utmost respect for human life; even under threat, I will not use my medical knowledge contrary to the laws of humanity;

I make these promises solemnly, freely and upon my honor.

The 1998 Version

Aware of the importance and solemnity of the act I perform and the commitment I undertake, I swear to practice medicine in freedom and independence of judgment and behavior;

- *to pursue as exclusive purposes the defense of life, the protection of physical and mental health of man and the relief of suffering, which I will inspire with responsibility and constant scientific, cultural and social commitment, all my professional acts;*
- *never to perform acts capable of deliberately causing the death of a patient;*
- *to adhere in my activity to the ethical principles of human solidarity, against which, in respect for life and for the person, I will never use my knowledge;*
- *to perform my work with diligence, expertise and prudence according to science and conscience and observing the ethical rules that govern the practice of medicine and the legal ones that do not conflict with the purposes of my profession;*
- *to entrust my reputation exclusively to my professional skills and my moral skills;*
- *to avoid, even outside the professional practice, any act and behavior that could harm the prestige and dignity of the profession;*
- *to respect colleagues even in the event of conflicting opinions;*
- *to treat all my patients with equal care and commitment regardless of the feelings they inspire in me and regardless of any difference of race, religion, nationality, social condition and political ideology;*
- *to provide emergency assistance to any sick person who needs it and to make myself available to the competent authority in case of public calamity;*
- *to respect and facilitate in any case the patient's right to free choice of doctor, taking into account that the relationship between doctor and patient is based on trust and in any case on mutual respect;*
- *"to observe the secrecy of everything that is confided to me, that I see or that I have seen, understood or sensed in the exercise of my profession or because of my state."*

A Later Version (March 2007)

Aware of the importance and solemnity of the act I perform and the commitment I undertake, I swear:

- *to practice medicine in freedom and independence of judgment and behavior, avoiding any undue influence and conditioning;*
- *to pursue the defense of life, the protection of human physical and mental health and the relief of suffering, to which I will inspire all my professional work with responsibility and constant scientific, cultural and social commitment;*
- *never to do anything deliberately causing the death of a person;*
- *to adhere in my activity to the ethical principles of human solidarity against which, in respect for life and for the person, I will never use my knowledge;*
- *to conduct my work, in science and conscience, with diligence, expertise and prudence and according to fairness, observing the deontological rules that*

regulate the practice of medicine and all legal ones that do not conflict with the purposes of my profession;

- *to entrust my professional reputation exclusively to my competence and my moral skills;*
- *to avoid, even outside professional practice, any act and behavior that could harm the decorum and dignity of the profession;*
- *to respect colleagues even in the event of conflicting opinions;*
- *to treat each patient with equal care and commitment, regardless of ethnicity, religion, nationality, social condition and political ideology and promoting the elimination of all forms of discrimination in the health care;*
- *to provide emergency assistance to those in need and to make myself available to the appropriate authority in the event of a public calamity;*
- *to respect and facilitate the right to free choice of doctor;*
- *to promote a therapeutic alliance with the patient based on trust and mutual information, respecting and sharing the principles that inspire medical art;*
- *to observe professional secrecy and to protect the confidentiality of all that is confided to me, that I see or I have seen, understood or sensed in the exercise of my profession or by reason of my status;*
- *to refrain from any diagnostic and therapeutic persistence;*
- *to make my knowledge available to medical progress.*

Hippocratic Oath and Code of Ethics [12]

The Hippocratic Oath enabled medicine to become a rational science even though it has never been a definitive document over all these years. It begins with an invocation addressed to each god and goddess, all the enlightened gods starting with Apollo the doctor: Asclepius, Hygieia, Panacea, and so on. In the Jewish, Christian, and Muslim versions, this list has been partially substituted or extended depending on the deities worshiped in these religions.

The Arab oath, for example, begins with an invocation to Allah, the Lord of life and death, giver of health, creator of healing and all care. Several extant manuscripts are accompanied by explanatory notes. At the time of Hippocrates, there were many uneducated charlatans posing as doctors.

The oath was a way to identify medicine people could trust and also to distinguish true doctors from fakes.

The text may sound surprising when it lingers on condemning some practices (then already in use) such as abortion and euthanasia, or surgical malpractice, which seemed to precede contemporary medical ethics. But, putting such "prohibitions" in their historical context, they make sense, serving as a guide against physicians who put their patients at undue risk.

[12] Huber (2003), Rothstein (2001), Sritharan et al. (2001), Stevenson (2002), Veatch (2002) and Wear (1998).

The oath describes what doctors should do, not just what they should not do. It really seems to uphold its position as a model of a code of professional ethics, a guide to entering the profession, especially since doctors have the obligation to "teach the art of medicine." The oath sets up medical knowledge not just as knowledge that is positive in itself, but as knowledge that "engenders obligations to those who possess it."

To sum up, the original oath consists of two portions. The first defines the teacher-pupil relationship and the second sets out the ethical code of medicine.

The main solemn promises the new doctor makes can be summarized:

1. Administer the best medical care and medicines, only for the benefit of patients.
2. Do not provide any deadly drugs, even if asked for or advice on how to procure them (suicide).
3. Do not procure an abortion.
4. Keep both your existence and your art pure and clean.
5. Do not operate for a kidney stone (meaning he must not use unfamiliar techniques).
6. Refrain from deliberately causing injustice or harm.
7. Do not have sexual intercourse with your patients.
8. Observe medical confidentiality (secrecy).

Comments and Considerations

The "ancient" version is markedly different from the others. In some Greek manuscripts the oath is written in the shape of a "cross" and in others it unites Christian and pagan divinities. This indicates, once again, that the oath has never been a fixed and unalterable document. The Hippocratic Oath was later translated in all the languages of those times. The Christian version included some changes. The prohibition of abortions, for example, was reinforced, eliminating any mention of the use of an abortive pessary. However, abortion was not prohibited in ancient times, and in fact various methods are described in the Corpus Hippocraticum, including the use of drugs. Although written in antiquity, its principles are still held sacred by doctors today: treat the patient to the best of your abilities, preserve the patient's privacy, pass on the secrets of medicine for future generations. The prohibition for a physician to cause the death of a person deliberately or on request: "I will not give anyone a deadly drug, even if requested, nor will I suggest such advice; similarly to no woman will I give an abortive drug" is currently interpreted as a reference to assisted suicide, while the original probably included both euthanasia and the participation of a doctor in torture, acts of brutality or murder. The statement "I will not operate on those who suffer from the disease of the stone, but I will turn to those who are experts in this activity," constitutes a ban on any type of surgery, not only lithotomy. Certainly 2500 years ago the risks far outweighed the benefits in complex surgical operations!

In the modern Hippocratic Oath, the doctor undertakes, in what they call the "therapeutic alliance," to defend life, never to perform acts capable of promoting death, to found care relationships on trust and mutual information. It is the human and ethical dimension that must guide the doctor's conduct. Anyone who participates in any inhuman practice, voluntarily or involuntarily, on patients or other individuals, such as prisoners or convicts, degrades the whole profession. The loss of the "human" component seems to be related to the continuous request for specialization that conditions the doctor's attitude, preventing the establishment of a solid personal relationship based on trust with the patient.

In conclusion, the Hippocratic Oath covers some important issues in the relationship between doctors and patients. One of the main points it makes is that the doctor is responsible for his work in case of difficulty.

Furthermore, the Oath has a particularly individualistic perspective: it provides ethical indications for the important relationship, particularly compared to earlier codes. This individualistic aspect changed with the "medical experiments" conducted during the Second World War.

The oaths were summed up as "a solemn promise" of:

– solidarity with teachers and other doctors;
– charity (to do good or avoid evil);
– to do nothing evil to patients (so as not to cause harm);
– do not assist in suicide or abortion;
– entrust surgery to surgeons;
– do not seduce patients;
– to maintain the appropriate confidentiality.

The religious and/or "pagan" basis of the oath has been revisited to achieve a new modern and universal formulation. For example, in recent times, the World Medical Association (W.M.A.) pleaded for the Oath, in order to "serve humanity, striving to achieve the highest international standards in Medical Education, Medicine, Ethics and Care for all people in the world." The Oath establishes first of all that the medical professional must give credit to their teachers and also to their students. This ensures that the doctor does not forget the traditions and customs of those who accompanied and guided him in this career. Another important moral principle is the maintenance of integrity. Doctors must always ensure the consent of patients, never exploiting them, respecting their privacy; never using deadly drugs, never inducing abortions, and, ultimately, "not playing God." The Oath has been subject to revisions and renovations that have downsized the style and, perhaps, somewhat altered its message.

Importance in Time

Hippocrates made such an impression on medical history that his name has been associated with medicine over the centuries and today doctors still consider him as the "father" of modern medicine, even though he was born around 430 years before Christ.

Some share his belief that the observation of a patient and his symptoms ("clinical observation") are a vital aspect of medical care and predict the course of the disease. Others, however, oppose his convictions, as expressed in his Oath and in "On forecasting diseases" in his "Corpus." The ideas of Hippocrates and others nevertheless spread to the eastern Mediterranean, and others began to record what they saw about disease. Those of these writings that have survived have given historians a vast resource to study. The assumption was that all diseases had a natural rather than a supernatural cause. Hippocrates' ideas were a strange mixture of common sense and factual inaccuracies. His suggestions on diet and exercise are as valid today as they were 2500 years ago and so is his use of clinical observation. His theory of the "four humors" dominated medical treatments until the seventeenth century!

Hippocrates' most important contributions were in the development of the medical profession and in a code of conduct for physicians, with current, unambiguous arguments. [13]

Some of His Aphorisms

- In any disease it is a good sign if the patient maintains lucidity and appetite, a bad sign if the opposite happens.
- Old people generally get sick less than young people, but if their illnesses become chronic, they almost always last until death.
- Any disease can happen in any season, but some are more likely to occur and get worse in certain seasons.
- Those who are used to putting up with jobs that are familiar to them, even if they are weak and old, do them more easily than those who are not used to them even if they are strong and young.
- Do not disturb the patient during or immediately after a crisis and do not experiment on him with purges or other irritants, but leave him alone.
- The elderly tolerate fasting better than middle-aged men and the young bear it badly and worse than smaller children, especially very lively ones.

[13] Carrick (2001), Couch (1934), Mastrangelo (2010), Ogunbanjo et al. (2009), Orr et al. (1997) and Tyson (2001).

Hippocrates in Recent Times

Dante Alighieri mentioned Hippocrates, in verse 143 of the fourth canto of Hell, together with other eminent scientists and historical figures who occupy the first circle of Dante's Hell (Limbo) for not having had the good fortune to know Christ.

Hippocrates was mentioned in the Patristics and in the Scholastica by Cyprian of Carthage (+258 A.D.), Gregory of Nazianzo (+390 A.D), Gregory of Nyssa (+395 A.D.), and Eusebius of Caesarea (+339 A.D.) who supported a theory of the natural sciences, as a remedy for illnesses and also magical and demonic implications. The Didache (Doctrine of the Twelve Apostles) of the first century A.D. asserted: "You must not induce an abortion, you must not kill a baby."

Honorius Augustodunensis (1080–1154) agrees with Hippocrates that "The healing of the body leads to a cure of the soul."

Knowledge about Hippocrates and the *Corpus hippocraticum* spread through Nestorian-Syrian Christianity. Thomas of Aquinas also mentioned Hippocrates a few times.

Both the Canadian and the US "Hippocratic Registry" are organizations of doctors who uphold the original principles of the Oath as inviolable over time.

Hippocrates in Ecclesiastical Writings[14]

Among the works of Petrus Hispanus (ca. 1205–1277), a physician with academic degrees, who later became Pope John XXI, there are two comments on Hippocrates in the text *De regimine auctorum et Prognostica.*

Pope Pius XII (1876–1958) in 1954 defined the ethical-medical significance of Hippocrates' works: "The works of Hippocrates are undoubtedly the noblest expression of a professional conscience that first of all requires respect for life and sacrifice for the sick."

Pope Paul VI (1897–1978) reminded doctors to be faithful to the Hippocratic Oath handed down over the years as the "defender of life."

Pope John Paul I (1912–1978) wrote imaginary letters to historical figures, including Hippocrates, with the title "Illustrissimi."

Pope Saint John Paul II (1920–2005), in 1978, on the occasion of the audience with the Association of Italian Catholic Doctors, cited the Hippocratic recommendations not to use medicines that contradicted not only Christian ethics, but all natural ethics, and were in open contradiction to the professional duties expressed in the famous Oath of the old pagan doctor:

"May all doctors be faithful to the Hippocratic Oath they take when they are awarded their degree." He also exhorted doctors to consciously serve their duty to men: "Be deeply convinced of this truth because of the long tradition that goes back to the intuitions of Hippocrates himself".

[14] Couch (1934), Lowes (1995), Ogunbanjo (2009), Orr (1997), Roth (n.d.), Tyson (2001) and Woodbury (2012).

In the ceremony appointing the members of the Pontifical Academy for Life, *Expressis Verbis* is mentioned and Pope Benedict XVI, in his speech to surgeons in 2008, cited Hippocrates as the crucial point of bioethics.

Pope Francis also spoke about Hippocrates, on the occasion of the 70th anniversary of the Catholic Doctors Association, on November15, 2014.

Oppositions to the Oath [15]

Since 1181, the year it was first presented, at the University of Montpellier, in France, the Hippocratic Oath has been an ethical model for doctors and a basis for medicine and it is also rooted in myth.[16]

In medical schools thousands of novice doctors are invited to take an oath that often draws its origin and formulation from a Greek doctor who practiced and taught more than 24 centuries ago![17]

The ancient Greek world and Christianity present points of agreement and offer a common approach to the ethical questions arising in the practice of modern medicine.

Physicians today face a number of important ethical issues that are not covered in the Oath. For example, the following are not mentioned, among other things:

- honor patient preferences
- sharing medical information with patients
- avoiding conflicts of interest, such as profit, by ordering unnecessary evidence or treatment
- protecting patients enrolling in research studies
- treating all patients equally, regardless of economic status, social class, education, race or suspected potential bias
- how to avoid the practice of medicine, when it is compromised, due to physical or mental illness.

Recent biomedical advances and changing social needs have raised a number of new moral questions and doubts, for which the traditional ethical guidelines, set in the Hippocratic *Corpus*, are no longer adequate.

However, the other ethical values and principles established by the *Corpus* and its supporters over the centuries are still respected. In modern times, society has questioned the paternalism expressly advocated in the document.

This challenge, however, does not diminish its historical and ethical value. On the contrary, it demonstrates that certain timeless values evolve in line with social change.

[15] Colburn (1991), Lowes (1995) and Woodbury (2012).

[16] Shmerling (2015).

[17] Hurwitz and Richardson (1997).

Increasing numbers of doctors are convinced that the Oath is inadequate to face the realities of a medical world that has seen enormous scientific, economic, political and social changes; a world of legalized abortion, assisted suicide, and various calamities unforeseeable at the time of Hippocrates. It is seen as little more than a pro-forma ritual with scant value beyond defending tradition.

Some doctors argue classical Oath makes no mention of such contemporary issues as the ethics of experimentation, care in a team, or the social and legal responsibilities of a doctor. Furthermore, most modern oaths do not mention penalties, there is no risk of "losing face" for potential offenders.

Moreover, is the "Oath" still relevant in the era of AIDS, assisted suicide, in vitro micro-surgery, genetic pharmacology and the management of many other treatments?

The heated debate sees both those who always believe that its principles are well founded and those who now consider them obsolete and inadequate to modern medicine. Many people believe that the whole document not only needs to be updated, but could also in fact be eliminated altogether.

Fortunately, there are many other useful resources beyond the Hippocratic Oath to guide doctors in the right direction. No doctor has ever stubbornly adhered to it and it has never been legally binding.

Some, moreover, maintain that it has the same relevance today as ever: a public declaration of the social contract between the medical profession, its individual members, and society as a whole. These doctors simply believe he is independent to behave morally and ethically towards patients, overlooking the roles of the healthcare industry, employers, the pharmaceutical industry, etc. Furthermore, should the Hippocratic Oath continue to set the ethical standard of patient care for doctors today or is it an anachronism that should be eliminated? Many doctors disagree on the answer.

Since the 1950s there have been repeated efforts to modernize the oath and to keep it relevant. Various versions have been suggested, especially in the USA, and other oaths have been consulted, such as the original Hippocratic Oath, the Hippocratic Oath revised by the World Health Organization or Lasagna, the Maimonides prayer, the declaration of Geneva, the declaration of the University of Naples, and the Duties of the General Medical Council, "Not one has proved to be a relevant substitute that we are aware of," family doctors have replied. It is not only the subjects of the oath that matter, but the oath itself: the doctor swears to behave morally and honestly.

Some criticisms refer to the invocation of "all the Gods and Goddesses" since this, with its pagan character, inserts a religious element into medical ethics to which many doctors are opposed. Women were not doctors in ancient Greece, so the oath is intended only for men—an unwelcome reminder. Doctors are prohibited from administering "poisons" to patients.

Other Comments

If this warning were taken literally today, pharmacotherapy, chemotherapy, and radiotherapy would be prohibited. Abortion is prohibited, as is assisted suicide. Any concept of death is absent. Some doctors find the promise of respecting ethical standards written for times past hypocritical—a seemingly useless undertaking. In conclusion, however, the Hippocratic Oath remains very relevant, not only on account of its longevity but, above all, the spirit it generates. However, when asked, "Still relevant?", another doctor replied: "Absolutely no, not in a medical world controlled by unknown administrators, none of whom see patients or realize what it takes to treat patients every day. Hippocrates would have turned over in his grave." Doctors also wonder if the original oath or an alternative version, should the older version be withdrawn, always has the same relevance, because Hippocrates summarized the best of medicine known to him and opened a new era of clinical practice.[18] The oath is basically a set of rules by that all doctors must respect.

Hippocrates marked the ethical guidelines in relation to his profession. Every life must be worshiped and preserved, whether it is that of a king or a slave and no practitioner can abuse its power, so today's doctors must adhere to the same standards. As already mentioned, it is often considered to have lapsed[19] but the alternatives have never been accepted as definitive, even revising the classic text, eliminating suspicious language and appealing to the doctor's duty as such. Hippocratic ethics must be emphasized more than the oath itself, rather than the "anti-historical" banality of dedications to deities no longer recognizable or the respect reflecting the surgical incompetence of the time.

The Hippocratic Oath maintains its application for "how a doctor should behave towards patients and colleagues and his responsibilities towards society."

The *art* consists of three things: the disease, the patient, and the doctor, with the underlying premise of "doing no harm," say the Hippocratic treatises. It is reported that "The oath has been administered to medical graduates in many European universities for centuries" and there is widespread public opinion that the oath should still be administered to all doctors upon graduation. [20] About 98% of Americans and nearly 50% of British medical students swear an oath, both upon entering medical school and upon graduation, even if its use has not been constant or continuous. In the UK, the General Medical Council [21] revived its professional code along with the British Medical Association (BMA), Royal Colleges and other organizations.

---

[18] Chesanow (2017).

[19] Medscape (2016).

[20] Rosenhek (2009).

There were many comments, from all over the world and based on various cultures and traditions.

Comment on the Oath: "It explains well how a doctor should behave towards patients and colleagues and his responsibilities towards society. I don't care much for language; it's the thought behind it that matters."

[21] Crawshaw (1994), Crashaw and Linn (1996), Garrison (1929) and Loudon (1994).

Review of the Hippocratic Oath ?

The practice of medicine is a privilege that leads to important responsibilities. "I promise that my medical knowledge will be used to benefit people's health: My professional judgment will be exercised independently as far as possible and will not be influenced by political pressures or factors such as the patient's social status. I will not put personal profit or career above my duty to patients."

"I want to ensure that patients receive the information and support they need to make decisions about disease prevention and improve their health. I will try to change laws that are contrary to the interests of patients or my professional ethics."

It is not clear whether the oath has greatly influenced the competence of doctors to debate effectively on ethical questions. The main focus of a medical oath appears to be the core values of the profession, to generate or strengthen the necessary resolution in doctors. Oaths exemplify professional integrity and traditional moral virtues such as compassion and honesty and also provide moral guidance.

The first ceremony of "**Affirmation of a new doctor,**" declaring the commitment to take on the responsibilities and obligations of the medical profession, took place at Imperial College London on 27 July 2001, attended by friends and family: all the newly qualified doctors confirmed their commitment. The final report below shows some of the positive statements, which simply reaffirm the truths of the medical profession: A promise is read out:

"Now, as a new Doctor, I solemnly promise that"

I will act to the best of my ability to serve humanity, care for the sick, promote good health and relieve pain and suffering. I recognize that the practice of medicine is a privilege that requires great responsibility and I do not want to abuse my position.

I will practice medicine with integrity, humility, honesty and compassion, working with my fellow Doctors and other colleagues to meet the needs of my patients.

I will never intentionally do or administer anything that causes overall harm to my patients.

I will not allow considerations of gender, race, religion, political affiliation, sexual orientation, nationality, or social status to influence my duty of care.

I will oppose policies that violate human rights and will not participate in them.

I will strive to change any laws that are contrary to the ethics of my profession and I will work for a more equitable distribution of health resources.

I will assist my patients in making informed decisions that coincide with their values and beliefs and will support patient confidentiality.

I will recognize the limits of my knowledge and will try to maintain and increase my understanding and ability throughout my professional life. I will acknowledge and try to right my mistakes and honestly evaluate others to answer for them.

I will try to promote the advancement of medical knowledge, through teaching and research.

"I make this declaration solemnly, freely and on my honor."

In addition: ***"Affirmations in the present"***

I listen to the mind—I am sincere—I have dedicated myself to my patients—I give my patients the time they need—I am selfless when it comes to my work—I am dedicated to helping others—I am confident about my abilities—I enjoy helping others—I love my work—I am an intuitive doctor

"Affirmations for the Future"

I will focus—on the needs of my patients—I will only think about my patients—I will stop feeling insecure—Others will see me as a brilliant—doctor.—I will overcome any doubts about myself—I will be efficient with my time—I will be patient with others—I will be attentive and understanding—I will bring relief for the pain of others—My medical skills will develop incredibly.

" Natural claims "

I am naturally genuine—I was meant to be a doctor—Helping others is my calling—I have a thorough knowledge of the human body—I am excellent in my profession—I always know how to handle medical situations.

In 1992, a BMA working group indicated that the "doctor's statement" could reinforce the decision to behave with integrity and therefore recommended that "medical schools incorporate Medical Ethics in the core curriculum and that all medical graduates commit themselves to observing a code of ethics."

A review of the international bibliography reveals the extent to which the Hippocratic Oath has influenced medical ethics over the centuries. The Oath specifically mentions two of the four principles of bioethics: non-evil and beneficence.

The first significant revision of the Oath began in 1948, when the newly established World Medical Association adopted, together with the Geneva Declaration, an oath with no reference to religious principles, and which was drafted to be adequate for medical practice in different cultures. The Hippocratic Oath has also appeared in Muslim literature, where the only significant changes are that of having replaced references to Greek deities with statements conforming to Islamic theology.

Today the issues related to medical ethics are related to the deontological ones and finally also to the legal ones. It is particularly encouraging that bioethics committees have been jointly established by various bodies, such as ministries, scientific institutes, and the church. We can therefore distinguish legal duties, for which the doctor is obliged by law to observe a given behavior; deontological duties, disciplinary rules suggested (imposed?) by the Order of Physicians-Surgeons.

In Conclusion

Although the Oath is not part of any specific ethical doctrine, it was widely accepted by Greece and then around the world as the basic text of medical ethics. The principles of charity and non-maleficence and the protection of life in general formed the common ground of the Oath and Christian ethics, laying solid foundations for ethics and bioethics. The Oath influenced ethical thought, typically Greek, not only in ancient times, but also in the early Christian and Byzantine periods, right up to the modern era.

I have already mentioned that particular attention will be paid to other documents, containing concepts unknown to most people, and clear allusions to an often forgotten medical practice. The content of these "historical" oaths has been and still is debated in the light of scientific advances and discoveries.

Then too, even if the current oaths seem, at least partly, a mere formality, the statements expressed are a necessary part of correct ethical education. They highlight a series of norms centered on the concept *primum non nocere;* recognizing the patient an autonomous and responsible individual who has the faculty to make free decisions about his own medical treatment.

One of the most controversial issues concerns the legal consequences deriving from possible non-observance of the oath, if dictated by religious, social or economic reasons, and there are numerous ethical concepts on how to overcome this problem, in order not to deviate from the moral norms outlined in the oath.

A compromise is often reached between respecting the patient's autonomy and upholding the moral standards established for the doctor.

The patient and doctor must discuss the matter in depth, to reach a rational, independent decision that can be shared. A rational but "paternalistic" approach can offer a good solution to this problem.

References

Aristotle. Italian encyclopedia Treccani; 2009.

Aristotle. Etica Nicomachea, traduzione, introduzione e note di C. Natali. (IT. Nicomachean ethics, translation, introduction and notes by C. Natali). Rome: Laterza; 2014.

Armocida G, Zanobio B. History of medicine. Amsterdam: Elsevier; 2002. Chap. I.

Behringer W. Storia culturale del clima. Dall'era glaciale al Riscaldamento globale. (IT. Cultural history of climate. From the ice age to global warming). 3rd ed. Gravellona Toce (VB): Bollati Boringhieri; 2014. p. 349.

Berdine G. The Hippocratic Oath and principles of medical ethics, Southwest Respir Crit Care Chronicles. 2016;4(16).

Boylan M. Hippocrates, internet encyclopedia of philosophy. 2002. Accessed 28 Sep 2006.

Carrick PJ. Medical ethics in the ancient world. Washington, DC: Georgetown University Press; 2001. Pt. 1–2: 11–108.

Cartwright M. "Greek medicine," ancient history encyclopedia, last modified Sep 12, 2013.

Cavalli F. Breve storia della medicina. Antichità e Medioevo. (IT. A brief history of medicine. Antiquity and the middle ages). Anno Accademico; 2013-2014.

Chesanow N. Is it time to retire the Hippocratic Oath? Medscape, 2017.

Colburn D. Under oath. The Washington Post, 1991.
Cosmacini G. Guerra e Medicina. Dall'antichità a oggi. (IT. War and medicine. From antiquity to today) (Chap. I). Bari: Laterza; 2011.
Couch HN. The Hippocratean patient and his physician. Trans Proc Am Philos Assoc. 1934;65:138–62.
Crashaw R, Linn C. Evolution of form and circumstance in medical oaths. West J Med. 1996;164:453–6.
Crawshaw R. The Hippocratic Oath is alive and well in North America. BMJ. 1994;309:952.
Ede A, Cormack LB. A history of science in society: from the ancient Greeks to the scientific revolution. North York, ON: University of Toronto Press; 2012.
Fioranelli M, Zullino P. I, Ippocrate di Kos. (IT. Hippocrates of Kos). Bari: Laterza; 2008.
Garrison FH. An introduction to the history of medicine. 4th ed. Philadelphia: WB Saunders; 1929. p. 96.
Gosić N. The Hippocratic Oath a historical perspective in bioethical education. Synth Philos. 2008;46(2):225–38.
Guinan P. Hippocrates and natural law. Catholic Med Q. 2012;63(1).
Hellenic, Hellenistic, and Roman Medicine. Fifth century BC to third century AC (Ch 1). In: A short history of medical ethics. Oxford: Oxford University Press; 2000. p. 1–12.
Huber S. The white coat ceremony: a contemporary medical ritual. J Med Ethics. 2003;29(6):364–6.
Hulkower R. The history of the Hippocratic oath: outdated, inauthentic, and yet still relevant. Einstein J Biol Med. 2010;25:41–4.
Hurwitz B, Richardson R. Swearing to care: the resurgence in medical oaths. BMJ. 1997;316: 1671–4.
Jacques J. Hippocrates (trad. It.). Turin: SEI; 1994.
Jones WHS. The doctor's oath. The early forms of the Hippocratic oath. New York: Cambridge University Press; 1923.
Jones DA. The Hippocratic Oath: I—its content and the limits of its adaptation. Catholic Med Q. 2003;54(3):9–17.
Jones WHS, Withington ET. Hippocrates' collected works I. Hippocrates, De Prisca medicina. Cambridge: Harvard University Press; 1868.
Jonsen AR. Medical history in India and China (Chap. 3). In: A short history of medical ethics. Oxford: Oxford University Press; 2000. p. 27–41.
Jori A. Medicina e medici nell'antica Grecia.Saggio sul "Perì téchnes" Ippocratico. (IT. Medicine and doctors in ancient Greece. Essay on the Hippocratic "Perì téchnes"). Bologna: Il Mulino Publisher; 1996.
Jouanna J. Greek medicine from Hippocrates to Galen: selected papers. Leiden: Koninklijke Brill; 2012.
Kantarjian H, Steensa DP. Relevance of the Hippocratic Oath in the 21st century. The ASCO Post, 2014.
Koios N, Veloyanni L, Alvanos D. Evolution of medical ethics and bioethics in Greece: "ancient-Christian-contemporary Greece". Eleftherna—scientific yearbook, vol. III; 2006.
Lanata G. Ippocrate. Opere. (IT. Translation and commentary), Hippocrates. Works. Turin: Boringhieri; 1961.
Littrè E. FR. Oeuvres complete with Hippocrates. I. Imprimerie Moquet et Compe Paris, chez J.P. Bailliere, 10 vol. Recuperati da Concetto de Luca in "Ippocrate ed il Corpus Hippocraticum (tratti dalle "Opere Complete" del Littrè) (IT. Recovered from Concepts de Luca in "Hippocrates and the Corpus Hippocraticum (from the *Complete Works* of Littré) Trad. in Italian, 1839-1841.
Loewy EH. Textbook of medical ethics. New York: Plenum Publishing Co.; 1989. Chapter 1: 1–6; Chapter 2: 16–17.
Loudon I. The Hippocratic Oath. BMJ. 1994;309:414.
Lowes RL. Is the Hippocratic Oath still relevant? Med Econ. 1995;72(11):197.
Mantovanelli L. Scribonio Largo, Ricette mediche. (IT. Scribonio Largo, medical recipes). Padova: Sargon Ed; 2012. p. VII–XV.

Mastrangelo D. Il Tradimento di Ippocrate, La medicina degli affari. (IT. Hippocrates' betrayal, business medicine). Salus Infirmorum Ed., 2010.
Medscape. Is the Hippocratic Oath still relevant? 2016.
Nordqvist C. Medical News Today, 9 Aug 2012.
Nutton V. The Hippocratic Oath. Med Surg. 2013;58:2609–16.
Ogunbanjo GA, van Bogaert KD, Biko S. The Hippocratic Oath: revisited. SA Fam Pract. 2009;51(1):30–1.
Orr RD, Pang N, Pellegrino ED, Siegler M. Use of the Hippocratic Oath: a review of twentieth-century practice and a content analysis of oaths administered in medical schools in the U.S. and Canada in 1993. J Clin Ethics. 1997;8:377–88.
Pellegrino E. The medical profession as a moral community. Bull N Y Acad Med. 1990;66(2):221–32.
Reich WT, editor. Encyclopedia of bioethics—revised edition. New York: Macmillan; 1995. 2950 pp.
Rosenhek J. Is the Oath outdated? Doctor's review, 2009.
Roth G. Ippocrate nei documenti ecclesiastici e nelle opere Teologiche. (IT. Hippocrates in ecclesiastical documents and theological works). n.d.. http://www.vaticva/roman_curia/pontifical_councils/hlthwork/documents/rc_pc_hlthwork_doc_0 5101997_roth_it.html.
Rothstein RM. The white coat ceremony. Mt Sinai J Med. 2001;68(3):224–5.
Russo RG. Il codice di Ippocrate. (IT. The Hippocratic Code), SSFA Oggi, nos. 40–42; 2014.
Shmerling RH. The myth of the Hippocratic Oath. Harvard Health Blog, Nov 25–28, 2015.
Sprengel C. Storia prammatica della medicina. (Pragmatic history of medicine). Translated from the German. Chapter IV—Raffaele Miranda, Naples; 1814.
Sritharan K, Russell G, Fritz Z. Medical oaths and declarations. BMJ. 2001;323(7327):1440–1.
Sterpellone L. I grandi della medicina, Le scoperte che hanno cambiato la qualità della vita. (IT. The greats of medicine. The discoveries that have changed the quality of life). Rome: Donzelli, Virgola Ed; 2004. p. 27–36.
Stevenson WT. Declarations for new doctors are unnecessary. BMJ. 2002;324(7341):8511.
Trueman CN. "Hippocrates" the history learning site; 2015.
Tyson P. The Hippocratic Oath Today, NOVA, 2001.
Veatch RM, editor. Cross cultural perspectives in medical ethics. 2nd ed. Boston: Jones and Bartlett Publishers; 2000. p. 240–58.
Veatch RM. White coat ceremonies: a second opinion. J Med Ethics. 2002;28(1):5–9.
Vegetti M. Etica degli Antichi. (IT. Ethics of the ancients). Rome: Ed. Laterza; 2006. Chaps. 1–2.
Wear D. On white coats and professional development: the formal and the hidden curricula. Ann Intern Med. 1998;129(9):734–7.
Woodbury E. The fall of the Hippocratic Oath: why the Hippocratic Oath should be discarded in favor of a modified version of Pellegrino's precepts. GUJHS. 2012;6(2):9–17.

4 Rome, Barbarians, and Medieval Codes

Roman medicine, from its birth until the second century B.C., was of an empirical nature and was based for at least five centuries on the teachings of the Etruscans.[1]

"Grecia capta ferum victorem coepit et artes intulit agresti Latio" [The conquered Greece conquered (in turn) the fierce winner and introduced the arts into rural Lazio].

However, this was how Quintus Horatius Flaccus (Horace 65–8 B.C.) reiterated in the Epistles (II, 1, 156) how much Rome depended on Greece for religious, artistic, health, and medical questions.[2]

There were three schools with different medical approaches in Rome at that time:

1. Methodical medicine, founded by Asclepiades from Bithynia (first century B.C.). He based his teachings on the "atomistic" theory and did not believe in the Hippocratic humoral theory, thus avoiding drastic remedies and surgery: he preferred to heal with gymnastics and diets. He is credited with the motto "cito, tuto, jucunde" (quick, safe, joyful), related to methods for treating diseases.

[1] The Etruscans were profound connoisseurs of medicinal plants and the preparation of medicaments; they used castor oil (purgative), myrtle (astringent), camomile (calming), garlic and onion (purifying and to get rid of intestinal parasites), scammony (jaundice), thyme (vermifuge), cabbage leaves (rheumatism), wine (tonic) and some minerals, such as iron filings and iron oxide (anemia) and copper (inflammation). Etruscan medicine also had religious leanings: the head and hearing were under the tutelage of Tinia (Jupiter), the eyes of Uni (Juno), the hips of Laran (Mars); the fingers, feeling and touch were the realm of Minerva (Athena), the genitals Turan (Venus), the feet Mercury. The mysterious civilization of the Etruscans, who lived in the Italian peninsula for almost a Millennium revealed very little about this, however. We only know that it was not based on magic and tended more towards reality. In fact, for at least five centuries the doctors in Rome were mainly of Etruscan origin and enjoyed high esteem even among neighboring populations, especially in dentistry, surgery and orthopedics.

Cavalli (2013-2014), pp. 32–44.

[2] Quinto Orazio Flacco (2006).

R. G. Russo, *Medical Ethics*, https://doi.org/10.1007/978-3-031-42444-1_4

2. Pneumatic medicine: this was a return to Hippocrates and its founder was Athenaeus of Attaleia (50 A.D.), known for his studies on semeiotics and on the wrist.
3. Eclectic medicine, using the experiences of the other two schools; it boasted Agatino of Sparta (90 A.D.) and Areteo of Cappadocia, famous for his anatomical descriptions and various pathological pictures (diabetes, celiac diathesis, vertigo, melancholy, mania, etc.).

Medical knowledge[3] came from the medical treatises and methods of the Greeks, Etruscans, Egyptians, Persians, and other conquered peoples. A doctor in ancient Rome was usually a "generic" professional who did not have any particular specialization, with few exceptions: surgery (surgus), ophthalmology (ocularius), and otolaryngology (auricularius). The best known doctors were:

- Aulus Cornelius Celsus, although not in fact a doctor, referred to the teachings of Hippocrates and Asclepiades. Of his encyclopedic work "*De Artibus*" only an eight-volume section, "*De Medicina*" has survived. The text (like Hippocrates) makes no claim that contemporary medicine is better or worse than its predecessors. This attitude became typical of doctors in the Middle Ages and the early modern age, alongside the idea of the possible evolution of medicine. Celsus was open to an ethical approach, with the definition of the physical and moral qualities that make an excellent surgeon: young and strong, firm-handed and courageous, compassionate towards the sick, and aiming to achieve recovery.
- Antonio Musa, physician, and botanist during the reign of Emperor Augustus, set up the first public hospitals, *valetudinaria*, mainly used for the care of the military.
- Sorano, a Greek physician, lived during the reigns of Trajan and Hadrian. He was the main representative of the Methodical school and laid the foundations of scientific gynecology and obstetrics. His treatise "Gynecology" was published again in 1838. He dealt with ethical and philosophical reflections.
- Great authority was always attributed to Claudius Galen of Pergamon, who lived in the second century A.D. and above all in Rome, as a doctor for the Stoic emperor and philosopher Marcus Aurelius. He studied in Corinth, Smyrna, and Alexandria and then worked as a surgeon for the gladiators, and this enabled him to study physiology and the human body. He became an "expert doctor" and his

[3] There was still no scientific basis for medicine: it consisted therefore mainly of previous "ancient" information (Hippocrates, Galen) and religious influences, while the philosophical concepts of "soul" (immaterial) and "body" gradually lost ground (mortal and material). The medical texts that circulated between the fifth and tenth centuries A.D. in the great monasteries and the rare schools were in fact compilations of widely disparate materials, mostly intended for teaching: short theoretical-practical works, collections of pharmacopoeias or, often, practical manuals where the various diseases were described briefly with an indication of the relative therapy. In addition to the Hippocratic texts and some rare Galenic texts, there were reworks of works by Mustio, Aureliano Celio, Sereno Psammonico and others (including Paul of Aegina and Oribasius).

patients included the consul Flavius Boethius, the emperors Marcus Aurelius, Lucio Vero, Commodus, and Septimius Severus.

He supported the doctrine of the four temperaments (sanguine, phlegmatic, choleric, melancholic), formulated by Hippocrates. He dealt with the *materiae peccans* (material error, including pus), blood-letting, the function of the ureters and the "recurrent nerve", willow bark (aspirin) and laudanum (tincture of opium). Galen maintained that a physician should also be qualified in three branches of philosophy: logic, the science of how to think; physics, the science of "nature", and ethics, the science of what to do.

Many of the doctors who came from Greece to Rome[4] proved disappointing on the professional and moral levels, often revealing themselves to be charlatans or scammers.

Besides private medicine, Rome established a community of hygiene and sanitary services to prevent disease by improving health conditions, thanks to the construction of aqueducts to bring water to the city, public baths, and wastewater networks. Rome became a model of social hygiene in the world: its aqueducts, spas, parks, hygienic surveillance of food, sewers and sanitary laws, all in defense of public health, and beds of health-giving plants were known and renowned throughout the Empire.

Morals and Medical Ethics

In ancient times, many medical societies were gradually obliged to practice their profession in an appropriate and ethical manner, often adopting a code of conduct or taking an oath. Every culture and every social system served as a setting for the definition of health and disease, as well as therapeutic methods, and physicians' behavior.

These commitments eventually acquired an ethical aspect of dominant morality. In ancient Greece, and in particular from the classical period onwards, the Greeks had apparently already associated with this important science a number of ethical rules to ensure service for others, in the best possible way.

[4] Other doctors in Rome were Antillo, Oribasius, Julian the Apostate (the most important Roman author after Galen), Paul of Aegina, Cassius, Calpetanus, Arruntius, Rubrius, Quintus Sterninius Xenofons, Charmis and Alcon. Each city had some public doctors (archiatroi) who stood out on account of their specializations. Martial, for example, mentioned Cascellius (dentist), Hyginus (ophthalmologist), Fannius (ear, nose and throat), Eros (cosmetic surgery) and Hermes (hernias).

Medicine began to be studied on more scientific lines, though the citizens still trusted in simple herbalremedies (scientia herbarum), the intervention of minor deities, the protective power of amulets and the recitation of magical formulas. The (modern) concept of "prevention is better than cure" was clear, with diet therapy, exercise, hydrotherapy, bloodletting, purgatives and enemas.

Bresadola (2014), Cosmacini and Menghi (2012), Galen (1490), Russo (2007a) and Xenophontos (2014).

The Romans had a relatively strict and formal code of conduct, codified in the laws of the time. Religion and Divinity guided and pervaded their morality throughout the history of ancient Rome. Religion and morals were the foundations of society and had a fundamental influence in the government of ancient Rome, starting with the first kings who, together with the various divinities, based their right to govern on personal qualities.

In a simplistic way it can be assumed that morality, as in other ancient civilizations, was based on the rights of the strongest, "the victor."

Cicero (106–43 B.C.) succinctly stated that: "*Salus populi suprema lex esto*" (The welfare of the people must be the supreme law. Cicero, De Leg., IV). This is a perfect example of practicality and pragmatism that marked Roman culture even with respect to moral issues. In classical antiquity the practice of medicine was a right, not a privilege. No official license was required to practice medicine and anyone who wanted could establish himself as a practitioner of the healing arts—a doctor. Consequently, this term covered all those who called themselves doctors. The phrase "professional ethics" can be misleading if reported in those times, since there were no professional standards applied by law or by any medical organization, or any swearing of oaths or acceptance of a formal code of ethics.

This does not mean there were no ethical norms; several examples are evident both in medicine and in classical literature. But what might appear to be in tune with modern models of medicine may well have been the prerogative of only a minority, not representative, of the doctors of the time. The emergence of medical ethics almost coincided with the early stages of medical science. As there was no system for medical authorizations or licenses, there were also no applicable professional rules or sanctions against doctors who were "unethical." However, doctors who carefully and rigorously followed their commitments earned a good reputation, essential for gaining customers and profits.

With the first century A.D., however, a new culture began to be felt in the classical Roman world: Christian culture[5] revolutionized morality and behavior and Christian charity revolutionized society's attitudes towards the sick, as illustrated on a large scale in the great plague that raged in Rome in the third century A.D.

Although the ethical rules of the Hippocratic Oath were in force throughout the Roman period, no particular system of medical ethics surfaced.

Nevertheless some historical references indicate that Christian communities became involved later in issues such as the doctor-patient relationship, the social

[5]Greek prisoners of war, hired as useful craftsmen, were among the first doctors who practiced in Rome, as slaves or freedmen. The first Greek physician who operated in Rome was Archagathus, in 219 B.C.; some wealthy families of the time welcomed them into their homes as personal physicians. Many treatments were still based on superstition and had little practical use; in this regard some satirists (Martial and Pliny) derided and mocked them. Roman medicine, especially in the countryside, was initially the prerogative of women. Empirical cures were handed down from mother to daughter and were mostly based on healing herbs. The doctor (curator), who came later as a professional, was instead only male, recognized in wars or plagues.

Davies (1971), Galen (1490), Jackson (1988), Jonsen (2000), Ch. 1, pp. 1–12, Kroeber (1910), Marasco (1997) and Veith (1957).

behavior of doctors, and professional conduct. Christian teaching seemed to change the entire spectrum of medical treatment, taking charity as the guiding light. During and after this period there were various versions of the Hippocratic Oath, some of which had already been around a long time.

Romans: Public and Private Health[6]

Unlike Greek society, which considered health a private and personal matter, the Roman government protected and encouraged the improvement of public health. The organism, if kept in good shape, would be able to fight disease: a healthy mind in a healthy body (*mens sana in corpore sano*), according to Juvenal, second century A.D., Satire, X, 356.

The vespasians (public urinals), aqueducts, and public hospitals, that have remained unsurpassed until modern times, also contributed to the progress of medicine, especially in the field of public health and hygiene. The Romans did not have the knowledge to understand the exact mechanisms behind diseases, but their personal hygiene and obsession with cleanliness probably helped limit the spread of epidemics in major cities, despite fact that the level of health care was pretty poor overall. Aqueducts were built to bring water to the city, to public baths and to sewage networks. In Rome there were 144 public baths; in every house: not only in those of the rich but also in the *insulae* (the poorest quarters) there was a fountain and clean running water.

When a Greek spoke of *iatroi* or a Roman of *medici*, each was using a word loaded with significance. Both indicated a selfless and compassionate goal. With the fifth century B.C. the term *iatros* was used to signify "the good ruler" of the body, just as philosophers had been described as "doctors of the soul."

The culture of the first three centuries of the empire is appropriately labeled Greco-Roman. Many doctors in Rome believed they could restore the right balance of the "four humors" in patients and felt that medicine was sufficiently advanced.[7]

By the fourth century, after Constantine the Great, Christianity had added its theological virtues of faith, hope and charity to the list of human virtues, together with the paradigmatic one of compassion, which came partly from Christianity's emphasis on how to help others. The etymological root of "compassion" in fact means "to suffer with". A good Christian physician took care of the poor as part of his duties. With the flourishing of Christianity, the cult of Aesculapius-savior was replaced by Christ, the physician of body and soul.

Rome was a thriving civilization that existed for about 1200 years. According to the various periods of its existence, the customs and therefore ethical attitudes also varied considerably.

---

[6] Amundsen (1977, 1986), Brandon (1965), Encyclopedia of Bioethics (2016), Macer (1990), Pelàez (2002) and Ostrowski (2006).

[7] Castiglioni (1946), Penso (1991), Russo (2007a) and Wazer (2016).

With the fall of the Roman Empire, Roman medicine declined too and the Middle Ages took shape, with great epidemics and plagues and hundreds of thousands of victims.

Religious-Christian medicine fought the magic formulas and promoted prayers, the laying on of hands and anointing with holy oil. Folk medicine, over time and with the Byzantine influence, became conventual and this, with the use of medicinal herbs and the re-discovery of ancient medical texts, marked the beginning of a new medical science. The Gospel addressed the sick and spoke of healing as divine intervention. Christianity united morality and ethics in the various fields of human society in a single set of values. Unlike the Greeks, again, who hospitalized their patients in temples in the hope that the gods could cure them, the Romans built hospitals specifically for their care. The first "hospitals" were founded in the fourth century and were soon run by monastic orders.

Barbarians

An unexpected event shocked the civilized world when the Barbarians occupied much of the Empire. Their invasions followed incessantly from 166 A.D., initially for looting but later with the transmigration of entire populations.

There was, however, an unexpected positive side, as a "medical culture" also existed among the invaders. Ostrogoths, Visigoths, Longobards, Merovingians, and Carolingians produced, like other "barbarians," precise and innovative legislation in the health field, including the first rudiments of (medical) ethics—still to be better defined.[8]

The Roman Empire fell apart under the blows of the barbarians who attacked its borders starting from the second half of the third century and finally settled on its lands in the west for ever longer periods, at times launching decisive attacks on the center of the peninsula and increasingly mixing with the Italic population. As early as 276 A.D. the Franks and the Alemanni had crossed the Rhine and entered Roman Gaul. From 375 came the Huns, the Ostrogoths, the Visigoths and then the Vandals, the Swabians, again the Visigoths, and the Ostrogoths. Angles, Frisians, Saxons, and Jutes settled in Great Britain, while the Longobards took over almost the whole of Italy.[9]

[8] After the breakdown of the Roman Empire, starting from 476 AD—a period of about a thousand years assigned by historians to the Middle Ages, the new Christian religion began to grow (rising to state religion after 325). Morality had a rational basis among the barbarians, who personalized and modified it in various ways, also in the light of historical events.

Religion became associated with ethics in health practices.

Castiglioni (1946), Pelàez (2002), I think, 1991, already cited. Russo (2007a). Op-cit., Hubert et al. (1967) and Koios (2006), already cited.

[9] Bird (1989), Horse et al. (2008), Crisciani (2010) and Jonsen (2000).

Wikipedia, Medieval Medicine Fifth to Fourteen Centuries CE Chap. 2: 13–26.

Liguori et al. (2011), Pelàez (2002), Regimen Sanitatis Salernitanum (2007-2016), Robert (1753) and Zardo (2012).

In the Ostrogothic Kingdom of Italy, Flavius the Great, Aurelio Cassiodoro wrote to a doctor in relation to "certain sacred oaths of a priestly character" which medical students were obliged to recite, a clear reference to the Hippocratic Oath.[10] Frequent struggles for power also brought renewals in social, economic and medical and hygiene regulations, by the Visigoths and Ostrogoths. Very significant was the establishment of the famous "Visigothic Code of Eurico" (*Codex Euricianus*), which can be interpreted as a writing on forensic medicine, divided into 12 books, with numerous innovative laws and regulations.[11]

The code was compiled around 470–480, under the reign of Alaric II, and brought together the laws that governed the Visigoths. It was intended to regulate the life of the Romans, based on existing imperial laws. This "Alaric's Breviary" was promulgated during a meeting of the Visigoth nobles in Toulouse, France, on February 2, 506. The Visigothic Code (*Forum Judicum*) is a set of laws promulgated for the first time by King Chindasuinth in 642–643 and only fragments survive. In 654 his son, King Recceswinth, published an expanded code of laws that first applied equally to Goths and Romans, abolishing the old tradition of separate laws for Romans and Barbarians. Book XI, Title I: Doctors and the Sick, described the regulations, thus resembling an ethical code.[12]

A few fragments are worth reporting:

1. No doctor will take blood from a woman in the absence of her relatives (father, mother brother, son, uncle or other) unless there is an urgent need; if none of the above persons can be present, the woman must be subjected to bleeding in the presence of respectable neighbors or slaves of both sexes, depending on the nature of her illness. If a doctor does it without the presence of any of the aforementioned persons, he will be obliged to pay ten "solids" to that woman's husband or relatives; it is by no means unlikely that irregularities will sometimes occur on such an occasion.
2. No doctor should visit people in prison. No doctor will enter a prison when the governors, tribunes or deputies are also excluded from them, without being accompanied by the jailer, so that the prisoners, influenced by fear,

[10] Bird (1989), Cavalli (2022), already cited, Crisciani (2010), Jonsen (2000), Chap. 2, pp. 13–26, Liguori (2011), already cited, Pelàez (2002), Regimen Sanitatis Salernitanum (2007-2016), Robert (1753) and Zardo (2012).

[11] The Visigoths, a population of Scandinavian origin, reached Italy on several occasions. They looted Rome in 410. After the fall of the Western Roman Empire in 476, they played a very important role for two and a half centuries. They were different from other barbarians in that in legislation and in the management of their civil affairs they manifested a sense of humanity and true philosophy, rarely seen even in other civilized nations.

Amundsen (1980, 2004), Hubert (1967), already cited and Scott (1910).

Wikipedia, Cassiodorus.

[12] Nemec (1976).

cannot obtain the means to commit suicide from the doctor. If poison were to be given or administered by doctor under such circumstances the course of justice would be greatly impeded. If a doctor is guilty of this infraction, he will be liable for the same punishment.

3. When a person requests that a doctor treats him for his illness or heals his wound under a contract, after the doctor has seen the wound or diagnosed the illness, he can undertake the treatment of that sick person as agreed and reported in writing.
4. If a doctor takes on the treatment of a sick person under a contract, he is expected to restore the person's health. But if the patient dies, the doctor will not be entitled to the fee stipulated in the contract and no responsibility can be attributed to either party
5. If a doctor eliminates a cataract from a person's eye and makes the person whole, he is entitled to five "solids" for his services.
6. When a doctor takes blood from the patient and the patient is severely weakened as a result, the doctor will be obliged to pay him 40 "solids." If the patient dies as a result of this, the doctor will be dealt with by the patient's relatives, as they see fit. If the patient is a slave and severely weakened or dies, the physician must give his master a slave of equal value in his place.
7. If a doctor is given a slave to teach about medicine, he is entitled to 12 "solids" as a fee.
8. No doctor should be imprisoned without a hearing, except in the case of murder. If he is indebted, a guarantee must be provided.

The practice of medicine was not highly regarded by the Visigoths, a nation of warriors, and was often practiced by slaves, as before in Rome and later by barbers and charlatans during the Middle Ages.

Malpractice was a broad term: the risks taken by the practitioner, even in ordinary cases, were not compensated by the fees he could receive if he was successful.

The danger of harms and sanctions in the event that a patient died did not make the profession very attractive. Even after he had carried out his task conscientiously and assiduously, the doctor could be found guilty of murder and be handed over to the exasperated relatives of the deceased, for the wild excesses of vengeance—the *Lex Talionis*.

This was not an attractive prospect to further the interests of medical science. The first code of Medical Ethics (or its initial draft), Formula Comitis Archiatrorum (register of the main doctors), was drawn up by Cassiodorus (484–490 to 577–590)[13] for Theodoric the Great (454–526). This thus appears as the first code of medical ethics, the archetype for contemporary ones, among the first codes of Christian

[13] Afshar (2016), Motamedi (2014), Nemec (1976) and Rajala (2015, 2016).
Wikipedia, Cassiodorus.

medical ethics. The whole Formula bears the Hippocratic medical signature. This is not surprising because Hippocratic medicine was a practice accepted in Italy at the time. Theodoric had in effect restored an ancient Roman institution and prescribed the wording of the oath that people appointed to that position were to recite.

It was inspired by Cassiodorus's *magister officiorum*; Doctors were thus able to broaden and deepen their knowledge and also consult colleagues. It was then confirmed that all those who took care of human health had to refer to the people listed in the Comitis Archiatrorum.

A few regulatory references are indicated:

- Medicine must not be defined by a change of idea based on the event but on the doctor's experience.
- After their training doctors should refer to books, specially old ones, whether or not they deal with medicine.
- Doctors should give up on disagreements that harm patients; if no agreement can be reached, they should seek advice from someone, without envy because a prudent man is willing to seek advice.
- Doctors are consecrated by oaths: they must promise their teachers to hate iniquity and love honesty.
- Doctors are not allowed to fail in their duty and must diligently seek whatever cures the sick and strengthens the weak.
- Although mistakes may be the cause, a sin against human health is a crime of murder.

- In medieval Europe, medicine[14] generally operated under the umbrella of the Church. Hospitals that cared for the elderly and the sick were often run by religious orders, which could also maintain the infirmaries. When medicine could not help, the faithful often turned to the saints and visited shrines in the hope of miraculous cures. The Church was the only dominant institution in medieval life; his influence pervaded almost every aspect of people's lives: his teachings supported traditional beliefs about ethics, the meaning of life and the afterlife.

[14] In 476 the Barbarian king of the Eruli, Odoacre, deposed the last Roman emperor, Romolo Augustolo and proclaimed himself king of the Eruli, Sciri, Rugi, Gepidi and Turcilingi. The Ostrogoths overcame Odoacre, and he, with his family and followers, was killed by Teodorico.

Cavalli (2013-2014), pp. 52–67.

Cosmacini (1977), already cited, Dyer (2002), Eco (2010), Mount (2016) and Prioreschi (2003).

Wikipedia, Medieval medicine of Western Europe.

Woodbury (2012).

During the reign of the Emperor Nero (54–68) Andromachus the Old the Emperor's personal physician, was appointed *archiatra*. This was the position assigned to those who looked after the health of the Romans and the population of other cities.

Causes of medical stagnation in the Middle Ages included:

- the loss of medical knowledge and the presence of bad doctors and charlatans
- the Church's ban on dissecting corpses and encouraging prayer and superstition to cure diseases
- the emphasis on authority rather than observation and investigation
- the lack of resources to form appropriate public health systems
- social unrest and wars, with consequent interruptions in communication and learning
- the insistence on Galen's writings and the belief that illness was a punishment from God.

However, the Church encouraged people to participate in the Crusades, thus coming into contact with Muslim doctors, who were significantly more skilled than their European counterparts. It was only under Moorish rule that doctors and surgeons acquired extensive knowledge and achieved professional eminence.[15]

Medical-Assistential Codes in the Middle Ages[16]

Fourth to Fifteenth Century A.D.

With the fall of the Roman Empire, Roman medicine also declined; the Middle Ages began with real epidemics and pestilences and hundreds of thousands of victims. The Middle Ages are generally divided into high (476–1050), low (1051–1340), and late (1341–1492).

The oldest medical practices were a mixture of empirical interventions, because nobody knew the real reasons for their effectiveness or failure, and the effects of magic and mysterious external forces, which were believed to be the causes of pain and illness itself.

There were enigmatic procedures reserved for some, properly initiated, who could boast special healing powers.

The ability to purchase medical care was generally limited to the king, the aristocracy, or the wealthy upper classes, while middle-class merchants, city workers, day laborers, peasants, serfs, and the poor had to rely on home remedies, astrologers, bone manipulators, barber-surgeons, and charity from the Academy.

Clearly, medical ethics was largely unknown, without prejudice to the desire, not adequately met, to heal and overcome disease, while closely following a variety of "prescriptions." In fact, the true doctors were considered to be those who presented

[15] von Engelhardt (2010), Kroeber (1910), Russo (2007b) and Ostrowski (2006).

Wikipedia, Chirurgia, anatomia e Chiesa cattolica nel Medioevo. Medicina medievale—(Notes and bibliography attached).

[16] Amundsen (1977, 1986), Brandon (1965), Encyclopedia of Bioethics (2016), Mount (2016) and Veith (1957), already cited.

themselves as representatives of the Church, or a theologically neutral alternative, such as the *incantatores* (enchanters), doctors who were always condemned in the literature, and considered diabolical practitioners of illicit arts, contrary to ecclesiastical morality.

Throughout the Middle Ages, as we already said, there was no specialization in medicine so almost every family needed to maintain someone who dealt with the simplest health problems and someone entrusted with more complex problems: these included midwives, tooth-pullers, experts in the use of herbs, bone-setters, etc. In the cities, those who treated wounds and provided certain types of surgery (hernias, removal of kidney stones, incision of abscesses) could be found. Those suffering illness or trauma could in the end turn to rural medicine, priests, astrologers, witches, mystics or even a doctor (properly so-called), if one was available. The boundaries between these "professional figures" were blurred and indistinct.[17]

Doctors and Patients[18]

Most people in the Middle Ages had never seen a doctor. The cures were a mixture of superstition (magic stones and spells were very popular) or self-declared men (or women) of faith, to exorcise evil spirits from allegedly mentally ill people or to prepare herbal remedies (some of which are still in use today).

In the early Middle Ages, caring for people was often linked to magic and witchcraft (white or black), accepted as "part of life," although there were also some Medici (who mainly treated the rich and powerful) who had even received a qualification in Bologna or Montpellier. Through medical schools, Europeans begun to learn about Arab cultures or ancient Greek medicine. Compared to the knowledge of the Arabs, for example, European medicine was not advanced.

Doctors, for their part, were generally not very reliable and therefore ethics and strategies did not differ much from the traditional uses which included blood-letting

[17] On the heels of the various Barbarian cultures, medicine too had to align itself with classical thought and with religion, Latin and Greek science and the teachings of the Bible. This is illustrated in the booklet of medicine, in verse, Commentario Medicinale, written by the Archbishop of Milan, Benedetto Crespo (681–723). The described remedies employed in folk medicine, with extracts from Plinio and Dioscoride.

Hippocrates' Theory of the Four Humors, put forward, generated and upheld for almost a thousand years, was increasingly hard to follow, and less clinically acceptable as scientific progress proceeded! The translation of these texts opened the way to a new literatary tradition, right up to the first century A.D. It was often preceded by a thorough philological analysis of the features of each work, including the extra-linguistic and extra-literal contexts.

Bird (1989), Carrick (2001), Cavalli (2013-2014), Jonsen (2000), Maion (1999) and Regimen Sanitatis Salernitanum (2007-2016).

[18] Magic and witchcraft, in their various forms, formed a sort of crossroads for medieval culture. The main "influences" of the time met and clashed there: religion, science; popular culture and higher culture; imagination and reality.

Crisciani (2010), Kieckhefer (2004), Liguori (2011), already cited, Morpurgo (2013) and Russo (2007a, b).

(which probably made patients even weaker) and "magic potions." It is therefore quite likely that the peasants (who knew nothing of the "cultural" side), with their magic stones, herbal drinks and prayers enjoyed better effects.

Barbers, working as doctors, offered various surgical operations and, considering the times and general conditions, were often successful. They had ample practice in treating wounds and broken bones due to the many wars of the time. They knew how to use casts and how to seal wounds with egg-white or to stop infection with old wine.

They knew how to use alcohol or plants like mandrake to put people to sleep or to relieve pain during operations. They could even remove the gallbladder or do a Cesarean section.

The teachings of Christianity almost always included due assistance to the sick inside and outside the cloister and brought about the first changes already in the late Middle Ages.

All the monastic regulations specified that assistance to the sick was part of a monk's duties, reflecting their ethics and rules of conduct.

The Beginnings of Medical Ethics[19]

Medieval medical ethics initially developed as a combination of classical medical etiquette and Christian ethics. The treatment of the most serious and even desperate cases was generally not discouraged, and anyhow a doctor who refused a case was dishonored.

The Hippocratic Oath nevertheless prevailed in the following centuries (partly due to the lack of a valid alternative), and then passed from the obligation (or challenge?) for monks to treat even the most serious diseases, thus making it a subject of general appreciation and consideration and significantly affecting the application of medical ethics. They were not allowed alcohol, should never be arrogant and were not expected to believe they offered the only solutions to disease.

A new medical culture took form, based on morality but also on religious teachings; therefore the rules of conduct were dictated by theology or by other colleagues who had distinguished themselves in the community.

Medical texts in Latin could not be ignored and in the ninth and tenth centuries they dealt with the beginnings of medical ethics, albeit still "incorrect and discrepant," as defined at the time.

[19] The history of the three main foundations of medical ethics (moral, ethics and religion) is complex. Religion for the most part has always been intrinsically associated with ethics. If to start with it was purely instinctive, it later became a social standard: though there were broad divergences of teaching, in different times and places, the underlying moral impulses were similar. When religion began to influence morality, ethics became surrounded by rules and recommendations that rested on ceremonial grounds. The "codes" were, at least initially, largely ritualistic.

The main points were:

1. "Of those who undertake medical studies"—this was a preparation for the Hippocratic Oath, from which some sections and teachings were picked up, but with no comment. Rules of conduct for one's own person are reaffirmed, and in relationships with others, with the sick, with women, and with medicines.
2. "Doctor Teodoro's instruction"—the doctor is encouraged to keep up to date, not to be indolent, to visit patients, to reflect on what is the best treatment, to be chaste, to respect confidentiality, to receive payment, and to trust in God and in the Muse of Medicine.
3. "Arsenius's letter to Nepoziano"—Arsenius, a doctor, teaches his son the qualities of a valorous doctor. In addition to good intentions, he is exhorted to keep morality in mind and to develop knowledge in the sciences and the main specializations. The letter (eighth century) ends with: "The doctor is defined as a master or liberator in health, a providential architect who frees people from suffering."
4. "Letter on the teaching of medical art"—Referring to Hippocrates' teachings, "the doctor must be able to absorb a large amount of doctrine." The physician must not reveal the secrets of the profession, nor speak evasively or "be slow of mind." Conduct and manners with men or women are described, the procedure to be followed in taking the pulse and other professional procedures.
5. "Letter on what the doctor should be like"—Repeats all the information and suggestions already listed, including the best technique for checking the pulse.
6. "How the doctor should approach the patient": "... with measured steps, looking without speaking ... and not keeping your head down and your eyes lowered ..."
7. "Dioclete's letter to Pamperio"—The doctor is reminded to approach the patient with a happy, sober, attentive face; not to practice harmful treatments, to use bloodletting. "We must combat the ailment as soon as it arises: the need cannot wait."
8. "How should you visit the sick person?"—some procedures should be followed in order to assign the right treatment. First the doctor asks the patient some specific questions, about any pain and its intensity; he checks his pulse and then questions the patient about feces and urine, even if other doctors have already visited him.
9. "The beginnings of medicine"—the tradition and history of the earliest medicine is narrated: Apollo, Aesculapius and particularly Hippocrates. Surgery, dietetics, and drugs are discussed.
10. "Hippocrates' origins, life and doctrine"—details are given about his family, his doctrine, and his disciples—starting with his Oath and moving on gradually to the other books and studies.

Many "Rules"[20] were codified between the twelfth and fourteenth centuries: they too provided doctors and surgeons with details of the codes of professional conduct and assistance. But not only this: the attitudes towards God, towards oneself, patients and their relatives were all specified—a veritable formulation of medical ethics and healthcare etiquette.

The question of information to the patient—the basis for the doctor's correct conduct (ethical for those times), had its origins in the Corpus Hippocraticum, where it was suggested not to reveal anything to the patient. This concept was repeated in the Middle Ages by Henri de Mondeville (c. 1260–1316) who asserted that "the patient needed to know nothing." There was therefore growing interest in a topic of basic importance: everyone's health.

Below are the main points set down in the continuous updating of medical ethics:

Rule of St. Benedict (534 AD)—Chap. 36—The sick brothers

1. Care for the sick must take precedence over everything, so they are truly served as if they were Christ himself.
2. The sick, however, should bear in mind that they are served out of love for God, and must not oppress the brothers who care for them with excessive demands.
3. One must assist them with great patience, because through them great merit is acquired.
4. There should be a dedicated room and a God-fearing, diligent and caring nurse for sick monks.
5. They are allowed to use the baths as often as necessary for therapeutic purposes; the healthy, on the other hand, especially the younger ones, are allowed to use them more rarely.
6. The weakest patients will be allowed to eat meat in order to recover their strength.

Rule of San Pacomio (third century AD) and Precepts

… The sick patients are assisted with special care and given various abundant foods

[40] If an illness arises, the person in charge of the house will turn to those who serve the sick to receive what is needed.

[46] If one of those sent outside falls ill on the road or in a boat and has a desire for fish broth or something that is not usually consumed in the monastery, he will

[20] There are about 30 Regulae, of Western and Latin origin, with legislative aspects for monastic life. The rules differ widely in length, form and structure; the later ones depend on the earlier ones and some were intended for a particular monastery, although they spread elsewhere later, while others originally had a general character. However, a monastery could pass from one rule to another or even use several, as needed: regulae mixtae. Each rule had its own history: some were used mainly local, while others were adopted more widely. However, the custom arose to collect several rules together, especially the shorter ones (corpora regularum), often in chronological order, sometimes in order of importance, and they were read together and used in the same monastery. By Bernardino A. Monastic rules from: "Patrologia. Vol. 4"- Ed. Marietti 1996; Chapter VIII. Canonistic, Penitential and Liturgical Literature. August 20, 2015.

not sit at the table with the other brothers, but the nurses in charge will give it to the sick brother somewhere apart, in abundance, so as not to disappoint him.

Rule of Saint Augustine (written around 400)—Chap. 5

[37] The care of the sick, convalescents and any others who suffer some indisposition even without fever should be entrusted to a single person who has the task of personally withdrawing from the dispensary whatever he deems necessary for the purpose.

Rule of the Order of the Templars (1242)—according to St. Bernard

[52] Special attention should be paid to the sick. Brothers who are ill must be given very close care, as if Christ himself were being served. One must recall the Gospel saying "I was sick and you visited me."

They must be treated patiently, because through them one acquires greater (celestial) retribution.

[53] The sick are always given whatever they need. To the assistants of the sick we recommend every observance and careful care for the different diseases. Depending on what is available in the house, meat, poultry and anything else are to be provided until recovery.

Saint Francis of Assisi—Rule with no seal (1221)—Chapter X

[34] Should a friar fall ill, wherever he may be, the other friars are not to leave him without first appointing one or more confrères to serve him as they would like to be treated themselves. In case of extreme necessity, other people may be called in. All this comes from the "evil one" and he is a carnal man; he does not seem to be a friar, since he loves the body more than the soul.

Salerno Medical School

The beginning of medieval medicine in Italy coincides with the establishment of the Salerno School, cultural components of the time coexisted.

The Salerno School was the first and most important medical institution in Europe, the forerunner of modern universities. The next ones arrived only after the year 1000 (Paris 1100, Bologna 1150, Montpellier 1181). This school brought together the best of the Latin, Greek, Arabic and Hebrew traditions in medicine. The school based its principles on Hippocrates' humoral theories (for which Salerno earned the title of Hippocratica Civitas).

In the twelfth to thirteenth century, the *Regimen Sanitatis Salernitanum* was published, which collected together other indications that were ahead of the times:

Si tibi deficiant medici, medici tibi fiant hæc tria: mens laeta, requies, moderata diæta.	If you lack doctors, May these three things be doctors for you: A happy soul, quietude and a moderate diet.

"Oh doctor, when you are called to the sick person ... look at the pulse, but do not be deceived by the numerous pulsations, due to the joy at your arrival ... wait until it has calmed down, up to a hundred you will listen to the pulsations, so that you can understand the nature ... Order that you have brought the urine ... you'll look at the color, the substance and the amount ... "

Health and Disease

Health, sickness, and healing are part of the universal eschatological process, along the path to salvation.

The transit from health to sickness, or from sickness to health, was interpreted on the basis of the categories of constitution (the heavenly condition), fallen (the earthly condition), and restored (the resurrection).

The patient and the doctor saw their actions and their life in this perspective. For the sick person in the Middle Ages, disease was a manifestation of earthly existence; for the physician, his actions were part of the salvation. The seven virtues[21] included the behavior of the doctor and the patient, and respect for health and illness. The seven works of mercy included visiting the sick—for patients, doctors, and also society.

The Apothecaries

Collecting herbs and formulating preparations, with real or presumed therapeutic activity, has been going on for more than a millennium. Already among the Romans there were people who manufactured and dispensed remedies prepared with spices, medicinal herbs, extracts or animal skins (vipers, lizards, and scorpions) in the *tabernae medicinae* (*pharmacies*). There the pharmacotriba formulated and sold the medicinal remedies prescribed by doctors.

The Greeks called the apothecary a rhizotome (referring perhaps to collecting roots of plants). The pharmacists of the Medical School of Salerno were the forerunners of a new medical profession: the pharmacist.

The first pharmacies were set up in ground-floor rooms fitted with shelves displaying various medicinal herbs, plant roots, plant and animal extracts, in clay pots and jars, as well as other mineral products employed as needed in decoctions, infusions, ointments, poultices, etc. These "chemist' shops or apothecaries" were called *jatrie* and politicians, curious people and men of culture met up there. They prepared and sold poultices, syrups, elixirs, etc. The first work describing various 'recipes', or prescriptions, is attributable to Galen (129–201 AD.).

Later, towards the sixth century, pharmaceutical methodology started to become more rational. A first distinction between the apothecary and the doctor was made by Frederick II (c. 1235) who carried out a health "reform" in Italy. In 1240, an ordinance established that only a pharmacist, bound by an oath, could open a pharmacy, and only in a specific place. In other places there were different laws. In the Middle Ages the apothecaries' guilds were born and their qualifications and roles were identified better and recognized.

[21] Theological Virtues: Faith, Hope, Charity: Cardinal Virtues: Prudence, Justice, Strength, Temperance. Works of mercy: Burying the dead, Visiting prisoners, Feeding the hungry, Clothing the naked, Healing the sick, Giving drink to the thirsty, Hosting pilgrims.

Thus it was that Nicolò Salernitano could write his famous treatise "Antidotarium" which Emperor Frederick II raised to the status of an official pharmacopoeia throughout Europe. However, the fundamental work on medieval medicinal botany remains the treatise "*De Medicinis Simplicibus,*" attributed to Matteo Plateario (known as Arcimatteo). Before starting their work, apothecaries had to take an oath, undertaking to observe all the rules for the preparation of medicines, for their genuineness and for the sales prices.

The **Venetian Apothecaries' Oath** (1111 A.C.) solemnly testifies and promises to the Creator of all, God in the Trinity, whom, he said "I worship with candid faith, to observe all the following rules to the full and constantly, by my own strength and judgment":

- I will always live and die in the Christian Faith.
- I will give due reverence to the Doctors and faithfully honor my Tutors, respecting my elders, and especially to the others who use my Art.
- I will preserve the dignity of this Art as far as I can.
- I will not do anything without taking advice, or without manifest reason, or even less for mere gain.
- I will not give purgative medicines without the order and agreement of the Doctors.
- I will not give poison, or advise anyone about this.
- I will not give anything that can cause abortion and could harm others.
- I will not modify any order from a Doctor.
- I will not use a substitute without the advice and permission of the Doctor.
- I will not carry out the harmful orders from the Empirics.
- I will give the Sick all the help I can with my Art.
- I will not keep in my shop any medicine of any sort that is not perfectly good, nor will I allow my young administrators to violate this oath.
- Herewith I swear to the praise and glory of our Savior Jesus Christ Protector of this Sacred College.[22]

It took a few centuries before the first "*spezieria*, apothecaire, apothecary" was accepted and became the "pharmacy" we know and appreciate today.

From the eleventh to twelfth century Western medical ethics had more firmly adopted the moral values of the catholic religion and the emphasis was shifting to the duties and principles of a good doctor, meaning the professional dimension. The pragmatic concept that the practice of medicine was a privilege that required

[22] Similar procedures, or at least initial historical documentation, are included for Naples (twelfth century), Genoa (1227), Catania (1240), Venice (1258), Florence (1310), Asti (1322), Brescia (1524), (Santa Severina, Crotone, 1525), Palermo (1543), Bologna (1574), Mantua (1583), Rome (1583), Ferrara (1595). Later, the apothecaries appeared in other cities such as Paris, London, Barcelona, Valencia, Montpellier and Marseille, and soon throughout Europe.

Ciasca R., The art of doctors and apothecaries in Florentine history and trade, from the twelfth to the fifteenth century, Florence - Leo S. Olschki, Ed. 01/01/1927.

Vecchiato (2013).

training and skills therefore implied clear responsibilities, specially when the doctor had to deal with serious or hopeless cases.

Several factors had always to be assessed:

1. the disease is due to recognizable natural factors, such as infection;
2. therapy is based on the recognition of these factors and on therapies linked to the causes of pathogenic events;
3. healing depends on the doctor and death is sometimes due to inadequate or inappropriate action by the doctor;
4. the good doctor is the one who heals often ... and who makes the fewest mistakes ...

After the year 1000, medicine began to apply the results of reason with caution and to detach itself from the teachings of the Ancients. However, we have to wait for the innovative work of extraordinary figures, such as Theophrastus, Paracelsus, and Andrea Vesalius, to see a significant break with the positions of the past.

From the eighth to the fourteenth centuries, many endemic diseases appeared in Europe alongside the increasingly precarious health conditions linked to hunger and malnutrition. The most important infectious diseases in Europe that persisted at the end of the fourteenth century were: dysentery; ergot poisoning (also known as St. Anthony's Fire); gonorrhea; influenza; leprosy; malaria; measles; plague; puerperal fever; smallpox; typhus; and typhoid fever.

Some were epidemic, others endemic. The young, the elderly and the weak were most vulnerable, because of poor nutrition, heavy work, or previous illnesses. Medieval doctors treated these diseases one symptom at a time, with separate prescriptions for fever, cough, chills, and so on.

It is therefore clear that the development of medicine ground to a halt, accompanied by diminished attention to the rules and codes of conduct of doctors.

The end of the Middle Ages marked the beginning of the early modern age, followed in much of Europe: the Renaissance. The birth of experimental science in the seventeenth century and its subsequent evolution changed the figure of the doctor and led to his shifting towards an increasingly shrewd and reliable definition of pathologies and possible treatments.

References

Afshar L. Medical oath: the educational impact. J Med Educ. 2016;15(1):1–3.

Amundsen DW. Medical deontology and pestilential disease in the late middle ages. J Hist Med Allied Sci. 1977;XXXII(4):403–21.

Amundsen DW. The development of medical ethics. Vancouver: The University of British Columbia; 1980.

Amundsen DW. The medieval Catholic tradition. In: Numbers RL, Amundsen DW, editors. Caring and curing: health and medicine in the western religious traditions. New York: Macmillan; 1986. p. 65–107.

Amundsen DW. Medical ethics, history of Europe: I. Ancient and medieval. A. Greece and Rome, encyclopedia of bioethics. 2004. http://www.encyclopedia.com.

Bird LP. Medical ethics. In: Bird L, Barlow J, editors. Oaths & prayers, an anthology. Richardson, TX: Christian Medical & Dental Society; 1989. p. 1–15.

Brandon SGF. B.C. and A.D.: the Christian philosophy of history. Hist Today. 1965;15(3).

Bresadola M. Dioscorides's De materia medica. Wall Street International, 2014.

Carrick PJ. Medical ethics in the ancient world. Washington, DC: Georgetown University Press; 2001. Pt. 1–2: 11–108.

Castiglioni A. History of medicine. Milan: A. Mondadori Ed; 1946. p. 7–11.

Cavalli F. Breve storia della medicina. Antichità e Medioevo. (IT. A brief history of medicine. Antiquity and the middle ages). Anno Accademico; 2013-2014.

Cavalli F. Breve storia della medicina. Dalla preistoria al medioevo. (IT: Brief history of medicine. From prehistory to the Middle Ages). Edit. Accademia Jaufré Rudel di studi medievali, Gorizia; 26, 2022.

Cosmacini G. L'arte lunga – Storia della medicina dall'antichità today), II Mondo Classico, Laterza, Rome-Bari. 1977;51–100.

Cosmacini G, Menghi M. Galen and Galenism. Health science and ideas. Milan: FrancoAngeli; 2012. p. 93–7.

Crisciani C. The training of doctors in the Middle Ages: doctrine and ethics. In: Formare alle Professioni. Figures of health. Milan: Franco Angeli Ed; 2010. p. 51–7.

Davies RW. Medicine in ancient Rome. Hist Today. 1971;21(11):770–8.

Dyer C. Europe in the middle ages. In: Making a living in the middle ages: the people of Britain 850-1520. New Haven: Yale University Press; 2002.

Eco U. Il Medioevo-Barbari, Cristiani, Musulmani. Milano: EncycloMedia Pub.; 2010.

Encyclopedia of Bioethics. Medical ethics, history of Europe: I. Ancient and medieval Christian Europe, 2004 & Encyclopedia.com. 2016.

Galen. De partibus artis medicae translated by Niccolò da Reggio: De partibus artis meditative, 3, 1, 19th century - Ed. Pinzi, Venezia; 1490.

Horse P, Proto MC, Patruno C, Del Sorbo A, Bifulco M. The first cosmetic treatise. A female point of view. Int J Cosmet Sci. 2008;30(2):79–86.

Hubert J, Porcher J, Volbach WF. The Europe of the Barbarian Invasions. Milan: Rizzoli Ed; 1967. p. IX–XIV; 1–3.

Jackson R. Doctors and diseases in the Roman Empire (Chap. 1). London: British Museum Press; 1988.

Jonsen AR. Medical history in India and China (Chap. 3). In: A short history of medical ethics. Oxford: Oxford University Press; 2000. p. 27–41.

Kieckhefer R. Magic in the middle ages, trans. by Federico Corradi, GLF ed. Rome: Laterza; 2004.

Koios N., Veloyanni L., Alvanos D. Evolution of Medical Ethics Cavalli F. Breve storia della medicina. Antichità e Medioevo Anno Accademico. 2006;2013–2014.

Kroeber AL. The morals of uncivilized people. Am Anthropol. 1910;12(3):437–47.

Liguori M, Cannavò G, Orrico M. Chap. IV—The obligation to inform. In: Medical responsibility: from theory to procedural practice. Maggioli Ed.; 2011. p. 129–30.

Macer DRJ. Shaping genes: ethics, law and science of using new genetic technology in medicine and agriculture. Christchurch: Eubios Ethics Institute; 1990. p. 348–92.

Maion D. The old English medical treatise, Peri Didaxeon, translation, society and culture (10); 1999.

Marasco G. Medici at the court of the Caesars: functions and therapeutic methods. Med Hist J. 1997;32(3/4):279–97.

Morpurgo P. Medieval medicine and the Salerno school. The Italian contribution to the history of thought, sciences; 2013.

Motamedi MHK. Breaching medical ethics in research. Trauma Mon. 2014;19(2):e17112.

Mount T. Medieval medicine: its mysteries and science. Stroud: Amberley Press; 2016.

Nemec J. Highlights in medicolegal relations. Bethesda: U.S. Dept. of Health, Education, and Welfare, Public Health Service, National Institutes of Health, National Library of Medicine; 1976. p. 10–1.

Ostrowski, M. The Church in the middle ages. Hist Rev. 2006;56.

Pelàez M. DISF. Org, Chap. II—Medicine and Christianity; Chapter III—the birth of hospitals in the bosom of Christianity; 2002.
Penso G. The medieval medicine. Ciba-Geigy Ed.; 1991. p. 19–26.
Prioreschi P. Medieval medicine (Ch. I-V). In: A history of medicine, vol. V. Omaha: Horatius Press; 2003.
Quinto Orazio Flacco. Satire, Rizzoli Universal Library. 2006. https://it.wikipedia.
Rajala AI. The elusive Formula Comitis Archiatrorum—the first medical ethics code? 2015.
Rajala AI. Following up on Formula Comitis Archiatrorum—still not convinced; 2016.
Regimen Sanitatis Salernitanum. Superintendence for the BAP of Salerno and Avellino. Copyright 2007-2016. http://www.ambientesa.beniculturali.it/.
Robert J. Mr. James's universal dictionary of medicine. Giambattista Pasquali ed. Venezia; 1753. p. 47.
Russo RG. Medieval history, middle ages and medicine. 2007a. http://www.mondimedievali.net/Medicina/storiachirurgia.htm.
Russo RG. Medioevo e medicina, La medicina nell'alto Medioevo. Maggio. 2007b. http://www.Mondimedievali.net/Medicina/indice.htm.
Scott CP, editor. The Visigothic code (Forum Judicum). Boston: The Boston Book Company; 1910.
Vecchiato R. Gli Speziali in Venezia. (IT. The apothecaries in Venice). Order of Pharmacists of the Province of Venice, Mazzanti Libri; 2013.
Veith L. Medical ethics throughout the ages. Q Bull Northwest Univ Med Sch. 1957;31(4):351–8.
von Engelhardt D. Etica Medica. 2010. http://www.webethics.net/filosofando_etica_medica.
Wazer C. The cutthroat politics of public health in ancient Rome. And what we can learn from it today. The Atlantic, Apr 22, 2016.
Woodbury E. The fall of the Hippocratic Oath: why the Hippocratic Oath should be discarded in favor of a modified version of Pellegrino's precepts. GUJHS. 2012;6(2):9–17.
Xenophontos S. Psychotherapy and moralising rhetoric in Galen's newly discovered avoiding distress (Peri Alypias). Med Hist. 2014;58(4):585–603.
Zardo N. A dip in the hygiene of the ancient Mediterranean civilizations. Perini J. 2012;38.

Far East: China

5

The history of Chinese medical ethics can be viewed in the light of medical advances and its concomitant appearance on the world stage. However, in all probability its long journey really started about 4500 years ago. Here is a possible sequence of the main events:

1. Traditional Chinese medicine (TCM)
2. Confucius and Confucianism + Ancient Chinese medical ethics (ACME)
3. Sun Simiao (fifth to sixth century)
4. Chang Kao (twelfth century)
5. Kung Hsin (sixteenth century)
6. Chen Shih-kung and Chang-Lu (sixteenth century)
7. More recent times

1. Historical Summary of Traditional Chinese Medicine (TCM) [1]

TCM encompasses a wide range of holistic therapies, originally gradually developed in ancient China from Paleolithic times, which were used globally for the treatment of a large number of diseases.

The principle of TCM is ***qi***, a vital force said to circulate in the body, that can lead to disease when its flow is obstructed. TCM is used in various forms, including herbal medicine, acupuncture, and physical exercises such as t'ai chi, with the aim of boosting the circulation of ***qi*** and relieving symptoms of disease. Other aspects may include the manipulation of *yin* and *yang*[2] which lead to health and well-being

[1] Jingfeng (1998), Chen (2002, 2005), Layne and Ferro (2017) and Veatch (2000), pp. 303–307.

[2] The universe, created spontaneously by its Tao (eternal, essential principle and fundamental force), is composed of two souls, the Yang and the Yin. When the body is in balance between Yang and Yin, health predominates. When Yang and Yin are unbalanced, sickness occurs. Yang represents light, heat, production and life; Yin is the dark, the cold, death and the earth. Yang and Yin

R. G. Russo, *Medical Ethics*, https://doi.org/10.1007/978-3-031-42444-1_5

when in harmony and disease when disrupted. These concepts are still not fully recognized in pharmaceutical medicine, where there is greater focus on achieving physiological and symptomatic goals with pharmacological agents. TCM focuses on actually relieving symptoms rather than just improving the clinical signs of the disease, and assesses the most appropriate therapy for comorbidities.

TCM is one of the unconventional medicines and is believed to be the oldest known medical system. In the twenty-fifth century B.C. the first monograph on medical theory was compiled (The Yellow Emperor Huang Di Classic, (2697–2597 B.C.) which laid the foundations for medical theory, composed of ***yin-yang*** and principles, which explained physiology, pathology, and etiology, guiding the diagnosis, treatment, and prevention of diseases, together with the application of drugs.[3]

Some dynasties followed:

Xia (2207–1766 B.C.),
Shang (1766–1120 B.C.), and
Zhou (1065–771 B.C.)

in which shamanic medicine was practiced and oracular inscriptions have been found. They spoke for the first time of the concept of disease, believed to be linked to an evil influence that could be eradicated with divinatory practices. The first medicinal substances were introduced: infusions, poultices to be applied to the skin and, above all, elixirs. The first outlines of pharmacology also appeared (pills and potions, herbal and mineral remedies) in addition to acupuncture and moxibustion. Later the idea of an independent medical profession gained favor and the medical system was formed around four main aspects: diet, internal, surgery, and veterinary. Doctors wore different uniforms in different groups, depending on their responsibility and "speciality." For example, *ji yi* doctors treated internal disease, *yan yi* doctors dealt with external disorders, *shou yi* were veterinarians and *shi yi* were dietary practitioners.

---

are divided into an infinite number of good and bad spirits called respectively Shen and Kwei. The Chinese doctor must consider the interdependence between organs and functions of the body, emotions, climatic and seasonal situations in order to understand the mechanisms to influence and increase vital functions. In summary: without Yang there is no Yin, without Yin there is no Yang.

[3] The origins of diseases were believed to be due to various causes, mainly external:

- Celestial, coming directly from the will of the emperor or through the rain;
- Malefic influence of the Gui, the spirit of the dead;
- Parasites and insect bites.

Demonic medicine considered that the concept of illness was based on the principle of the nefarious influence of evil spirits that had to be neutralized by the shaman with prayers, talismans and magic potions. The first steps in pharmacology, involving pills and potions, herbal and mineral remedies, were employed in addition to acupuncture and moxibustion. The reward system was: full fee for a 100% cure; reduction in the fee in relation to the percentage of treatment failure. Doctors were encouraged to improve their medical skills in order to earn better remuneration.

Pugliarello et al. (2000).

The Editors of the Encyclopædia Britannica, Traditional Chinese medicine. 10-20-2017.

Unschuld (1990) and Tsuei (1989).

In the period from 770 to 476 B.C. and the period of the Warring States (475–221 B.C.) medicine began to detach itself from witchcraft and magic and became based more on experience and professional competence.[4]

- Doctors did not have any concept of clinics or hospitals, but went round from one place to another practicing freely.
- They had no formal training and did not need a specific license, but applied their own skills and worked according to their consciences.
- Medicine was not to be practiced in six circumstances:

1. people who showed unreasonable arrogance or indulgence,
2. people who valued wealth more than life,
3. people who did not consider body and soul together,
4. people who suffered from the *yin-yang* connection,
5. people who were too weak to take medicines, and
6. people who did not believe in medicine, but in witchcraft.

In the animistic religion of China, a group of people known as Wu exercised (in the spirit world) abilities and powers not possessed by the rest of men. Many Wu practitioners were doctors who used medicinal herbs, besides charms and spells, to ward off death.

Divination and exorcism can be traced back to the fifth and sixth centuries B.C.

Zhang Zhongjing (150–c.219 A.D.),[5] who lived during the Eastern Han Dynasty, was the most eminent physician, often regarded as the Hippocrates of China, not only for his medical skills, but also for his high standards of medical ethics. At that time epidemics (especially typhus) were frequent and widespread due to civil wars. In 205 A.D. he wrote a Treatise on Cold Diseases and Various Diseases in which he included his decades of collected clinical cases, elaborating causes, pathologies, principles, and methods of treatment.

Pharmacology is another important contribution of TCM. The Classics of Materia Medica is the first pharmacological work (no longer available), composed

[4] It was believed that there were five physical states represented graphically in a circle, according to Tao symbols: wood, depicted in green—the vegetation that come to life in the spring, Yang; the fire that burns and disappears, colored red and associated with summer—the expression of Yang par excellence; the earth, symbol of the end of summer, Yin; metal, representing hardness and also autumn; Yin: water, the maximum of Yin—it is black and expresses winter. Apart of the human body is associated with each phase: wood to the liver, fire to the heart, earth to the spleen and pancreas, metal to the lungs, water to the kidneys. Curiously similar to the almost contemporary Theory of the Four Moods, indicated above (Wikipedia, Warring States Period).

[5] In this period (already after 300 B.C.) all the main theories of Chinese medicine appear: yin-yang, wu-hsing (5 phases), 5 flavors, 5 colors, the system of correspondence, Qi, diagnosis of the pulse, channels or meridians, acupuncture points. The roles of the doctor and the shaman become separate and the Six Philosophical Schools develop: Dao, Yin-yang (Naturalist), Confucian, Mohist, Legalist, of Names.

Oakes and Zhongjing (2017) and Wu and Zhongjing (2012).

around the second century A.D. During the Han Dynasty (206 B.C.–220 A.D.) the fundamental cultural values formed, thanks to the assumption that medicine is a human art that emphasizes the care of patients and self-training in virtues for doctors.

Ge Hong (281–341 A.D.) proposed some methods for the treatment of infectious diseases. Often these were based on the then archaic concept of *similia similibus curantur* (healing like with like—perhaps anticipating immunotherapy?).

At the beginning of the Jin dynasty (third century A.D.),Wang Shuhe declared that the Cunkou is the point of the pulse where the radial artery can be felt throbbing.[6]

During the Ming dynasty[7] (1368–1644) medical knowledge progressed significantly and the numbers of doctors grew rapidly, particularly in the more prosperous regions, parallel to the growth of the population, the spread of the press, conomic dynamism and the consolidation of a wealthy urban elite. The Ming dynasty had a cultured and complex medical tradition (in addition to the popular one) and benefited from advances in the publication of previous medical texts and from the theoretical advances made in during the Jin and Yuan dynasties. Professional conscience grew with the increasing influence of Confucian morality on medical ethics.

The study of medical material peaked with the publication in 1596 of the reasoned classification of the Pharmacopoeia and in 1593 with the Compendium of Medical Matter, concerning 1892 types of herbal drugs.

The works of the doctor Li Shizhen (1518–1593)[8] were fundamental; he anticipated the phenomenon of genetics, the variations related to it, and the adaptation of animals to their environment. A professional code for doctors was drafted by the surgeon Chen Shi Gong (1555–1636), and included Five Prohibitions in the Standard Surgery Textbook:

- Never be late when called by a patient, be he poor or rich, and administer the necessary medications and provide treatment, whether paid or not.
- Do not visit a woman, a girl or a nun without the presence of a third person, and observe the obligation of confidentiality.

[6] At that time, 24 different different types of wrist heart rate were distinguished: fu (floating), kou (hollow), hong (full), hua (smooth), su (quick), cu (running), xian (tight string), jin (tight string), chen (depth), fù (hidden), ge (hard and empty), shi (forced), wei (weak), se (slow or hesitant), xi (minute), ruan (soft), ruo (weak), xù (weak), san (scattered), huan (moderate), chi (slow), jie (slow with irregular intervals), dai (intermittent) and dong (tremulous).

[7] Ki Che Leung (2001) and Will (2001).

The Compendium of Materia Medica comprised 16 categories: water, fire, earth, metal and stone, grass, cereals, vegetables, fruit, wood, tools, worms, scales, shells, birds, beasts and man. Other writings followed: (Wan-ping hui-ch'un, 1587); return to life after illness (Chen Shih-kung, 1605 A.C);

Bird (1989), p. 39;

– (Wai-ko Cheng-Tsung: 1627–1707);

– A manual of surgery (Chang-Lu, 1627–1707);

Ten Commandments for Doctors (Chang-shih-i-tung: 1555–1636);

Bird (1989), pp 40–41.

[8] Nappi and Shizhen (2010).

- Never replace valuable components of a medicine with components of little value.
- Never leave the doctor's office during opening hours to have free time to devote to fun, and present treatments and prescriptions to patients in an accurate and legible way.
- Never harbor immoral thoughts if the patient is a prostitute or a man's lover; treat these people as worthy people, leave the patient's home immediately after treatment, and return to visit only if called again.

More Data on TCM [9]

TCM argued that the causes of all diseases can be divided into three categories:

- exogenous (e.g., unseasonal climate changes, such as strong wind, cold, summer heat, humidity, drought, and fires);
- endogenous (e.g., joy, anger, melancholy, fear, meditation, and pain);
- intermediate (e.g., burns, frostbite, snake, insect or other animal bites, metal injuries, food abuse, excessive drinking or sexual activities).

There were eight key principles for diagnosis: superficial, internal, cold, hot, strength, asthenia, yin and yang. There were also four types of medical method: inspection, investigation, auscultation, smell and palpation. The three main concepts can be summarized as follows:

(a) Professional ethics: those who practice this medicine consider man at the center of the world around them.
(b) Prevention: this was based on a balanced diet and included energy diagnostics (wrist, eye, tongue, and skin study), acupuncture, pharmacology, gymnastics, and massage.
(c) Synergy of forces between man and the social environment, which are interdependent, influencing each other.

These commandments remind physicians to follow standards of care, competence, and prudent practice to avoid the risk of harm to patients. They interpret the principle of non-male-ficence in a comprehensive way. Ancient Chinese ethics attached great importance to the virtue of charity and the value of free service to the poor. The concept of medical ethics or the reflection on moral issues in medicine probably dates back to the Axial Age, [10] when the first Chinese works on disease and

---

[9] The Editors of Encyclopaedia Britannica, Traditional Chinese medicine. Encyclopedia Britannica, Oct. 20, 2017.
Wikipedia (n.d.).

[10] The Axial Age refers to the period of time from 800 B.C. to 200 B.C. It was a time when many new and important ideas (independently) arose in various places around the world: India, the West and China. It was proposed by the German philosopher Karl Jaspers (1883–1969).

healing were produced, and in fact they are still essential readings in today's TCM. The basic vocabulary also grew up through the teachings of the main schools of thought including Confucianism, Taoism, and the Yin-Yang theory itself.

2. **Confucius + ACME**

Confucius was born in 551 B.C. in the Kong[11] family and given the name Kong Fuzi (Master Kong); this was Latinized as Confucius (or Confutius) in 1687, by the first Jesuit missionaries in China. His profound culture, rich in content and meaning, exerted a decisive influence on the thought, culture and political life on the Chinese of the time. Confucius was the first to found a private school in China; Confucian culture at that time spread widely, embracing the social, political, cultural, educational, ethical, and moral aspects of life. His theories of morality and ethics with goodness as the core, and rituals, served as keynotes for the development of Chinese medical ethics. Confucius formulated the concept of conscience and emphasized self-control, introspection and self-respect together with self-blame in case of errors.[12]

Medical ethics in China therefore has a very long tradition and the values of ancient Chinese medicine grew up alongside the development of the same medical professionalism: the profession meant one's duties. Ethical knowledge in the medical world before Confucius was far from complete or systematic, but was fragmented and considered almost a banality. However, many scholars[13] were already practicing healing arts and formulating professional ethics. To summarize: the four principles are clearly identifiable in Ancient Chinese Medical Ethics—ACME: (1) charity and (2) non-maleficence have always been the main points, based on humanity (Jen), which is the central theme of Confucianism. Medical ethics is also supported by (3) yi, justice and autonomy (4). ACME required doctors to maintain a respectful attitude and to examine all patients equally and assist them with relentless fatigue to the point of self-sacrifice. ACME attached great importance to the virtue of charity and the value of free service to the poor. Confucius preached universal love for all patients, regardless of social status, family background, appearance or age, etc. He also believed that everybody had a conscience—an innate sense of right and wrong. This was to lead doctors to four other senses:

1. The sense of Piety: compassion and love for the patient.
2. The sense of Shame: The doctor would feel sinful if ever:
   (a) he put his interests before those of his patient,

Jaspers (1949) and Bellah (2005).

[11] Confucius, Wikipedia.
Guo (1995).

[12] Nie (2011), Tsai (1999) and Veatch (2000), pp. 292–303.

[13] Bird (1989), pp. 39–41, Kao (1979), Dharmananda (2010), Doering (2002), Feldman (1985), Tsai (1999), Jonsen 2000, Chap. 3, pp. 27–41, Lee (1943), Qiu (1988), Tsai (1999), Unschuld (1979) and Ming et al. (2015).

   (b) he reached a diagnosis without employing all four methods of physical examination,
   (c) he abused drugs, or
   (d) deceived a patient.
3. The sense of Respect
4. The sense of Right and Wrong.

Confucius's enthusiasm was neither shared nor understood by either the rulers or the people, and he was often the object of slander and harassment. The solution he proposed was simple: to save society: man had to be saved. He therefore arranged that instead of imposing a universal code of conduct everyone should examine himself. This is one of the main reasons for the initial lack of codified medical ethics in Chinese medicine.

He also maintained that morality is inherent to human nature and is expressed as *ren* or humanity, and benevolence. From this origin of morality some more concrete principles are generated such as *ren*, *yi*, *li* and *zhi*, or benevolence, justice, correctness, and moral conscience: these form the main guiding principles for our life. This is the principle of the moral mentality, together with concern for the suffering of others.

Man has always been the object of Confucius' teaching and the focus of his interest. An individual is a superior man if he possesses wisdom, humanity, courage, filial piety, liberality, diligence, humility, sincerity, and many other virtues. The basic principle was do not do to others what you would not want them to do to you. Confucius contrasts the superior man with the inferior man, the first motivated by impeccable moral conduct and the second by profit. For 2500 years Confucian scriptures were the basis of the ethics, moral philosophy, and ideology of Chinese medical culture. Hand in hand with the advent of medical activities in remote antiquity, ethical issues started to appear in daily practice, albeit in a primitive form, and the concept of medical ethics began to take shape.

Confucianism[14]

"You have to understand Confucianism before you can really understand what medicine really is," Confucius said. The set of doctrines of Confucius and his successors, which form the foundation of classical Chinese thought, consists of moral, social, and political reflections. Despite the failure and persecutions that accompanied Confucius in life, starting from the Han dynasty (206 B.C.–220 A.D.), Confucian thought was adopted as a state ethics. The main texts were fixed by tradition in five classics "*Wujing*" and in four books "*Sishu.*" These are texts of various kinds (history, philosophy, poetry) that collect the most ancient knowledge of Chinese civilization, from the ninth to the fourth century B.C.

[14] Veatch (2000) and Chai and Yang (2006), pp. 366–381.

Confucianism was the philosophical guide of Chinese feudal society for over 2000 years and contributed to the guiding principles of Medical Ethics. Obviously Confucianism was opposed by some illustrious doctors, supporters of an opposite medicine or of witchcraft. Later the system was followed and even partially modified by medical professionals of all generations throughout Chinese history.

This system involved concepts such as the need to attach great importance to life and to give the best of oneself to save the dying and to heal the wounded.

Doctors had to show concern for those who suffered from diseases and practiced the profession honestly, opposing an imprudent and undignified style; they had to be equally gentle in treating both noble and humble patients and respect the results obtained by other professionals.

Over the course of China's long history, this appeared to be a rather evolved system of Medical Ethics. Confucianism held a dominant position for a long time in ancient China, with objective, function, and structure centered on ethics and morals. Its main promoter of this was Sun Simiao.

Influence of Confucianism in Chinese Medical Ethics

Confucius was the helm and ideological guide of the philosophy of Chinese feudal society for over 2000 years. He was a great pedagogue, thinker, and philosopher, the common thread of medical ethics in ancient China.

The core of Confucian thought is "benevolence" or "love and goodness of heart" and "humanity." He argued that "those who are kindhearted" are good to the people. In other words, all people should love each other, not just doctors for their patients. Benevolence: it is the core of Confucian ethics. The Confucians believed that medicine (with the primary purpose of saving lives) had its highest expression in love. Zhang Zhongjing (150–219 A.D.), physician and writer of the first systematic text on herbal treatment, said that Confucians could realize their goal of loving people only if, thanks to medical theory, they treated people with benevolence. This is the origin of the saying "Medicine is the art of humanity." It required the worship of human life and nothing was more precious than that (see Footnote 14).

Thus, even Mencius (third century A.D.) had said: "In medicine, benevolence means that no harm is done to patients; it would be inconvenient for the doctor to act as if he were doing his patients a favor; care is his duty, the main expression of humanity. The request for money or sex for the treatment is inadmissible." Confucianism also suggested a universality of the cure. No patient should be given better or worse care based on the circumstances or the (unacceptable) will of the health care worker. The Confucians were rigorous and scrupulous in their diagnosis to avoid doing harm.

Tianchen Li, a Ming Dynasty physician, suggested "We should treat patients like our mothers."

Moral Education

The emphasis placed by the Confucians on education and moral growth also had a direct bearing on the promotion of traditional medical ethics and on the enhancement of the moral advancement of doctors. As a motto, Confucian doctors argue that "medicine is a benevolent art" or a technical art to save life and cure diseases. Confucius also stressed that those who lack perseverance are not qualified to become a doctor: this art embodies the spirit of Man and reflects social responsibility and the characteristics of the medical profession. Based on the Buddhist concept of "samsara," the medical profession is an ideal profession to fulfill the mission of doing only good deeds in this world. This new idea helped to form a primitive standard for Medical Ethics between the third and fifth centuries A.D., for which the following were recommended:

1. careful consideration and consideration when it comes to the disease;
2. a diligent way when it comes to medical art
3. careful and appropriate management when prescribing a prescription or medication.

Ancient Chinese Medical Ethics (ACME)

ACME requires doctors to respect patients, with a sincere, decorous and disinterested attitude toward medical practice; it requires their further enhancement with a respectful attitude.

The literature, also regarding Medical Ethics, can be summarized in the following principles:

- Appreciate the value of life[15] and practical medicine with compassion and humanity
- Master Confucianism before learning medicine
- Master medical knowledge by studying valid sources, with diligent and extensive study
- Improve clinical skills and maintain a high professional standard
- Be frugal, not greedy for wealth and fame
- Treat patients equally and as if they were family members
- Be sincere, decent, dedicated, attentive and selfless in the treatment of patients
- Treat female patients only in the presence of an assistant; respecting their privacy and without any lust

[15]The value of life was determined by doctors who had to: (1) appreciate life, save from death and heal the wounded with all available means; (2) be concerned about the suffering of patients and practice medicine with honesty; (3) diligently improve medical skills and counter imprudent work styles; (4) act with decorum, decency and courtesy; (5) recognize that all patients are equal before the doctor; (6) respect the results of other people and the ethics of academics.

- Be modest and prudent toward other doctors, so as not to belittle them and not to criticize them.

These principles indicate that the ACME is established on the basis of Confucian ethics: for 2500 years Confucian scriptures have been essential teaching materials for students and the dominant moral philosophy of Chinese cultural ideology. Medical practice was regarded as one of its many functions.

ACME has a strong deontological function: it reveals the nature of ethics based on duty because of its emphasis on the responsibility of doctors to treat and help their patients and not only to seek profit and fame or to give space to selfish desires.

ACME is an ethics based on virtue: Confucian philosophy holds that the moral growth of an individual is the key to achieving a social order and the flourishing of human beings.

If doctors cultivated virtue this would ensure that their medical practice is ethical. Humanity, compassion, justice, sincerity, truth, modesty, frugality, moderation, diligence, altruism, determination and wisdom, etc., appear several times in the AEMC codes, which seem reveal that "only a virtuous doctor is a good doctor".[16]

Other Notes

The discussion relating to Medical Ethics subsequently involved many doctors:

Hsu Chun-fu in 1556 compiled a section of his book "The Via Medica" on this subject. At the same time **Kung Hsin** wrote a maxim for the most reliable doctors. This was later used as a motto (slogan) in the baccalaureate of Peking Union Medical College (Beijing, 1939).

The Ancient Chinese Medical Ethics was a body of rules weighed down by idealism and it was also the practice that doctors accepted as their moral standard. The standard of ethical medicine varied according to races, uses, customs and times. An action considered moral by one people might not be moral for others; its purpose was to promote the medical profession as a service to humanity and also to regulate its practice. Particular considerations had to be given in relation to:

1. Treatment of female patients. "Men and women, in giving and receiving, must not touch each other" (Mencius third century BC, C.)
2. Free Service (most Chinese doctors were retired government officials or scholars with no imperial examination; the practice of medicine was a philanthropic enterprise or benevolent act with no financial return).
3. Origin of the disease (most Chinese believed that sickness and suffering were the punishment for sins committed and that health and happiness were the reward for the virtues expressed).
4. Social relations (a social service was set up in many hospitals to assist patients in need).

[16] Lee (1943), Tsai (1999) and Veatch (2000), pp. 308–316, 318–337.

5. Difference between the doctor of the nobility and the common people (it was believed that the physical constitution of a noble was delicate, while that of the common citizen was more resistant; different classes of doctors were established for each category of patients).
6. Secret prescriptions. (The dispensing of secret prescriptions was never considered immoral in China. Some even considered it an honor to be aware of a secret formula. Secret remedies still exist today.)

3. **Sun Simiao (Sixth Sec.)**[17]

Sun Simiao was born around 581 A.D., at the beginning of the short Sui dynasty (581–618 A.D.) and shortly before the unification of northern and southern China (589 A.D.). He worked as a doctor during the Tang dynasty (618–907) and died in 682, having completed 2 books of a 30-volume encyclopedia on medical practice that would establish his place as a central figure in the field of herbal medicine. At the time of the Ming Dynasty, in 1527, eight stone tablets bearing quotes from his works were exhibited in Huayuan, his hometown. In Beijing a "Temple of the King of Medicine" was dedicated, and in his hometown celebrations are still held to commemorate his life every year. He was considered and esteemed like a Buddha and as the King of medicine. His biography (in The Standard Histories of the Tang Dynasty) highlights his interests in philosophy, following his study of Yi jing, Daode jing, works related to the yin-yang theory and *shu shu* numerical calculations.

Sun Simiao's code is found in the first book of his encyclopedia which he titled "Recipes are worth a thousand pieces of gold."

This is the first complete record of Chinese medical practice ever written and is still studied today. It lists thousands of herbal recipes and information on the many health benefits of acupuncture, massage, nutrition, and exercise. The code is often referred to as the Chinese Hippocratic Oath. This oath is unique in that it is based on the principles of Daoism, Confucianism, and Mahayana Buddhism, in particular with the concepts of universal compassion and love. The Recipes are worth a thousand pieces of gold, printed in 652, was a complete treatise on the practice of medicine in 30 chapters. It describes the characteristics of a great doctor and what behaviors are inappropriate, such as the desire for wealth or fame.

According to Sun Simiao, a great doctor should not pay attention to status, wealth or age; he should not care if a person was attractive, friend or foe, if he was Chinese (*Han*), or if he was educated. The doctor must meet everyone on an equal basis and should always act as if he were thinking of them as next of kin. The text includes chapters on diet, nourishing life (*yang xing*), pulse diagnosis, acumoxa (a combination of acupuncture and moxibustion), massage, and exercise. His interests included the treatment of women and children. The chapters relating to the month of May dealt with herbal food recipes.

---

[17] Dharmananda (2010), Hyton (2010), Li and Liang (2016), Raphals (2017) and Wilms (2010).

The second book is virtually a supplement to the first. It adds about 800 recipes for prescriptions, with details on gathering and preparing for another 200. Some are new herbs, including some from India. It also refers to many mystical and magical practices, including exorcisms, talismans, spells and descriptions of acumoxa points, effective against demons. Sun Simiao was the first Chinese doctor to write extensively on medical ethics.

His philosophical concerns span several medical areas, in particular the practices for feeding life (yang sheng), first described in philosophical texts bu elaborate in great practical detail by doctors and alchemists such as Ge Hong and Tao Hongjing. Sun Simiao's point of view on medical ethics is extremely important in the history of Chinese medicine.

In his Qianjin Yaofang (Essential Recipes, or Prescriptions), he proposed for the first time the notion of good faith for a great doctor, offering a comprehensive argument on the guiding rules of medical ethics for the profession. Human life is of fundamental importance—more precious than a thousand pieces of gold; saving it with a single prescription means showing great virtue. His book was only a manifestation of a noble moral character. The concept *Rén*, a fundamental virtue of Confucianism, refers to benevolence, charity, humanity, love, and kindness.

Confucius also defined the *Aì Rén* principles relating to love of your neighbor. *Yì* involves right conduct, morality, duty toward neighbors, and justice, while *Lì* implies profit, gain, and advantage, which are not the right motivation for actions that concern others.

It is explained thus: "The gentleman (*junzi*) understands Yì; the little man (*xiaoren*) understands something."

"Yì can be divided into two components: *zhōng* (doing the best, conscientiousness, loyalty) and *shù* (reciprocity, altruism, consideration for others). The goal of Chinese medicine is to heal ailing bodies. Sun Simiao has convincingly argued for a radical extension of the doctor's role: every time he treats a disease, he must calm down and stabilize his will; he must be free from desires and voluptuousness and must first develop a heart filled with great compassion and empathy. He must commit himself to dedicating himself completely to alleviate suffering. When he sees the suffering and pain of others he must behave as if it were his own and open his heart deeply to their misery.

He must not "avoid dangerous mountains with rugged cliffs," at any time of day or night, in the cold of winter or in the heat of summer, hunger or thirst, fatigue or tiredness. He must immediately witness their rescue without thinking of effort or appearances. By acting in this way, he can serve as a great physician to the masses; acting against this, he is a gigantic thief to all sentient beings. Finally this is what is meant as the meaning of "feeding life" in Sun Simiao's work: cultivating "*qi*" in balance with the macrocosm for the benefit of the individual body, the body of the family (in particular his: women, children and the elderly), the political body and the "Body" of the cosmos. He was an excellent doctor with first level experience in Chinese Medical Ethics. In the preface of his Inestimable "Formulas for emergencies," with the title of "Importance of medical knowledge and medical ethics," he dealt with what a doctor with a deep knowledge of medicine and with a noble character should be like.

He summarized Medical Ethics as follows:

1. The duty of doctors is to heal the wounded, save the dying and alleviate their suffering. No matter how rich or poor they are, patients need to be treated equally.
2. He must never be afraid of difficulties and danger and must help patients with all his heart.
3. He must never feel disgusted with how much and what stink there is in the treatment of patients.
4. Make an accurate diagnosis, stay calm and pay attention to patient safety.
5. Show great respect for peers and never be jealous of others.

Today, even in China, medical ethics has a social value and, moreover, it practices what Sun Simiao preached and has always patiently treated those who have suffered from injuries or dysentery with a bad smell or infectious diseases. He himself has treated several hundred leprosy-like cases and brought them to recovery. His monograph "On the absolute sincerity of the great Doctors" is often called the "Hippocratic Oath of China." It emphasizes compassion as a basic practice that treats the patient as if he were a relative. It is based on the concepts of universal compassion and love of Confucianism and Mahayana Buddhism.

Sun Simiao also argued also on the absolute sincerity of great doctors, and stated:

> I promise to follow the path of the great doctor. I will serve and live in harmony with nature and teach patients to do the same. Whenever I treat an illness, I first relax my spirit and then solve the question. I will not give in to desires, but will first develop an attitude of compassion. I swear to save the suffering of all sentient beings.
>
> If someone comes for help, I will not ask whether the patient is noble or common, rich or poor, old or young, beautiful or ugly. Enemies, relatives, good friends, Chinese or foreign, foolish or wise - are all the same. I will consider them like my closest relatives. I will not be overly circumspect and worry about omens or my own life. I will look at the sufferings of others as if they were my own and I will worry a lot. I will not hide in the mountains. Day and night, in cold and heat, with hunger, thirst and fatigue, I will resolutely go to the rescue. It will be my duty to diagnose suffering and cure disease. I will not be proud of my abilities and I will not be driven by greed for material things. Above all, I shall keep an open heart. As I move on the right path I will receive great happiness as a reward without asking for anything in return.
>
> Anyone who acts contrary to this is a gross thief for those who still maintain their spirit. Anyone who does this is a great doctor for the living.

He then added:

- I will not worry about my own life or fortunes or misfortunes. My purpose is to preserve the lives of others.
- If I am able to do this, I realize that I am a great doctor for those who are sick. If I act contrary to these precepts, I am nothing but a great thief to those who are alive.
- People too often look with contempt on those who suffer from abominable ailments, such as ulcers or diarrhea, but I will maintain an attitude of compassion, understanding and care. A great doctor should never adopt an attitude of refusal.

- I will not discredit other doctors and boast of my own reputation.
- Doing this I will fulfill my responsibilities and my destiny as a doctor, until I am no longer able to respect my obligations, or until the end of my life.

Sun Simiao stressed the need for thorough training, rigorous conscience, and self-discipline. He also explained that compassion and humanity (jen) are the basic values of the practice of medicine.

Medical Writings and Medical Ethics

Sun Simiao's most important achievements dating from before the Tang Dynasty are: "Prescriptions for Emergencies worth a Thousand Gold Pieces," containing many medical prescriptions, and a second work containing another number of recipes.

Sun Simiao, for the first time in China, proposed ethical rules that a doctor should observe: "Human life is of fundamental importance, more precious than a thousand pieces of gold," and "Medicine is a hard art to master," he wrote, then added: "If he does not receive divine guidance, the doctor will not understand the dark points." To summarize, one can conclude that he set out the fundamental aims of medical ethics as follows:

1. The goal is to help, without seeking material goods.
2. Save life and do not kill any living thing.
3. Do not seek fame: virtuous behavior will be rewarded by Man and the spirits.

From other doctors, to ensure your own progress—only charlatans are jealous of the superb skills of other doctors. These moral doctrines lay stress on the obligation to help others.

Sun Simiao refused official positions offered by the Wendi emperor of the Sui Dynasty and the Taizong and Gaozong emperors of the Tang Dynasty. He preferred to devote himself to the care of ordinary people as a general practitioner, always maintaining that patients should be treated regardless of rank, wealth, age or beauty.

He considered health care a medical duty and proposed measures to maintain health. He also argued that actions such as massaging the scalp, rolling the eyes, squeezing the head, and walking brought health.

Teaching

Sun Simiao devoted himself to the teachings of I-Ching and yang-yin philosophy. He studied the human body and its functioning and was a medical specialist who possessed great skill and observed high medical ethics, of which he was certainly the founder in China. In summary, (as a repetitive issue) he introduced and spread the following principles:

The Purpose of Medical Practice

1. The aim is to help, without obtaining material goods.
2. Save life and do not kill any living thing.
3. Do not seek fame: virtuous behavior will be rewarded by Man and the spirits.

What Is Required to Be a Great Doctor

1. Fully master the fundamentals of medicine, work hard and relentlessly.
2. Be calm and purposeful—don't give in to selfish desires.
3. Strive, with great compassion, to save every living creature.
   + MORALITY OF MEDICAL PRACTICE
4. Express yourself clearly and maintain a dignified appearance.
5. Do not be too talkative, and do not engage in provocative speech.
6. Do not draw attention and luck only to yourself; sympathize and help wholeheartedly.
7. Examine, diagnose, and prescribe treatments effectively.
   +ATTITUDE TOWARD PATIENTS
8. Treat everyone on an equal footing, rich and poor.
9. Do not reject or despise a patient suffering from repugnant diseases such as ulcers and diarrhea—be compassionate and understanding.
10. Don't brag about yourself in a sick patient's home.
    + ATTITUDE TOWARD OTHER DOCTORS
11. Do not belittle another doctor in order to exalt your own virtues.
12. Do not criticize the work of others and do not decide whether they are right or wrong.

After Sun Simiao

Chinese doctrines reached Europe in the eighteenth and nineteenth centuries: in 1700s and 1800s Commandments for the Chinese doctor:

1. Physicians must always be ready to answer all calls from patients, rich or poor. They should treat them equally and not worry about financial compensation.

   Thus their profession will naturally prosper day after day and their conscience will remain intact.
2. Doctors may visit a lady, widow or nun only with an accompanying person, never alone. Intimate diseases of female patients must be examined with the appropriate attitude and must not be disclosed to anyone, not even the doctor's wife.
3. Doctors should not ask patients to send them pearls, amber or other precious substances as payment for the preparation of medications. If necessary, patients

should be instructed on how to mix the prescriptions themselves in order to avoid errors. It is not appropriate to express admiration for the patient's possessions.
4. Doctors should not leave their office. Patients should be examined personally, at the prescribed times. To avoid disputes, prescriptions must be made according to the medical formula.
5. Prostitutes should be treated as if they were patients from a good family and free services should not be provided as if they were poor. Refrain from ironic comments toward the sick. After a home visit, the doctor must leave the house without delay. As the disease improves, medications may be sent, but doctors should not make additional visits for further fees.

4. **Chang Kao (XII Sec.)**

An important work on Medical Ethics was written by Chang Kao in 1189. In a chapter (Precautionary tales against professional errors in his text, "The Medical Colloquies"[18]), he collected 12 stories on incorrect remuneration received and/or request, with the express purpose of urging doctors to provide free services. Lust, getting rich at the expense of women and excessive wealth were considered immoral.[19]

Medical Ethics

The induction of artificial abortion was severely denounced; great emphasis was placed on the virtue of chastity. Most Chinese believed that sickness and suffering were in themselves the punishments to be "paid" for sins committed, while health and happiness were due rewards for the virtues encountered.

This is probably due to the Buddhist influence in China. The practice of medicine was considered as a non-profit act of benevolence and respect for professional ethics would only be rewarded by a rich harvest of blessings. For this reason, ancient Chinese doctors dared not do anything that was unethical or professionally immoral.

In the history of Chinese medicine, almost all practicing doctors were retired government officials or scholars who failed the "imperial" exam. The practice of medicine was to be understood as a philanthropic enterprise, a benevolent act to be practiced and passed on to all doctors, to serve the entire community and relieve it of suffering, without worrying about any financial return.

5. **Kung Hsin (Sixteenth century)**

Kung Hsin urges the physician to educate himself and specialize in the correct treatments to alleviate the sufferings of the patient (1556). His informative and

[18] Kao (1989) and Lee (1943).

[19] Bird (1989), pp. 39–41.

concise maxim has been used since 1939 as the motto for the baccalaureate of Peking Union Medical College. It is read:

> The good Doctor of today guards kindness and justice.
>
> - He must research and specialize in the arts of his profession.
> - He must use adequate treatment methods according to the different conditions of the patient.
> - He must not boast of the art he has lent, but be intent on alleviating the suffering of the sick regardless of their class.
> - He must assist the seriously ill and adopt every expedient to keep them alive: his goodness is equal to that of Providence.
>
> The doctor who works according to these principles will be remembered by future generations.

His son, **Kung Ting Hsien**,(1605) prepared the requirements for doctors in 1558, with content very similar to the above maxim. He wrote The Five Commandments and Ten requirements for Doctors.

6. **Chen Shih-Kung and Chang-Lu (1627–1707)**

Chen Shih-kung and Chang Lu wrote "General Medicine" in 1627. This last text also described the ten things from which a doctor must refrain in order to be ethically correct:

1. acquiring bad habits
2. excessive self-confidence
3. strong prejudices
4. imitating or showing little initiative
5. making a diagnosis carelessly
6. practicing 'magic' healing
7. treating nobility and common people alike
8. neglecting poor patients
9. extorting high compensation for critical cases
10. criticizing or defaming other doctors

The latter constitute the most comprehensive statement on Medical Ethics in China and also deal with professional secrecy, responsibilities, behaviors, and related remuneration. The importance of the advancement of medical knowledge is also recalled, as well as the rules for social coexistence (see Footnote 19).

It was believed that nobles had a delicate constitution, while the common people were hardier. Therefore they had to be treated differently.

10 Requirements of Chen Shih-Kung

1. A physician or surgeon must know the basic principles. He must study with deep dedication all the available texts, ancient and otherwise, and understand them properly so as not to make mistakes in the clinic.
2. Medicines must be carefully selected and prepared according to pharmaceutical formulas, but can be modified according to the patient's condition. The powders can be freely prepared. Pills and distilled medicines must be prepared well in advance. Gypsum can also be used. The effectiveness of tampons depends on posture. Do not discard valuable drugs, they can be used again.
3. A Doctor must not be presumptuous, nor criticize others operating in the area. He must be modest toward all other colleagues; he must respect the elderly, help the younger ones, learn from his superiors and not fight the arrogant; all this to ensure that hatred and slander do not have the upper hand.
4. Treating a disease is just like caring for the careful management of a family. If a man's body is not cared for properly, he will be prey to diseases; these will further weaken him, to the point of causing death in the most serious cases. If the family is in financial difficulty their reserves will gradually diminish until they suffer poverty.
5. Man receives his destiny from Heaven. He must not be ungrateful to the divine decree. Professional gains must be approved by conscience and must be in accordance with His will. Otherwise, the descendants will be condemned.
6. Gifts must be simple, except for weddings, funerals and to comfort the sick. One fish and one vegetable dish will be enough to donate a meal. A man's virtue lies not so much in giving exaggeratedly, as in prudent economy.
7. Medicines must be distributed free to the poor. Additional financial aid should be extended to indigent patients, if possible. Without food, medication alone cannot relieve the patient's discomfort.
8. Savings must be invested in real estate and not in superfluous, useless luxuries. Furthermore, the doctor must not go to taverns and gambling houses that could distract him from his practice. Hate and slander must be avoided.
9. The medical office and dispensary must be equipped with all necessary equipment. The physician should improve his knowledge by studying medical texts, old and new, and update himself with the most recent publications. This is a fundamental duty.
10. A physician must be ready to answer a call from government officials with respect and sincerity. He must tell them the cause of the illness and the required prescriptions. After healing, no further medicinal remedies of other origin should be sought. A law-abiding person must not antagonize officials.

Literature on the ethics of medical practice and the moral character of doctors appeared sporadically. Other most important works and main doctors were:

Chu Hui-ming (1590); **Tou Chuan Chen Xin Lu**: Medical treatments learned by heart; **Ming I Jen**: Exhortation for distant doctors; **Wan-hui ping-chun**: Coming back to life from a myriad of diseases; **Wai-Ko Cheng-Tsung**: Orthodox Manual of Surgery.

7. More Recent Data[20]

Medical ethics is currently taught in China as a compulsory course, to emphasize correct ideological thinking and educate doctors to be moral models of human behavior and to avoid conflict.

In August 2002 only about 19% of the students were interested in helping people and then it was believed that by overcoming the institutional and cultural issues in the different districts in China, difficulties could be reduced and Chinese teachers in Medical Ethics they could spur a better future together with the support and encouragement of the international community.

China has made substantial progress in medical research and patient care in recent decades, but its economic expansion, lifestyle changes and rapidly aging population have led to an increasing burden of chronic diseases, including cardiovascular disease and stroke, diabetes, and cancer.

Japan

The Seventeen Rules of Enjuin (Twenty-Fifth Century A.D.) and Notes of Medical Ethics

The Seventeen Rules of Enjuin[21] are a code of conduct developed for students of the Japanese school of medicine "Ri-shu," in the sixteenth century. They recall the same number of norms as in the "Prince Shotoku" constitution.[22] These norms require you to actively collaborate with other colleagues as in a brotherhood and not to practice euthanasia and abortion. The text reflects the priestly role of the doctor and underlines the belief, also found in the Hippocratic oath, that medical knowledge should not be disclosed outside the school.

The rules are similar to the Vejjavatapada, the Buddhist medical doctor's oath, the Oath of Asaph, and the Hippocratic Oath, in that they stress the rights of the

[20] Xiao et al. (2016).

[21] Reich (1995).

[22] Umayado, Crown Prince of Japan, also known as Shōtoku Taishi, Prince Toyotomimi and Prince Kamitsumiy (574–621–622) was one of the legendary sages of Japan and promoted reforms between the ancient and classical eras. He spread Buddhism; sent a delegation to China and adopted Chinese characters for writing; he was inspired by Confucianism, he supported meritocracy and not family lineages. In 604 he drafted the constitution of 17 articles, establishing codes of conduct for rulers and subjects, within a Buddhist society.

physicians' teachers, require the physician to respect the patient's privacy rights, and prohibit both euthanasia and abortion. They also emphasize that physicians should love their patients and that they should work together as a brotherhood.

Seventeen Rules of Enjuin

1. *Each person should follow the path designated by Heaven (Buddha, the Gods).*
2. *You should always be kind to people. You should always be devoted to loving people.*
3. *The teaching of Medicine should be restricted to selected persons.*
4. *You should not tell others what you are taught, regarding treatments without permission.*
5. *You should not establish association with doctors who do not belong to this school.*
6. *All the successors and descendants of the disciples of this school shall follow the teachers' ways.*
7. *If any disciples cease the practice of Medicine, or, if successors are not found at the death of the disciple, all the medical books of this school should be returned to the School of Enjuin.*
8. *You should not kill living creatures, nor should you admire hunting or fishing.*
9. *In our school, teaching about poisons is prohibited, nor should you receive instructions about poisons from other physicians. Moreover, you should not give abortives to the people.*
10. *You should rescue even such patients as you dislike or hate. You should do virtuous acts, but in such a way that they do not become known to people. To do good deeds secretly is a mark of virtue.*
11. *You should not exhibit avarice and you must not strain to become famous. You should not rebuke or reprove a patient, even if he does not present you with money or goods in gratitude.*
12. *You should be delighted if, after treating a patient without success, the patient receives medicine from another physician, and is cured.*
13. *You should not speak ill of other physicians.*
14. *You should not tell what you have learned from the time you enter a woman's room, and, moreover, you should not have obscene or immoral feelings when examining a woman.*
15. *Proper or not, you should not tell others what you have learned in lectures, or what you have learned about prescribing medicine.*
16. *You should not like undue extravagance. If you like such living, your avarice will increase, and you will lose the ability to be kind to others.*
17. *If you do not keep the rules and regulations of this school, then you will be cancelled as a disciple. In more severe cases, the punishment will be greater.*

The rules stress the rights of doctors' teachers, require the doctor to respect the patient's right to privacy, and prohibit euthanasia and abortion. They also stress that doctors should love their patients and that they should work together as a fraternity.

The Lord said, Health is the greatest gift. He also said, He who cares for me should care for the sick. I also think that health is the greatest gift and I would like to be managed according to the Buddha. Therefore:

(a) I will use my ability to restore the health of all beings with compassion and reflection.
(b) I will be able to prepare the drugs well.
(c) I know what a medicine is suitable for and what it is not for. I do not want to provide what is unsuitable, only what is appropriate.
(d) I care for the sick with love, not out of desire for gain.
(e) I remain indifferent when dealing with feces, urine, vomit or saliva.
(f) From time to time I will be able to instruct, inspire, excite, and delight the sick with the Teaching.
(g) Even if I cannot heal a patient with the correct diet and the proper medicine, I will still ensure compassionate care.

Ethics

Ethics in the medical field has no direct correspondence in Japan.[23] In fact, due to the tradition of Confucianism, medical paternalism has never been questioned.

The whole practice has been regarded for millennia as "Jin's art" (Confucian love and benevolence), so it reflected the benevolent action of the physician on whom the patient completely depended. No attention is paid to ethical programs in medicine and treatment. Doctors did not discuss their problems outside their offices.

Medical Ethics itself, as we know it in Europe, does not exist in Japan. The word "bioethics," which has recently become popular, is used extensively to describe the relationships between different forms of life. Now that humans possess the ability to manipulate life, it is believed that new social and medical (called ethical) conventions are possible. Almost no attention is given to the ethical question at the beginning of medical treatment. Philosophers, scientists, politicians, and anthropologists refer to the problem expressed by the traditional academy: doctors simply do not argue and few lawyers are interested in medical care. Although there are some indications that an interest in Medical Ethics is emerging, the number of people involved is still too small. The failure to provide medical information by Japanese doctors is the most widely discussed topic regarding Japanese Medical Ethics, with more than 3000 articles recently published on this topic.

Until the 1980s, the undisputed practice of Japanese doctors was in fact to withhold a wide range of patient information, particularly, but not limited to, regarding cancer and poor prognosis.

Japanese Medical Ethics is a mixture of Buddhist and Confucian influences in combination with Shinto influence and, more recently, with Hippocratic and

[23] Reich (2004), Feldman (1985) and Underwood and Rhodes (2016).

Christian teachings. From the fifth to sixth century, the medical profession was reserved for the privileged classes.

With the centralization of the government in the seventh and eighth centuries. an office of medicine was established, with its penal and civil codes, and an official medical class was created.

After the "Heian" period (800–1200), the government sponsored health service was replaced by medical professionals. In the sixteenth century, a code of conduct very similar to the Hippocratic code was elaborated, corresponding to the aforementioned "The Seventeen Rules of Enjuin," outlining an almost priestly role for doctors. The code also has the directive to keep the art secret and to worry about the presence of charlatans, as was the case in Hippocratic ethics.

Abortive drugs are not allowed and neither are poisons. Some virtuous rules are included, including: "You hould also save patients who do not like or hate you" and "You should be happy if, after unsuccessful treatment of a patient, the patient himself receives medicine from another doctor, and is benefited by it."

The Influence of Japanese Culture

Japanese habits in relation to controversial medical cases are strongly influenced by two cultural aspects.

1. The role of harmony and consent. The Japanese make every effort to maintain a peaceful balance of compatibility in interpersonal relationships, professional earnings, and government operations. All this based on true agreement or conformity.
2. Japanese doctors have considerable power, much more than in Western countries. They are highly respected by anyone and are not afraid to take on the role of shaman or technician.

References

Bellah RN. What is axial about the axial age? Eur J Sociol. 2005;46(1):69–89.
Bird LP. Medical ethics. In: Bird LP, Barlow J, editors. Oaths & prayers, an anthology. Richardson, TX: Christian Medical & Dental Society; 1989. p. 1–15.
Chai W, Yang X. Traditional Confucianism in modern China: Ma Yifu's ethical thought. Front Philos China. 2006;1(3):366–81.
Chen KJ. The principle and practice of integrative Chinese and Western medicine. Chin J Integr Tradit West Med. 2002;8(2):82–4.
Chen KJ. Study of Chinese medicine: which is after all the right way? Chin J Integr Tradit West Med. 2005;11(4):241–2.
Dharmananda S. Ethics in modern practice of traditional Chinese Medicine (TCM). 2010. www.itmonline.org/articles/ethics/ethics.htm.
Doering O. Teaching medical ethics in China. Cultural, social and ethical issues. In: Asian bioethics in the 21st century. Baltimore: EuBios Ethics Institute; 2002.
Feldman E. Medical ethics the Japanese way. Hastings Cent Rep. 1985;15(5):21–4.

Guo Z. Chinese Confucian culture and the medical ethical tradition. J Med Ethics. 1995;21(4):239–46.

Hyton N. Sun Simiao's ancient Chinese code of medical ethics. Ezine articles, Submitted July 12, 2010. http://EzineArticles.com/expert/Nancy_Hyton/701709.

Jaspers K. The origin and goal of history. New Haven: Yale University Press; 1949. p. 1–77.

Jingfeng C. A historical overview of traditional Chinese medicine and ancient Chinese medical ethics. Ethik in der Medizin. 1998;10(1):84–91.

Jonsen AR. Medical history in India and China (Chap. 3). In: A short history of medical ethics. Oxford: Oxford University Press; 2000. p. 27–41.

Kao C. Medical ethics in Imperial China. Berkeley: University of Californian Press; 1979.

Kao C. Medical Talks. 1989;10:31–9.

Ki Che Leung A. La medicina nella società Ming. (IT. Medicine in the Ming society) Enciclopedia Treccani, Storia della Scienza; 2001.

Layne K, Ferro A. Traditional Chinese medicines in the management of cardiovascular diseases: a comprehensive systematic review. BJCP. 2017;83(1):20–32.

Lee T. Medical ethics in ancient China. Bull Hist Med. 1943;13:268–77.

Li M, Liang Y. Sun Simiao, super physician of the Tang Dynasty. J Tradit Chin Med Sci. 2016;XX:1–2.

Ming X, Douglas D, Gurzawska A, Brey P. Satori, Ethics assessment in different countries, China. Enschede: University of Twente; 2015.

Nappi C, Shizhen L. Brief life of a pioneering naturalist: 1518-1593. Harvard Magazine, 2010.

Nie J-B. Medical ethics in China: a transcultural interpretation. London: Routledge; 2011.

Oakes W, Zhongjing Z. The traditional Chinese medicine sage. Vision Times, May 1, 2017.

Pugliarello R, Biolchi P, Cardini F. In: Bellavite P, et al., editors. Medicina Tradizionale Cinese in: Le Medicine Complementari. (IT. Traditional Chinese medicine in: complementary medicines). Milano: O.M.C.Verona © Utet Periodici; 2000.

Qiu R-Z. Medicine, the art of humaneness: on ethics of traditional Chinese medicine. J Med Philos. 1988;13(3):277–99.

Raphals L. Chinese philosophy and Chinese medicine. In: Zalta N, editor. The Stanford encyclopedia of philosophy; 2017.

Reich WT. The 17 rules of Enjuin. Encyclopedia of bioethics, vol. 5. New York: Simon & Schuster; 1995.

Reich WT. Japan through the nineteenth century. Encyclopedia of bioethics. Farmington Hills: The Gale Group Inc.; 2004.

Tsai DF. Ancient Chinese medical ethics and the four principles of biomedical ethics. J Med Ethics. 1999;25:315–21.

Tsuei W, editor. Roots of Chinese culture and medicine. Oakland, CA: Chinese Culture Books Co.; 1989.

Underwood EA, Rhodes P. Japan, Encyclopaedia Britannica; 2016.

Unschuld PU. Medical ethics in Imperial China: a study in historical anthropology. Berkeley, CA: University of California Press; 1979.

Unschuld PU. Forgotten traditions of ancient Chinese medicine. Brooklin, MA: Paradigm Publications; 1990.

Veatch RM, editor. Cross cultural perspectives in medical ethics. 2nd ed. Boston: Jones and Bartlett Publishers; 2000.

Wikipedia. Medicina tradizionale cinese, Appunti di storia della medicina cinese. (IT. Traditional Chinese Medicine, notes on the history of Chinese medicine).

Will P-É. Science in China: the Ming. The Ming dynasty: general features, Treccani, history of science; 2001.

Wilms S. Nurturing life in classical Chinese medicine: Sun Simiao on healing without drugs, transforming bodies and cultivating life. J Chin Med. 2010;93:5–13.

Wu D, Zhongjing Z. The traditional Chinese medicine sage. Epoch Times, Clearharmony, 2012.

Xiao R-P, Wong GWK, Prince JM, Gartside M, et al. An impact on clinical practice and research in China. N Engl J Med. 2016;375:2391–2.

Near and Middle East 6

This chapter deals with the emergence and acquisition of a moral mentality and therefore of medical ethics in the two main civilizations of the Near and Middle East: Jewish (1) and Islamic (2). Generally speaking, the term "Near and Middle East" encompasses a wide range of cultures—not only Sumerian-Mesopotamian, through the Babylonian period, but also those of Egypt and Israel. Israel had its own distinctive medical profession that developed later, in the second century B.C. In a later period Arab culture gave rise to a new medical literature.

No writer at that time and in that area seems to have addressed what we today call Medical Ethics as a specific area of discussion. Nobody seems to have even written about its precursor, referred to as "medical etiquette." However, medical ethics existed as much as in any other culture, in line with the moral perceptions of those societies. Medical ethics could seem simple or complex, like in any monolithic or pluralist culture. There was an ethical framework for the practice of medicine, wherever people treated diseases, even on a magical-religious basis. From the medical point of view, as in other respects, Egypt, Mesopotamia, and Israel were three completely different worlds. Although they had common origins, each developed independently. Mesopotamia and Egypt are sufficiently similar, while Israel took a different route, dictated by its unique religious and moral vision.

Israel

Jewish Medicine and Ethics

From the very beginning of Israel's history, ethics and medicine have been closely linked. Religion and ethics were inseparable: Yahweh laid the ethical basis for the laws of Israel. Medicine in the Jewish world was born and developed in close connection with the covenant entered by God with his people. The Israelites knew about

R. G. Russo, *Medical Ethics*, https://doi.org/10.1007/978-3-031-42444-1_6

the rudimentary treatment of wounds, and herbs that could be used to treat various ailments due to natural causes.

The first mention of a Jewish medical profession is in the Wisdom of Jesus Ben Sira (also known for having composed Ecclesiastes in the Bible, in Israel at the beginning of the second century B.C.). Ben Sira urges his readers to honor "the doctor" as a servant of God who has received His skill. Dependence on God is essential for the patient, because it is God who heals: only God can dispense joy and suffering. Disease therefore takes on a symbolic meaning in a person's relationship with God.[1]

The fundamental difference between the worldview of the Jews (circa 1300 to 70 B.C.) and that of the other peoples of the Near and Middle East reflected their religious perspective. Israel's religion was monotheistic, while that of its neighbors was polytheistic, focused on the worship of natural forces, particularly those relating to fertility. In the Hebrew Scriptures, the cosmos is perceived as being under the direction of Yahweh. Although there is a personal force of evil (Satan), it is subordinate to Yahweh and poses no significant challenge to His authority. While polytheism did not impose absolute moral standards, Israel's ethical beliefs were founded on Yahweh, the world's transcendent creator and sustainer. The Bible[2] includes among its religious obligations some revolutionary concepts of preventive medicine and public health.

It has been estimated that more than half of the best-known rabbinic scholars and authors, philosophers, poets, and exegetes were physicians in medieval times: Maimonides, Nachmanides, Ibn Ezras and Ibn Tibbons, to name just a few.

The Jewish Vision in Case of Illness

- The doctor's obligation to cure the sick
- The patient's obligation to seek treatment and follow medical advice
- Holiness of life is of absolute value
- Duty to relieve pain
- Do not hasten death (even if imminent and irreversible)
- Remove whatever prolongs suffering
- Doctor-patient relationship (and mutual trust) must be preserved
- Abuse or coercion must always be avoided

[1] Jews often say Ha Kadosh, Baruch Hu, meaning "the Holy One, blessed be He," in reference to God.

Bird (1989), p. 22 and Cosmacini (2001).

[2] Jewish ethics developed from the Hebrew Bible, rabbinic literature, and subsequent literature.

Holy Bible: Genesis 6: 1–4; Genesis 37: 1; 28; Deuteronomy 28: 22,27, 35; Leviticus 26:16; Numbers 12: 10–11.

- Errors or medical negligence must be limited
- Follow a detailed, conscious decision-making process
- Medical knowledge and experience must be integrated with the patient's psycho-social features
- The patient's autonomy must be respected (in any case the patient must be informed)
- Always tell the patient the truth

The Bible laid the foundation and upholds it: the sanctity and dignity of human life, the obligation to safeguard health and life itself, with no compromises to superstition or irrational care, maintenance of the faith, a strict code of sexual morality, and many basic definitions of moral imperatives in medical practice, including the rights of the dead. Fairness and justice must be upheld: the first involves the recognition of six fundamental rights: the right to live, to own, to work, to dress, to asylum, and finally the rights of the individual (to rest and be free, prohibition of hatred, revenge, and holding grudges). The second concerns the acceptance of duties, specially toward the poor, the weak, friends, or enemies. Justice must be established by scientific means and the process is slow and hard. On some topics, rigid monotheism was in force: for example, only God could be the source of medical insight—including ethics.[3]

In terms of ethics, Judaism was the first religion to insist on the dignity of the person and the sacredness of human life. Murder was considered not only a crime against man, but a sin against God. The Talmud teaches that the Almighty created humanity and taught us that whoever saves one life saves a world and he who destroys a single life destroys an entire world.[4]

Common to all humanity is the obligation to observe the "Seven precepts of the sons of Noah": abstention from (1) idolatry, (2) blasphemy, (3) incest, (4) murder, (5) theft, (6) eating a limb torn from a living creature, and (7) the commandment to practice justice. But for the sons of Israel the contribution must be broader and

[3] Super (1914).

[4] Sanhedrin 4:5 (Sinedrio). It is one of the ten treaties of the Order of Damages, a section of the Mishnah and the Talmud that deals with civil and criminal damages in judicial procedures.
Eisenberg (2017).

higher in character. Hence the respect for the 613 precepts of obedience set down in the Torah.[5]

Specific concern for the sick in the Israeli community was extended and developed in the Talmud (see Footnote 5).

Possession of material goods had to be considered a debt to God; bosses were forbidden to exploit workers (Leviticus: 19:13); creditors were forbidden to offend the debtor's dignity (Deuteronomy: 24.10–11); even the slave retained his rights as a person (Exodus: 21, 26–27). In the Hebrew scriptures disease was seen in its moral and spiritual dimensions rather than as a purely physical phenomenon. A close relationship between sin and sickness was believed to exist, on two levels: (1) physical evil, including sickness, entered the world as a result of sin and (2) sickness was sometimes visited on individuals and nations because of their sins. So sickness and wounds were a consequence of sin, but they were also under God's control. The Hebrew word for healer or doctor is part of the verb "rapha," whose original meaning seems to be "he who sews together" or "he who repairs."

Apart from the medical resources, which were limited, healing could only take place thanks to Yahweh, through confession of sin, supplication, and prayer (Job: 33, 19–30). The Torah rejects any distinction between king and noble, citizen and slave, native, or foreigner ("Love the stranger as yourself": Leviticus: 19:34), all being equal before the law of God! In Judaism the distinctions between Jews and non-Jews are only of a religious order, and there are no social or political distinctions. Although the Hebrew scriptures depict Yahweh as the sole healer (Exodus: 15:26) and command the Israelites to refrain from resorting to magical or pagan healing practices (Ezekiel: 13,17–23), the use of natural or medicinal means was not discouraged, and apparently miraculous healings were also acceptable (2 Kings: 20, 7).

Until the second century B.C. there is no evidence of a Jewish medical profession. However, the general approach was that: (1) Good ethics starts with good facts. (2) There is no distinction between Jewish law and ethics. It is not always

---

[5] **Haggadah** is a compendium of rabbinic homilies incorporating folklore, historical anecdotes, moral exhortations, and practical advice from business to medicine.

Halachah, a tradition of rabbinic religious law, examines numerous problems often associated with ethics, contemplates the practical application of the 613 mitzvòt ("commandments") set out in the Torah.

Musar comes from the Book of Proverbs (1: 2) and means "moral conduct," "education," or "discipline." The word is used to refer to the observance and development of ethical and moral discipline.

Pentateuch: first five books of the Bible (Genesis, Exodus, Leviticus, Numbers, Deuteronomy) revealed by God to Moses and the Jewish people on Mount Sinai.

Talmud = in Hebrew it means teaching, study, discussion from the Hebrew root. Sacred text of Judaism.

Muntner (1995).

Torah (or Torah) is translated "instruction," "teaching," or "law" Proverbs 1: 8, 3: 1, 28: 4). Often it indicates the biblical Pentateuch (Genesis, Exodus, Leviticus, Numbers, and Deuteronomy).

obvious what is ethical. From a traditional Jewish approach, Jewish law, Halakhah, defines ethics and code of conduct.

Jewish Medical Ethics

The central concept for understanding Jewish medical ethics is the image of God (imago Dei).[6] "Two of the most notable contributions of the Jewish people to the progress of humanity converge: medicine and ethics."[7]

Basic Principles

Jewish Medical Ethics began primarily as "applied ethics" based on Halakhah, then intertwined with biology, science, medicine, philosophy, and theology.[8]

Its fundamental principles are:

- Jewish ethics, from which medical ethics comes, are based upon duties, obligations, commandments and reciprocal responsibility, on the other hand, is based on rights and autonomy; human decisions are justified and cannot be criticized, as long as they do not harm others.
- The doctor–patient relationship in Judaism is an agreement supported by a divine commandment, therefore an obligation.
- The doctor is obliged to treat and heal patients. It is prohibited to rely on miracles, and he must do whatever is necessary to heal according to standard medical practice.
- The patient is instructed to seek healing by the physician and to prevent disease if possible. The patient is not free to refuse treatment that could be beneficial or save his life. The principles of charity and non-maleficence forbid intentionally harming another person, physically, emotionally, or financially, or even by defamation or attacking the property of others. Jewish law clearly requires not only avoiding harm to others, but actively doing good (see Footnote 8).

Sources of Medical Ethics[9]

Jewish medical ethics comes from two basic sources. The first is the Torah (see Footnote 5) which is the central text of Judaism and is known as the Written Law. It

---

[6] Amundsen and Ferngren (1982), Ferngren (1987), McMillan et al. (1987), and Filippi (1987).

[7] Jakobovitz (1983).

[8] Amundsen (1996), Kinzbrunner (2004), and Lavine (2016).

[9] Eiseneberg (2017).

[10] Steinberg (1998, 2003) and Veatch (2000), pp. 62–77.

lists 613 precepts that observant Jews believe to be absolutely binding, and states: "I am the Lord who heals you!" (Exodus: 15:26). The duty to save a man is well founded in the Pentateuch (see Footnote 5) and restrictions are discussed at length and applied on the basis of standard texts of Jewish law. The second source is the Talmud (see Footnote 5) also known as the Oral Law: it recalls the obligation to save a man in danger, including the prevention of accidents or injuries. Permission to heal is granted to a physician only when he can offer the patient a treatment (even an experimental one) that can reasonably be expected to be effective.

The Jewish view of medicine is perhaps best expressed by the Shulchan Aruch (code of Jewish law) when it explains the opportunities that are accorded to doctors, and their responsibilities. Jewish medical ethics is the application of Jewish law to medicine.

Distinctive Criteria

Judaism emphasizes individual obligations and responsibilities: it considers the value of life to be of fundamental importance, coming before almost all other values. In secular medical ethics doctors are obliged to treat the sick. Perhaps one could argue that some diseases are ordained by God and should not be interfered with. However, in Jewish medical ethics, there is no contradiction between providing medical care and God's plans.

Since Jewish ethics allows a doctor to treat a patient, the next step is to clarify whether there is an obligation to do so. Deuteronomy (22.1–3) states that "if anyone finds a lost object, he is obliged to return it to its original owner." Surely doctors therefore have an obligation to restore someone's health. This is not simply limited to saving lives, but also includes—when possible—the broader goal of restoring health. Secular medical ethics is based on four well-known main concepts: autonomy, beneficence, non-maleficence, and justice. In theory, none of these necessarily has priority over the others, but in practice autonomy has tended to dominate. Judaism is about commitments, obligations, duties, and commandments, rather than rights, hedonism, and selfishness.[10]

Halakhah

Modern Jewish medical ethics developed during the second half of the twentieth century, when the Western world had to face the horrors of the Second World War.

The term "Jewish medical ethics" was coined by Rabbi Lord Jakobovits, in England, around 1950, based on the application of traditional rabbinic law; this has expanded with bioethics and has also dealt with biology, science, philosophy, and theology. Halakhah therefore not only deals with religious practices and beliefs, but

[11] Halperin (2004).

with numerous aspects of daily life as well. Its most literal translation is "the way, the way to behave."

The goals of Jewish morality are set out in the 613 commandments in the Torah and some can be defined as moral or ethical commandments. These include acts of kindness and a correct and respectful attitude toward others, avoiding harming others through action, word, or thought. The Jewish approach to any ethical question is based on two fundamental concepts: good ethics stands out thanks to its good elements and there is no distinction between Jewish law and ethics.[11]

The "Principles of Jewish Medical Ethics" are proposed below:

"Love your neighbor as yourself"
"Do not do to others what you would not do to yourself"
"Do what is right and true in God's eyes"
"Keep the law and be charitable"
"Be just, good and humble in the sight of your God".

They can be compared with Maimonides' 13 Articles of Faith.[12]

1. Do everything possible for every patient, to preserve life, cure disease and alleviate suffering.
2. Prevention is the highest form of healing.
3. Nutrition is the primary determinant of health and the backbone of preventive medicine.
4. Jewish prayer must be recognized as the most important and most powerful healing tool.
5. The atmosphere in the doctor's office must stimulate health.
6. The physician must be regarded as the highest authority in all medical matters and must be primarily responsible for the care of each patient.
7. Medical quackery, or what is commonly called alternative medicine, which some, though not all, use, must not be integrated into scientific medical practice, in accordance with the Jewish tradition of respect for the opinion of educated people and legitimate authority.
8. "Managed care", as sometimes exercised, must be abolished if it works against the patient's primary interests.

[12] Halevi and Lavine (2008).

[13] Halevi and Lavine (2008).

9. The Tort reform[13] (or similar) is essential if doctors exercise their profession in the best possible way, treating each patient according to his specific needs, with no fear of legal action.
10. A doctor cannot become rich as a result of medical practice, but he has the right to earn a good living.
11. An ethical physician makes money by providing services, not by selling medical products.
12. A physician and his employees may not accept gifts or presents of any kind, including useful items that bear product or company names; free dinners and free services, from any individual, pharmaceutical company, optician, medical provider or other services that patients are referred to or whose products are used in patient care.
13. It is unethical for a doctor to advertise his services.

Judaism was the first religion to insist on the dignity of the person and the sacredness of human life.

Jewish medical ethics is applicable to current bioethical dilemmas in all fields of medicine. It obliges patients to seek medical care and physicians to provide it. It is argued that life is a divine gift of supreme importance. While the prolongation of life is therefore a central principle of Jewish bioethics, this principle can be balanced against the patient's suffering. The Holy Bible includes all the teachings and precepts recognized by the Jews as revealed by God through Moses. "You don't have to complete the task, but you aren't free to stop doing it" [Pirkei Avot (Chapters of the Fathers) II:16].

As a result of the Jewish view of mankind, the Torah shows greater humanity than other codes of the ancient Middle East (for example, the Code of Hammurabi). There are, for example, provisions that protect the rights of the blind and deaf (Leviticus:19, 14); the fetus was considered created by Yahweh (Psalms: 139, 13–16; Jeremiah: 1, 5; Isaiah: 49, 1); abortion was not explicitly forbidden either by the Torah or by rabbinic Judaism and was allowed in some circumstances. The infant deserved the same protection as an adult; infanticide, a common practice in the surrounding Canaanite culture, was expressly prohibited (Leviticus: 18, 21; 20.2). Castration was also prohibited and eunuchs were excluded from Jewish religious life (Deuteronomy: 23, 1). The Hebrew scriptures do not provide information on the correct behavior of Jewish doctors: together with their patients, they were dependent on the Creator, from whom all true and lawful healing came (Deuteronomy; 32, 39). Jewish medicine is based on an infinite respect for the sacredness of life. Jewish medical ethics implies the obligation to safeguard health, opposing irrational treatment, with strict dietary and sexual restrictions, and many fundamental

[14] Proposta operata dal Senatore USA Tort, per modificare la giustizia civile vs. gli illeciti sanitari.

statements of moral imperatives in medical practice. Neglecting the body and physical needs was to offend God.

Among the "good deeds" on which the Talmud lays particular importance are: (1) visiting the sick, (2) paying extreme honors to the dead, (3) consoling the afflicted. Everything must be done in the best interest of the patient, and everyone must recognize their limitations: non-doctors will not deal with treatments or post-operative care and doctors must maintain their role and not think of acting as technicians. Illness is viewed as a sign of the breakdown of that direct and privileged alliance that puts man in close relations with God. It is precisely in the context of the covenant between God and the children of Israel, granted through Moses, that a specific relationship of cause-effect is identified, where prosperity, wealth, and happiness will follow obedience and fidelity; war, hunger, and pestilence will be inflicted [on you] for disobedience to the four cardinal values (autonomy, charity, non-maleficence, and justice). Call on the assistance and advice of the rabbis to follow the law of God, as defined by the Bible (and post-biblical sources).

Law for Gentiles

Judaism has always maintained that non-Jewish people are only obliged to follow the Seven Laws of Noah, based on the covenant with God after the Flood. They concern the prohibitions of:

1. murder,
2. theft,
3. sexual immorality,
4. consuming meat cut from an animal that is still alive,
5. believing in and worshiping, or praying to, an idol,
6. blasphemy against God.
7. Moreover, society must establish a fair system of justice to administer the law honestly.

In Conclusion

Jewish medical ethics is one of the most important sectors of modern Jewish ethics. The goal is to adhere closely to the law. Jewish traditions and ethical thinking establish which medical therapies or technological innovations are moral, and when certain treatments may or may not be used.[14]

The Halachic construct to answer an ethical question involves patients and/or their family members, the doctor, and the rabbi. The patient is obliged to seek the

[15] Freedman (1999).

best possible medical care; he has the right to choose his doctor and his rabbi and the right to express his personal wishes. The doctor is obliged to treat the patient and must use the best diagnostic and therapeutic interventions based on his knowledge and judgment. All medical decisions must be properly evaluated and applied.

Oath of Asaph the Doctor and Yohanan Ben Zabda

It is assumed that Asaph Harofe[15] lived in Galilee and Syria in the sixth century. According to Jewish legend, he was one of the "Levites," prisoners in Assyria, and later Vizier of King Solomon.

Together with Yohanan Ben Zabda, perhaps from Jericho, he founded and ran a medical school. He wrote in Hebrew, Aramaic, Persian, Greek, and Latin. He is credited with a treatise on medicine, called "Sefer Refu'ot" (The Book of Medicines), also known as "The Book of Asaph" and considered the oldest of its kind in Hebrew. His manuscripts are kept in the libraries of Florence, Paris, Munich, Vienna, London, and Oxford. Several chapters are based on classical Hebrew texts written hundreds of years before his time.

The content deals with numerous fields: physiology, embryology, the four periods of human life, diseases of various organs, hygiene, medicinal plants, the medical calendar, the practice of medicine, urology, aphorisms, antidotes, and finally the Hippocratic Oath. Jewish doctors who prepared medicines in a professional and acceptable way to the Jewish community and Jewish wisdom are mentioned as well. The Book includes a doctor's oath that encompasses the substance of the Hippocratic Oath, where the doctor swears to serve patients and "prevent them from evil and injustice." According to Asaph, the doctor must not approach the patient with a haughty or vengeful attitude and must never harm him. Both oaths (Asaph and Hippocrates) restrict surgery and require respect for the patient's privacy, forbid "professional" sexual abuse, prohibit the use of deadly drugs, and limit abortion. Asaph, however, rewrites the Hippocratic Oath to create a suitable professional pact for Jewish doctors. The two oaths differ rigidly, not in actual professional practice but more in the structure of the ethical life.

The Book of Medicines divides humanity into distinct categories: the wicked and the just or the wise, in contrast with the foolish. A wise doctor knows the traditional science of diseases and pains and proposes a cure according to the medical ethics of the ancients and according to their scientific knowledge. The foolish doctor neglects medical ethics and causes more damage to the body than the disease itself. Wise doctors treat patients according to the four elements of the body (hot, cold, wet, and dry) and know the potency of roots and pharmaceutical compounds, mixing them together. Each organ is healed according to the power of the substances administered.

If a doctor did not follow the instructions in the book, he could cause damage or mutilation to the body or transform disease into other diseases. The patient's pains

[16] Galbi (2012), Muntner (1968), Rosner and Sussman (1965), and Pines (1975).

could be affected, to the point of death. Furthermore, a foolish doctor could torture a patient until he preferred to die rather than live with such a painful body. However, diseases were only cured with God's help. Many people died because they were "immoral beings": "God punishes with a disease those who do not follow His commandments."

> "The Lord will strike you with consumption, with fever, with inflammation, with burning heat, with drought, with sand and with mold ... The Lord will strike you with the ulcers of Egypt, with scurvy and itching, which you will not be able to heal. ... The Lord will hit you on the knees and legs with severe blisters from which you will not be able to recover, from the soles of the feet to the top of the head."

Asaph asserts, however, that disease is not only due to divine punishment: his preamble states that two causes of disease had already been found among Noah's children and grandchildren, after the Flood. The first cause is "the wickedness that the Flood has not been able to wash away." The second is "human transgression and sinful ways." God gave Noah the right knowledge for medical healing; Noah recorded the recommendations in a book where he listed drugs to be used. This was taken up by Asaph himself to widen medical knowledge. Asaph finally insisted that doctors could not cure all diseases, particularly those caused by immoral acts.

> "Despite our vast experience and extensive medical investigations, we know that doctors cannot cure all diseases; only a few patients will be cured. With the help of God all diseases can be cured. Many people die as immoral beings. They will live in sloth and weakness as they have not behaved according to religion, despite being healthy. Such behavior causes disease. When they fell ill, they did not consult wise doctors, as ordained by God. So they die in a state of immorality, while they proceeded blindly with bloodthirsty deeds, not resisting temptation."

The oath discusses diseases, their treatments and prevention. Some of the ideas are still valid today, such as exercise, eating healthy food and personal hygiene. Asaph's oath ends with an imperative to please God and be righteous: "Keep His orders and commandments and follow all His directions to please Him, be pure, true, righteous."

> "A wise doctor studies and understands the classical wisdom relating to diseases and treats them on the basis of ancient medical ethics and according to his own scientific knowledge.
> The foolish doctor who heals by neglecting medical ethic causes more damage to the body than the disease itself."

A Latin presentation of part of his work is found in a Paris manuscript, with the title "*Distinctio Mundi secundum Magistrum Asaph Hebraeum, Qualiter Terra Permanet Ordinata*" (The Distinction of the World According to the Hebrew Teacher Asaph, How the Earth Remains Ordained).

Asaph's Oath

This oath[16] was a code of conduct for young Jewish doctors upon graduation. It includes ethical standards regarding the sacredness of life (euthanasia and abortion), corruption, and doctor–patient confidentiality and is believed to have been passed down by doctors from generation to generation.

The text can be divided into three parts, made up of 58 articles. The first part (1–13) contains the Doctor's moral obligations toward the patient, paraphrasing Hippocrates. In the second (14–44) you are invited to trust in God and in his attributes as Creator and Healer, with quotes from the Pentateuch and the Psalms. The third part (45–58) lays emphasis on the rules of conduct between Doctor and Patient.[17]

First Part

1. This is the pact that Asaph ben Berakhyahu and Yohanan ben Zabda made with their pupils. It included the following recommendations: they had to swear the following:
2. Do not risk killing with a herbal potion
3. Do not make a pregnant prostitute take a drink in order to cause abortion
4. Do not desire the beauty of women in order to fornicate
5. Do not divulge the secret of a man who has trusted you
6. Do not take any reward offered in order to cause you to destroy and ruin
7. Do not be hard of heart towards the poor and needy
8. Do not say that what is good is bad, nor that what is bad is good
9. Do not adopt the behavior of sorcerers who resort (as really happens) to fascination, wishes and witchcraft to separate a man from his wife or a woman from the companion of her youth
10. Do not desire any wealth or reward offered to induce you to lust
11. Do not seek help in an idolatrous cult so as to heal by resorting to idols
12. Quite the contrary—you must detest, abhor and hate all those who indulge that cult or profess it
13. Idols are non-living, null, useless and demonic beings: they can never help those who are alive.

[17] Ben-Tov (2013), Bird (1989), pp. 25–27, and Veatch (2000), pp. 57–62.

Second Part

14. Place your trust in the Lord your God, who is a true God, a living God
15. For it is He who kills and brings to life, who hurts and heals
16. Who teaches people knowledge and how to make use of it
17. Who wounds with justice and righteousness, and heals with piety and compassion
18. There are no depictions of His acumen or His power
19. Nothing is hidden from His eyes
20. He makes healing plants grow
21. He makes doctors perspicacious so they can heal, through the abundance of His loving-kindness. Let every living thing know that he was created by Him and that there is no other Savior
22. Therefore those who trust in idolatry will never free themselves from distress and misfortune
23. Therefore their confidence and hope are dead
24. It is therefore best to keep away from them so as to be far from all the abominations of their idols
25. Keep close to the name of the Lord, God of the spirit of every human being
26. The soul of every living being is in His hand to kill or let live
27. And no one can free himself from His hand
28. Always remember Him and seek Him in truth, righteousness and justice in order to prosper in all your works
29. He will help you to prosper in what you do, so every man will consider himself happy
30. All will abandon their graven images and will want to worship God, as you do
31. Therefore they will know that their trust was in vain and their efforts useless
32. For they pray to a god who will do them no good and will not save them
33. As for you, be strong, do not let your hands be weak; you will be rewarded for your work
34. The Lord is with you while you are with him
35. To keep His covenant, follow His commandments and adhere to them
36. You will be rewarded like His saints. Every man will say:
37. Blessed are the people who enjoy such abundance, happy are the people whose God is the Lord.
38. His disciples answered:
39. We will do all that you have urged us and ordered us to do
40. Like the commandments of the Torah
41. And we must do it with all our heart, with all our soul and with all our strength
42. Do His will and obey
43. Do not deviate from the straight and narrow path
44. And they (Asaph and Yohanan) blessed them in the name of God Most High, creator of heaven and earth.

Third Part

45. And they kept repeating (the rules), saying:
46. The Lord God, His saints and His Torah bear witness; you must fear Him, you must not deviate from His commandments and you must loyally follow His laws
47. Do not accept money to help an unbeliever
48. Do not prepare a deadly drug, or give it to a man or woman who can use it to kill their companions
49. Do not speak of the herbs that compose it, nor give them to others
50. Do not talk about any matter related to this topic
51. Do not use blood in any medical practice
52. Do not cause discomfort by means of iron tools or by fire without having already done the necessary tests
53. Thus, having lifted your gaze and your heart, you will not be excluded from the benevolence of Heaven
54. Do not harbor hatred or desire revenge on a sick man
55. Do not have second thoughts
56. The Lord our God hates it when this is done
57. But abide by His orders and commandments; follow all His ways, to please Him and to be pure, true and upright
58. So Asaph and Yohanan exhorted and entreated their pupils

Abukrat (Hippocrates)'s Moral Precepts: Twelfth Century

This was a Hebrew adaptation of the Hippocratic oath (Abukrat is the name of Hippocrates in Hebrew).

It was found in a twelfth century manuscript under the title "Musar he-hasid Abukrat" and was transcribed by Dosa ben Joseph, in 1461 in Constantinople. The text reads:

The Moral Precepts Attributed to Hippocrates (Considered to Be the Right)

1. The Doctor is considered worthy to enter the science of medicine he who respects his teachers and praises his masters, as he does his parents. Parents must be respected because education starts with them. The teacher must be venerated to remove (from the student) the veil of worldliness and grant him the yoke (commitment) of reality; he must assess the choice of a pupil who is capable of these studies and virtuous in his behavior. He will firmly and resolutely reject anyone who is unsuited to this Science.

2. He will pass on his wisdom and knowledge. And he will promptly restore the sick person's health, without hoping for payment. He will refrain from pursuing further examinations in search of new symptoms that could justify the hope of a reward.
3. He will try not to give instructions for the preparation of potions that cause death or other injuries, nor must he be involved in procedures that weaken the patient, with or without his consent.
4. He must not be persuaded to cause a pregnant woman to abort.
5. When visiting a patient, the doctor should not look at his wife or daughter, or at the maid.
6. He will consider confidentiality among the best of his qualities, for fear of revealing a secret disease after it has been confided to him, because the patient often tells the doctor things he would be embarrassed to tell his parents or relatives.
7. He will surely know how to refrain from debauchery and the shame of drunkenness, because these create problems for the mind and lead the heart as tray.
8. Above all, he must keep continuously learning in order to help the body to health and must never be tired of referring to books.[18]

From this text one can deduce—among other things—that before teaching medicine, the Master wants his pupil to accept the absolute authority of the Almighty. The Teacher is invited to be prudent and not to accept a student who is not prepared to act according to the moral precepts. The main assumptions of the Hippocratic Oath are recalled and respected here: helping the sick, prohibiting poisoning, abortion and abuse of women, maintaining confidentiality. Other passages have been interpreted differently, added or omitted.

Comparison with the Original Hippocratic Text

Despite wanting only to be a Hebrew adaptation of the Hippocratic Oath, which was written about 1800 years earlier, the current text differs from it in many points. For example:

- The theological introduction of the Greek gods is not included here.
- Hippocrates recommends that a doctor should share his knowledge of the art with his children and his teachers' children; in this text instead the teacher chooses his own pupil and then instructs him.

- Hippocrates asks doctors to treat only the teacher's children for free; here this principle is applied to each pupil, who is considered like his own child.
- The first aim of medicine, however, is to restore the sick to health. The Hebrew comment adds: "not in the hope of money." Hippocrates had not mentioned this. In Jewish law, doctors are in fact classified in the same religious category as teachers and rabbis, who must not accept compensation for their services.
- Hippocrates says: "... I will not give anyone, even if requested, a deadly drug, nor will I suggest such advice." In the Hebrew version the doctor must not agree "if someone else suggests that he do such a wicked deed" (though unfortunately, throughout history, some Jewish doctors have been accused of poisoning!).
- The dissipations and intoxications that affect the mind and heart, as recalled in the Hebrew text, have no correspondence in Hippocrates who only warns that the doctor's life must be "pure and holy," with no more details.
- The importance of constant learning is not mentioned in the Hippocratic Oath, but it is mentioned here (see Footnote 18).
- The "conjuration" [swearing] at the end of Hippocrates' text is not contemplated.

Islam (2)

History and Ethics of Muslim Medicine, Eightieth to Twelfth Century

Background

Between the sixth and tenth centuries a new monotheistic religion with specific characteristics, Zoroastrianism, developed, starting in Iran, then spreading throughout Central Asia. It was based on the worship of (Ahura) Mazda. It was the religion founded by the prophet Zarathustra (or Zoroaster). It persisted and spread until the rapid establishment of the Islamic religion in the seventh century. Small Zoroastrian communities still remain today in Iran, Tajikistan, Azerbaijan, and India.

They are known as Parsi. They too did their utmost in the continuous struggle between Good and Evil and in the search for the values of medical ethics. Zoroastrian priests indicated in their sacred text Avesta, in the part headed Vendidae, what the characteristics of the physician must be. The passages are set out in the third book of the Sassanid Persian encyclopedia, the Dinkard: they describe in specific detail the qualities of the ideal doctor of the sixth century.

The optimal physician had to know the parts of the body and the joints well, and the remedies for the most frequent diseases; he had to be friendly without jealousy, kind in words and not slothful. An enemy of illness but friend for the sick, he had to be modest, free from crime, insults, and violence; by noble deeds he had to protect his good reputation, not for gain but for spiritual reward.

He had to be ready to listen, have authority and be philanthropic, able to prepare herbal medicines in order to free the body from disease, corruption and impurities, to bring peace, and "multiply the delights of life."[19]

The medical culture of Islam came from the Sassanid Empire of Persia, in particular from the academy and hospitals of Gondishapur (in the west of present-day Iran) which had many contacts with India and with the Eastern Roman Empire too. Much had also come from Syria and the school of Alexandria in Egypt. Some of Muhammad's (fifth to sixth century) great teachings were also addressed to the medical world. He upheld the fear of God and the final judgment, as well as goodness, fairness, compassion, mercy, generosity, austerity of morals, sincerity, fraternity among believers.

Historically, Islam was born in the seventh century but was recognized in international law following the Treaty of Westphalia (1648), and it was only really defined in the second half of the last century.[20]

From the seventh century, Islam spread from Arabia to much of the world known at that time. The history of Arab medicine is largely linked to Islam and incorporates the entire heritage of pre-Islamic knowledge (the so-called Medicine of the Prophet). Medieval Arab culture acted as a link between ancient and modern medical science. First it was the Syriac Christians who translated Greek medical literature, including the works of Galen, Aristotle, Plato, Dioscorides, Paul of Aegina, and Hippocrates. Their texts were saved, translated, and edited with great care and veneration (see Footnote 20).

Greek civilization allowed the Arabs to assimilate a medicine based on rational elements and neutral from the religious point of view. The Abbasid Caliph Al-Ma'Mun (786–833) is credited with having started the movement for the translation of Greek scientific and philosophical works, with the establishment of a library, with works in Greek, Syriac, Hebrew, Coptic, Middle-Persian, and Sanskrit. The translations provided ideological tools to combat the Byzantines, considered not only infidels, but also culturally inferior, unworthy of considering themselves heirs of the Greeks. The first translators into Arabic were "Nestorian" Christian doctors.[21] Perhaps the most illustrious of the Nestorians was Hunain ibn Ishaq, known as Giovannizio.[22]

---

[18] The translation has been forced sometimes to be more understandable to a contemporary reader: the original is even incomprehensible. We are in the sixth century. A.D., at the beginning of the Middle Ages. This historical period conditions a vision that has nothing poetic about it. There are no precise indications on what to do to improve the relationship between men and God. Information is listed on "things" not to do, such as idolatry and the roads not to be taken. In the light of a careful reading we realize that the destiny of man is strongly conditioned by the presence of God.

[19] The text anticipates the importance of continuous learning to promote the progress of medicine, as reported in the revision of the Hippocratic Oath made in 2007.

[20] Larijani and Zahedi (2006).

[21] Castiglioni (1946), Filosa (2016), and Veatch (2000), pp. 233–239.

[22] Nestorius followers, patriarch of Constantinople (ca. 381–451).

Even today, Islam profoundly influences the beliefs, values, and habits of about one-fifth of the human race. Yet it is still poorly understood. Its deepest principle is an absolute belief in monotheism, summarized in the declaration of faith: "There is no divinity but God and Mohammed is the messenger of God." The four primary sources of law, on which Islamic Medical Ethics is also based, are: The Koran—the Holy Text believed to be the direct word of God, the Sunna—of the Prophet Muhammad and incorporated into Islamic scriptures; and the Jtihad—the law of deductive logic.

Since Islam does not admit a clergy of its own, "Ulema" (scholars) are responsible for interpreting and contextualizing religious teachings. Islam provides for laws (Shari'a), ethics, duties, and beliefs. The guiding principles of Islamic law are:

- Maintenance of life,
- Protection of an individual's freedom of belief,
- Conservation of the intellect,
- Maintenance of honor and integrity, and
- Protection of property.

Moral Commandments of the Koran

In the 17th chapter the Koran sets down ten moral provisions which are "the precepts of wisdom," revealed by Allah (reported below), pointing out only the main assumptions:

1. Worship Allah only;
2. Be kind, honest and humble with parents;
3. Be neither stingy nor spendthrift in your shopping: Verily, the wasteful are brothers of the wicked and the evil one is their thankless lord;
4. Do not engage in "crimes out of piety," for fear of starving;
5. Do not commit adultery;
6. Do not kill unjustly: nor take a life that Allah has made sacred, unless there is just cause;
7. Look after orphaned children until they reach the age of full strength;
8. Keep your promises;
9. Be honest and fair in your relationships;
10. Do not be arrogant in your claims or beliefs, do not pursue what you have no knowledge of, do not walk the earth with insolence, because you cannot tear it apart, nor can you reach the top of mountains. On this basis it was necessary to expand the four fundamental principles of medical ethics (Autonomy, Charity, Non-Maleficence, Justice), linking them to human rights.

The principles were to include human dignity and human rights, benefits and harm, autonomy and individual responsibility, consent, special interest to people unable to understand, and allowing consent to therapy. Various societies differ in their practice of medical ethics: the differences are mostly founded on cultural, religious, social, bioethical, and legal norms; good medical ethics is meant to ensure that all human beings enjoy the best possible health, without any basic distinction.

Guiding Principles of Islamic Law

Maintenance of life, Protection of freedom of belief, Maintenance of the intellect, Preservation of honor and integrity and Protection of property.

Medicine

In the Koran we read: "... when I am sick, it is God who heals me." It is not uncommon for Muslim patients and their families to pray to God for a cure, as if He were their ultimate source of salvation. The role of a doctor in treatment is therefore a "practice" strongly conditioned by philosophical concepts, divided into "experimental" and "clinical methodology."

The modern person rarely thinks that medicine may have religious or ethnic limits. The most important factor in the concept of "Islamic medicine" is its perspective on the history, theory, and practice of medicine itself. Any medicine applicable through Islamic teachings can be labeled "Islamic." For many centuries the world, especially Europe, has benefited from the great contributions made by Muslim doctors. The Arabic language became for the East what Latin and Greek were for the West, the main scientific language of humanity. Islamic teachings made medical or surgical treatment compulsory, above all when it would have been harmful not to practice them.

Many terms such as alchemy, alcohol, alkali, alembic, and aldehyde are of Arabic origin. Arab pharmacists, or "sandeloni," introduced a large number of natural remedies: senna, camphor, musk, myrrh, tamarind, nutmeg, cloves, ambergris, mercury, and others. It was the Arabs who created new solvents such as rose and orange water, tragacanth (to prepare emulsions and with antiseptic, emollient, anorexic, and laxative properties); they already knew about the anesthetic effects of cannabis. Studies on alchemy developed, and though they failed to discover the "philosopher's stone" (a hypothetical substance capable of transforming metals into gold), alchemists were responsible for the discovery of chemicals such as mineral acids, bismuth, antimony, phosphorus, zinc, and ammonia. The word elisir comes from the Arabic al-iksir.

"Allah has created a cure for every disease," said Muhammad. The Creator is, in fact, the source of all disease and healing, while the physician remains essential to distribute remedies and cures. In many cases, people referred to doctors as "Hakim," i.e. "the person who knows the needs for man and for life."

One of the most important obligations for doctors was to care about their own body and the nourishment of the soul. Mental health was believed to be the most important part of well-being, and its violation led to physical disorders known today as psychosomatic illnesses. Physicians were never to ignore the symptoms described by the patient, because they were of great importance in the diagnosis, and because they favored mercy and understanding. Doctors also had a duty to tell the truth, consider the benefits of therapy, and act only for the good of all. In the Islamic worldview, guidance on human affairs, the laws and principles by which Muslims must govern themselves come from a divine source, present in the shari'a, the law. As such, the foundations of morality and ethics cannot be separated from the law and do not change according to time and place, but are absolute. Many topics, such as assisted reproduction, genetic testing, euthanasia, stem cell research, cosmetic surgery, and postmortem issues, were not yet known. Thus, without clear evidence or legal precedents on these issues, jurists, facing new ethical problems, resorted to *al maqaşid al sharı'a* (for the purposes of the law).

Ethics

A minimum level of cultural awareness is a prerequisite for addressing minority traditions, for learning some key teachings of Islamic medical ethics and exploring its applications.[23]

Verse 5:32 of the Koran is enlightening: "If someone killed a person, unless it was for murder or to prevent the spread of evil on earth, it would be as if he had killed all humanity. And if someone saved a life, it would be as if he had saved the life of all humanity."

The term ethics has no connection with the Western concept: shari'a includes and represents morality as "Islamic law," but also as an "Islamic moral imperative."[24]

Some of the issues discussed by the Islamic doctor are universally important: abortion, organ transplants, artificial insemination, cosmetic surgery, doctor–patient relationships, to state but a few.

Other questions are strictly Islamic: impediments to fasting in Ramadan, diseases and physical conditions that cause violation of the state of purity, medicines containing alcohol, etc.[25]

Origin of Ethical Principles

Islamic ethics contain pre-Islamic Arab traditions, Koranic teachings, Persian and even Hellenistic elements, but there has been no new source of Islamic doctrine since the Prophet Muhammad. Previous Syrian and Persian medical works were translated into Arabic and formed the basis of ethics. In fact, there was not even a term equivalent to the Greek *ethos*, so there is no exact word for "ethics." The

[23] Guidi (1933) and Pergola (2009).

[24] Gatrad and Sheikh (2001).

[25] Stokke (2014).

closest term could be "*khuluq*" which indicates moral behavior, behavior and courteous character. Two terms that roughly refer to its meaning are "*Akhlaq*" and "*Adab.*" Akhlaq means "to create" or "shape" things, implying that the Muslim believer is expected to behave with decency at all times and in all places. Adab has a broader, fuller meaning and aims to underline the behavior and conduct of the doctor, his clothing, even his good manners and his relationships with patients, colleagues, pharmacists, nurses, and visitors.

From all this came the significance of "good manners," "etiquette," "refinement." Adab represents "how learning and knowledge are linked to right and appropriate human conduct," and the character, the foundation of personality in the medical profession, including sincerity, honesty, truth, compassion and understanding, patience, tolerance, and humility.

In the Islamic world, ethics have a juridical and religious matrix, which guides the customs and attitudes of believers. Muhammad said, in relation to the responsibility of doctors: "A person who practices the art of healing when he does not know medicine will be responsible for his actions." He also said: "O servants of Allah, seek healing, as Allah did not bring sickness without also sending treatment."

Medical Ethics

The components of ethics are widespread in all Islamic sciences of Fiqh (including jurisdictional competence), of Tafsir (Koranic exegenesis) and of Kalam (scholastic theology). In medieval times many authors tackled issues that today we would say are questions of medical ethics, and the main Arab treatise specifically dedicated to this was Adab al-ţabīb: "The good conduct of the doctor" by Ishàq Ibn 'Alī al-Ruhāwī, at the end of the nineth century, largely inspired by a work by Rufus of Ephesus[26] (first to second century A.D.) and based on previous works by Hippocrates and Galen.[27]

Particular attention was paid to the moral ethics of Islam: doctors and their patients had the right to make independent decisions. The Code of Ethics was modeled with the participation of members of Islamic centers (especially in Iran). Medical ethics can be evaluated differently from one country to another in response to developments in science, medical technology, and social values.[28]

---

[26] Rispler-Chaim (1989).

[27] Rufus Ephesius, Greek physician who lived in the time of Trajan (second half of the first century A.D.). He lived in Egypt and for some time in Rome. He studied the anatomy of the bodies of slaves and monkeys. He studied the eye, the uterine tubes, distinguished the pancreas from the mesenteric glands. He wrote about dietetics, pathology, anatomy, and patient care but also about slaves and the elderly. He mainly followed Hippocratic instructions. He also studied in Alexandria but operated in Ephesus which was an important medical center.

Rufus Ephesius (1879) and Haleem (1993).

[28] Ahmad (2005), Amine and El Kadi (1988), Athar and Fadel (2005), Padela (2007), and Rispler-Chaim (1989).

Medical ethics in Islam and the related international code laid down the following obligations:

- The physician must always maintain the highest standards of professional conduct and must always continue his medical education.
- A doctor will not allow profit to influence the free and independent exercise of professional judgment.
- A physician, in all types of medical practice, must be dedicated to providing competent medical services with full technical and moral independence, compassion, and respect for human dignity.
- A physician must deal honestly with patients and colleagues and strive to identify any physicians who lack character or competence or who engage in fraud or deception.

Duties of doctors toward the sick:

- The doctor must always bear in mind the obligation to safeguard human life.
- A doctor owes complete loyalty to his patients, with all the resources of his science. Whenever an examination or treatment is beyond his knowledge he (or she) will consult another doctor who has the necessary skill.
- A physician must maintain absolute confidentiality about everything he knows about the patient even after the patient has died.
- A doctor must provide emergency assistance, as a humanitarian duty, unless he is sure that others are willing and able to provide it.

Duties of doctors among colleagues:

- A doctor will behave toward his colleagues as he would like them to behave toward him.
- A physician must not poach patients from his colleagues.
- A doctor must [nowadays] comply with the principles of the Geneva Declaration (approved by the World Medical Association in 1948).

As regard the teaching of medical ethics, the information must be adequate for the required application and the Code must be included in the university curriculum. The main principles of the Hippocratic Oath have been recognized for Muslims, but the invocation of many deities in the original (Greek) version and their exclusion in later (Western) versions led Muslims to appreciate more the Muslim doctor's oath invoking the name of Allah.

The road to moral and spiritual perfection is described as the "*search* for God." A correct definition of medical ethics implies an analytical approach in which concepts, hypotheses, beliefs, attitudes, emotions, reasons, and arguments that underpin medical-moral decisions are critically examined. There are many ways to understand it; some of them are: informed consent and refusal of treatment; clinical reports, truthfulness, trust and good communication; confidentiality and good clinical practice; medical research; health care for people with physical and mental disabilities. Its adherents consider Islam as a complete way of life; sickness and health are only part of the believer's journey through life. The *uşūlalfiqh* (principles of jurisprudence), the *maqāşid al sharı'a* (purposes of Islamic law), and the *qawā"id fiqhiyya* (Islamic juridical maxims) permit Islam to adapt to changes in ethics. In Islam, there are often different opinions on particular subjects related to medical ethics and these are evident in the collections of *fatāwa* (legal judgments).

In Conclusion

The main characteristics of Islamic medical ethics are:

(a) a constant attempt to ground modern medical treatments in the classical sources of Islamic law;
(b) problems are mainly relevant to Muslims or derive directly from the commandments and prohibitions of Islamic law;
(c) a fatāwa is indicated to mediate, when Islamic law and state law are contradictory on some medical ethical issue;.
(d) Islamic medical ethics tends to stress the superiority of its way of life over other societies, especially Western;
(e) Islamic medical ethics is often inseparable from social and political issues.

Although some questions dealt with in Islamic medical ethics are restricted to Islam and mainly concern Muslims, others are common to most religions. Islamic medical ethics shows a solid understanding of purely medical material and the most recent discoveries: Islamic medicine is constantly developing and its ethics follows progress and provides Muslims with legitimacy for the adoption or rejection of any innovation.

Those responsible for this formulation are religious or medical figures. In medical practice, a code of conduct must be followed that applies ethical and moral standards together with professional ones.[29]

In order to grasp the principles of Islamic medical ethics better, one must take a comprehensive view of the Islamic world and appreciate that Islam is considered a complete way of life; sickness and health are only part of the believer's journey through life. Generally, the term "morality" refers to rules of conduct that a person or group believes to be reliable for distinguishing good from evil.

Activities that require careful analysis in which the concepts, hypotheses, beliefs, behaviors, emotions, causes, and arguments that underline the doctor's moral processes are critically examined according to Shari'a in relation to the five essential elements of the person: life, religion, intellect, honor (with integrity), and property.

Islamic medical ethics comprise, for example, the following eight points:

[29] Ahmad (2005).

- informed consent and refusal of treatment
- clinical relationships, truthfulness, trust, and good communication
- confidentiality and good clinical practice
- medical research
- human reproduction and new genetics
- treatment of children
- care for physical and mental disabilities
- vulnerability of the duties of doctors, including their training and the allocation of resources and rights.

Allah has defined the standards of right and wrong, hence the corollary "that good deeds are good only because Allah commands it and evil is evil, as Allah forbids it." Muhammad said, "I was sent to perfect my manners and ethical conduct," thereby emphasizing that character formation is central to the moral life. Islamic ethics begins with the renunciation of all worship except Allah: this would include self-worship (selfishness), worship of man's own products (idols, superstitions, etc.) and the renunciation of all that degrades humanity (atheism, injustice, etc.). By abolishing the inevitable inequalities based on race, skin color, language, country of origin, Islam proclaims (and claims to have achieved) individual superiority based solely on ethical value, accessible to all without exception.

Muslim Doctors

For many centuries the world has witnessed and benefited from the great advances made by Muslim doctors in the field of health; ethical needs were mainly based on Koranic ethics. They include guidelines for physicians' behavior and attitudes, personally and professionally.[30]

Advanced technologies in all areas of medicine posed still unanswered questions to scientific society, constantly influencing perspectives.

Muslims are divided into two groups. One group is educated and modern and accepts news related to science, regardless of religious or moral laws; the other group, of Islamic scholars, knows all about Islam, but nothing of the medical sciences.

Islam places importance on saving lives (through medical treatment or otherwise) and makes it clear that death is a part of the contract (with Allah), and the end of life depends on Allah's will. The same moral and ethical standards must therefore guide doctors in their private life and profession. Muslim physicians must believe in God and Islamic teachings and practices; they must be humble, modest, kind, merciful, patient, and tolerant. These physicians must realize that God observes and monitors every thought and action.[31]

[30] Amine and El Kadi (1988) and Sonn (1996).

[31] Athar and Fadel (2005), Nanji (1991), Arawi (2010), and Padela (2007).

The Doctor–Patient Relationship

During diagnostic and therapeutic procedures, the doctor–patient relationship may prove problematic as the patient's freedom of self-determination is limited or even canceled, as in case of severe or terminal illness, since the seriously ill patient is considered physically morally infirm, and that status means he is unable to consciously organize his own life.[32]

In short, the Islamic doctor must:

- believe in Allah and obey His commandments
- be wise and noble-minded
- always use a calm tone of voice, show common sense and apply good manners towards others, regardless of their class
- be aware that Life and Death belong to Allah
- take care of oneself to give others an appropriate example and keep up to date on the progress of medical science
- be sincere, despise greed and foster friendship and respect for authority
- be informed about the legal and religious norms in force, in order to provide adequate answers to patients on religion, prayer, fasting, pilgrimage, family planning, etc.
- avoid the use of drugs or other methods of therapy not permitted by Islam
- preserve the life and health of others. The doctor is Allah's tool for relieving disease.
- be modest and avoid vanity.
- adapt to keep up with scientific progress and innovation for the well-being of patients
- bear in mind that research, besides its therapeutic purposes, responds to the will of Allah.

A significant aphorism of the Islamic tradition:

> Nothing is more harmful to the patient than a doctor who is more gifted in speaking than in providing medical assistance.[33]

New technologies in medicine in areas related to life support and maintenance, such as organ transplantation, bio-technical parenting, and acquired immune deficiency syndrome have posed new questions and influenced the perspective in medical ethics. Muslim patients, their families and their doctors have to update their current knowledge and outlook.

---

[32] Filosa (2001).

[33] Zunic et al. (2014).

The basic questions are: "Who is the giver of life and death? Is it lawful for man to control his life and death as well as that of other human beings?" It is essential to depend on the will of Allah.

Doctors' Ethics

Doctors were required to bathe, wash their mouth and teeth, cut their nails, cut their hair, use a deodorant, dress appropriately, and pray before seeing patients.

The main characteristics of Islamic medical ethics are:

(a) There is constant attention: the treatments of modern medicine are based on the classical sources of Islamic law.
(b) The issues raised are predominantly relevant to Muslims, or come directly from the commandments and prohibitions of Islamic law.
(c) When Islamic and State laws are contradictory on some medical ethical issues, a fatāwa is indicated to mediate.
(d) Islamic medical ethics is almost apologetic about showing the superiority of the Islamic way of life over other societies, especially Western ones
(e) Islamic medical ethics is often inseparable from social and political issues.

I. **The Doctor's Personality**
The doctor must be modest, virtuous, generous and not addicted to alcohol. He must wear clean clothes, be dignified and have well-groomed hair and beard. He must not join the wicked, nor sit at their table. He must limit his company to people of good repute and be careful what he says; he must not hesitate to ask for forgiveness if he has made a mistake. He must be tolerant and not seek revenge; be friendly and peace-loving. He should not crack jokes or laugh at an inopportune or wrong moment.

II. **The Doctor's Obligations towards Patients**
The doctor must avoid predicting life or death—only God (Allah) knows. He must have patience when the patient keeps asking questions, and answer with gentleness and compassion. He must treat the rich and the poor alike, the master and the servant, the powerful and the weak, the educated and the illiterate. God will reward him if he helps the needy. The doctor must be punctual and reliable for his visits. He must not argue about his fees. If the patient is very ill or in an emergency, he must be grateful to the doctor, regardless of his fee. The doctor must not give abortion drugs to a pregnant woman unless it is necessary for the mother's health. If you are prescribing a drug by mouth, you must make sure that the patient understands correctly the name of the product, in case he asks for the wrong drug and gets worse instead of better. The doctor must show respect towards women, and must not reveal his patients' secrets.

III. **The Doctor's Obligations towards the Community**
The doctor must not speak ill of people who are respected in the community, or criticize any religious faith.
The Doctor's Obligations towards Colleagues
The doctor must speak well of his acquaintances and colleagues.
He does not have to exalt himself, humiliating others. If another doctor has been called to treat his patient, the family doctor must not criticize his colleague, even if he makes a diagnosis and recommendations different from his own. His duty is to advise the patient as best he can. He must warn him when the combination of different treatments could be dangerous because some different drugs taken together can be incompatible and harmful.

IV. **The Doctor's Obligations towards his Assistant**
If his subordinate makes a mistake, the doctor must not scold him in front of others, but cordially in private.

List of (8) Major Muslim Doctors

Medicine in Islam has gone through various stages of development and many doctors have been mentioned in the literature. Eight of the most significant in the Muslim tradition are discussed here.[34]

The Ninth and Tenth Centuries correspond to the phase of excellence and to real contributions to medicine; Islamic doctors were the leaders of the new medical and surgical culture.

1. Ali Ibn Sahl Rabban, **Abu al-Hasan al-Tabari**[35] was born around 838 A.D. in Marw, Tabaristan (near today's Tehran), to a Syriac Christian intellectual family. He was a doctor, scientist, and philosopher, and wrote 12 books on philosophy, medicine, and religious issues.

He described what an Islamic code of ethics might be in his book "*Firdous al-Hikmat*" (Paradise of Wisdom), which appears as the first ever written encyclopedia of medical ethics that incorporates all branches of the medical sciences.

It recalls the Islamic codes of ethics such as the personal characteristics of the doctor, his obligation toward patients, and commitment to the community, obligations toward his colleagues and toward assistants.

The text also describes:

(a) The general causes of diseases;
(b) Diseases of the head and brain;
(c) Diseases of the eyes, nose, ears, mouth and teeth;
(d) Muscle diseases (paralysis and spasms);
(e) Diseases of the regions of the thorax, throat and lungs;
(f) Abdominal diseases;
(g) Liver disease;
(h) Diseases of the gallbladder and spleen;
(i) Intestinal diseases;
(j) Different types of fever;
(k) Brief explanation of the organs;
(l) Pulse and urine examination.

[34] "What is relevant to Islam": The noun "Muslim" means "devoted to God," since it derives from the Arabic verbal name "Muslim" that is "submissive (to God)."

[35] Osler (1913), Aboukleish (1979), Ardalan et al. (2015), and Zahedi (2005).

Tabari avoided prescribing treatments without having first investigated and examined the patient. Tabari was an encyclopedist and had a holistic view of medicine. From an investigation of the scientific and moral characteristics of this great Persian scholar, it appears that he was interested in philosophy and medical ethics, citing the works of other scholars of the same age, with attention to clinical and hospital training. He emphasized indigenous and scientific therapies and liability in case of medical error in treatment. He discovered the scabies mite (Sarcoptes scabiei) and is particularly famous for having written *al-Mu'alajat al-Buqratiya* (Hippocrates' treatments), an important encyclopedic work.

2. Abumakr Muhammad Ibn Zakaria Razi (865–925), also known as **al-Rhazes**,[36] was born in Ray, near Tehran. He was a doctor, teacher, alchemist, philosopher, mathematician, and also an astronomer.

One of his most important contributions to medicine was the scientific differentiation between measles and smallpox. He wrote more than 200 books including *Kitab al-Hawi* (Liber continens), an encyclopedic work on medical information which was translated into Latin in 1280 and joined the medical school in Paris.

Rhazes was the first to use neuroanatomy to locate lesions of the nervous system and correlate them with clinical signs; he described the motor and sensory functions of the nerves and listed seven cranial and 31 spinal nerves. He excluded the Galenic assumption of a bone at the base of the heart and was the first to describe the recurrent laryngeal nerve. He clearly established the importance of the doctor's commitment to ethical principles. For this reason he disapproved of doctors who "used their profession to blackmail patients or employed illegal and dishonorable means": he called them "pseudo-doctors." His output also included some manuscripts and a book "Spiritual Medicine," related to medical ethics.

He divided the issues related to medical ethics under three main headings:

(a) Professionals: the personality traits that doctors must acquire to achieve correct medical training, such as: an appropriate tone of voice, confidentiality, self-confidence, based on study and not on wasted time (!) Medicine does not have to be a business and patients must be respected.
(b) Research: references and citations are essential. He criticized and opposed plagiary by doctors, considering it inappropriate behavior.
(c) Treatment: in providing health care, Rhazes urged doctors to observe ethical standards, trust and commitment to patients. He emphasized that first of all a doctor must find the cause of the pain and only after that prescribe therapy. He refused to prescribe opium since it can cause blindness, or poly-pharmacy which may cause patients other harm.

[36] Tabatabai (2008).

Al-Rhazes is also remembered for an aphorism:

> Truth in medicine is a goal that cannot be reached and everything written in books is worth much less than a doctor who thinks and reasons.

3. Ishaq bin Ali **Al-Ruhawi**[37] was probably born in Al-Ruha, the modern Şanlıurfa in Turkey. He was a Christian, perhaps with Nestorian training, and may still have been a Christian when he composed his works.

Among them the most famous is "*Adab al-Tabib*" (Practical Ethics of the Doctor, or Practical Medical Deontology), perhaps the most significant and oldest and most detailed book that deals with medical ethics.

He revolutionized the medical world and his foresight made this a true deontological treatise.

The text is based on the works of Hippocrates and Galen, also containing extensive instructions on mutual respect and moral obligations of doctors, nurses, patients, and other health workers. This work encouraged doctors to avoid nefarious influences and to realize that good character is far more important than wealth, and that the wisdom to understand is found in moral and perfect people.

The Chapters of Adab al-Tabib by al-Ruhawi[38]

His book began with the words "In the name of Allah ...." Legislative practices and penalties for fake and incompetent doctors were also discussed in Adab al-Tabib, and, to eliminate charlatans, the author defended medical examinations and licenses, whose content should be profoundly influenced by Galen's works.

1. Of the fidelity and faith in which a doctor must believe and on the ethics that he must follow
2. On the means and measures with which the doctor treats his own body and limbs
3. Of the things a doctor must be aware of
4. On the directions a physician should give patients and servants
5. On the behavior of visitors to patients
6. On the simple and compound drugs that a physician must evaluate and on the corrective directions that may be made by a pharmacist or others.
7. On matters about which a physician should question patients or others
8. On the need for the sick and healthy to trust their doctor

[37] Levey (1967) and Aksoy (2004).

[38] Levey (1967), Serour (2014), and Zunic (2014).

9. On the agreement that patients must follow the doctor's instructions and the result when they fail to do this
10. On the patient's behavior with those who live with him, and his servants
11. On the patient's behavior towards his visitors
12. On the dignity of the medical profession
13. On the people who must respect a doctor based on his skill, as well as kings and other honorable men whom they must respect even more
14. Specific accidents involving doctors, i.e. those already known, so that the doctor can be forewarned. Some are just anecdotal but can help him find out about non-cooperative people before the consultation, so that he is not the cause of any harm.
15. On the subject that not everyone can practice the medical profession but only those who have a suitable nature and a moral character
16. On examination of the doctors
17. On the ways in which kings can eliminate the corruption of doctors and lead people to respect medicine, as in ancient times
18. On the need to warn against scoundrels who call themselves doctors and the difference between their deception and true medical art
19. On the bad habits that people are used to but which can harm both the sick and the healthy and lead to doctors being accused
20. On the issues that a doctor must observe and bear in mind in periods of health to prepare for periods of llness, and the time of youth with a view to old age.

He encouraged doctors to keep a record of their patients' symptoms, treatments, and progress, so this information could be reviewed by colleagues, to help them.

Al-Ruhawi regarded doctors as "guardians of bodies and souls" and wrote the "Assessment of the Doctors" where he stated that, in the first place, a doctor must believe in the Creator alone, Allah, in whom he must have firm faith and to whom he must devote himself with all his soul. The doctor is advised "not to be vindictive, envious, hasty, moody, greedy but—on the contrary—indulgent, humble, erudite, calm, clean inside and out.

His clothes and his person must always be clean and perfumed and at the bedside of a sick person he should go with a pleasant expression, saying a few kind words of comfort. Great emphasis was placed on the interaction of spiritual and physical powers, stating that mental health is the important part of health and its violation can lead to physical illnesses (today they would be called psychosomatic). Furthermore, the Doctor "must never exaggerate with too many medications." If, however, the patient's condition threatens to evade his control, the doctor must switch to vigorous remedies without wasting time with palliatives."

Between the tenth and twelfth centuries other authors looked into the subject of medical ethics.

Here are some of them:

4. Ali ibn-**al-'Abbas al-Majusi** (930–994), known in Europe as Haly Abbas, born in Ahvaz, Persia. He was a Zoroastrian doctor (in Arabic Majūs = Mago—magician), one of the greatest doctors of his time. In 980 he wrote "The Complete Book of Medical Art" (al-Kitab al-Maliki), an encyclopedic work on surgery and medicine.

The text is divided into 20 "discourses," the first ten expounding theory and the second ten dealing with medical practice. It was translated and used as a textbook in schools throughout Europe until the eighteenth century. It described capillary circulation, anatomical details, and diseases of the spinal and cranial nerves. These data were also used in the Salerno school.

Ali Abbas introduced new surgical techniques, such as the removal of spinal tumors, and goiter. He correctly explained the cardiac circulation which Galen and Avicenna had got wrong and described the structure of the pulmonary arteries. He defined medical ethics and the importance—and necessity—of the doctor–patient relationship. He also discussed neuroscience, psychology, metrology, hygiene, human behavior, birth, poisons and antidotes, drug abuse, addiction to medicaments and the pains of love, and confirmed the principles of the Hippocratic Oath.

5. **Avicenna** (Abu 'Ali al-Husain Ibn' Abdallah Ibn Sina or Ibn Sina, (980–1038 A.D.), was born in Afshan (or Balkh) near Bukhara, in Persia. He was an expert on Islamic laws and various sciences; at the age of ten he knew the Koran by heart and, at the age of 17 he cured Nooh Ibn Mansoor, king of Bukhara, of an unknown disease that other doctors had not been able to cure. He thus gained access to the royal library containing thousands of rare manuscripts. At 18 he was already recognized as a great doctor. His oldest surviving works date back to 1001 when he was only 21 years old.

He studied philosophy and medicine; after Bukhara he went to Jurjan, Ray, Hamadan and then Isfahan where he wrote his masterpiece, the "Canon of Medicine" which was not immediately and universally accepted: the iron logic which he demonstrated greatly disturbed readers, creating many perplexities. Then, gradually—thanks to numerous enthusiastic commentators—the many merits of the work were discovered, first of all the deeper study of themes barely mentioned by Galen.

Avicenna managed to blend the doctrine of Aristotle and the medical theories of Hippocrates. He described the three heart valves, muscle movements, pain perception and the nerves, liver, spleen, and kidneys.

He clarified the six extra-ocular muscles and nerves and tendons in different anatomical structures, in contrast to previous interpretations, the vertebrae, the cerebellum, and the caudate nucleus. It was translated into Latin by Gerardo di Sabbioneta, with the title Liber canonis medicinae. The Canon of Medicine was also translated into Hebrew and was used as a textbook until the mid-seventeenth century.

He wrote nearly 270 different treatises, many of them medical. He was a doctor, philosopher, encyclopedist, mathematician, astronomer, politician, governor, and administrator. His contributions on anatomy amount to the most important advances from Claudius Galen (120–200) to Andrea Vesalius (1514–1564).

He addressed fundamental philosophical questions such as the origin of the cosmos, the role of God in human existence and in the universe. His work was adopted by medieval Christian philosophers, including Thomas Aquinas. His best-known works are: Book of Salvation, Canon of Medicine, Book of Healing, Divine Wisdom, Book of Sum and Substance, Philosophy for Prosody, Book of Virtue and Sin.

He stated that "students should learn the general principles of medicine, and analyze diseases that affect different organs, so to do this first they must study anatomy." He died of a severe colic in 1037, at the age of 58, when he was known as one of the greatest philosophers of Islam and medical doctors.

He was buried in Hamadan, where his grave can still be seen today. August 23rd, his date of birth, is celebrated every year in Iran.

All previous medical books were overshadowed by his great Canon of Medicine, in five volumes, dealing with

1. Theoretical medicine,
2. Simple medicines,
3. Localized diseases and their treatment,
4. Generalized diseases,
5. Composition and preparation of drugs.

The book was called "the most famous medical text ever written," "the medical Bible for longer than any other work." He dealt with mineral, animal, and vegetable poisons, rabies, phlebotomy, breast cancer, skin and childbirth disorders, describing the use of forceps. He also gave an excellent clinical picture of meningitis, described chronic nephritis, facial paralysis, pyloric stenosis, and gastric ulcer. He dealt with jaundice, dilation, and narrowing of the iris, describing the six motor muscles of the eye and the functions of the tear ducts.

Although there is no chapter specifically devoted to medical ethics, there are numerous references that consider human beings as the focal point of medical activities. The first necessary condition for the practice of medicine is to know it. On the topic of scientific research, he provided an example of the moral progress that should always accompany science and the importance of ethics in science and technology.

6. Yusuf ibn Ismail **al-Kutubi** (known as Ibn al-Kabir) wrote a text related to pharmacology in the year 1311, entitled "What a doctor cannot afford to ignore" where he criticized some of his contemporaries, calling them "ignorant" because they had not been educated in ethics.

Any Muslim doctor must in fact abide by moral obligations; Islamic law, wrote Ibn al-Kabir, is also capable of addressing legal problems that arise in medicine.

Other Islamic Doctors, Subsequently

7. Ab**u 'Imran Musa ben Maimun ibn "Abd Allah" known as Maimonides**: among the many Jewish philosophers of the Middle Ages, who had close connection with Islamic medicine, primarily I indicate Maimonides, perhaps the most representative.

Musa (Moses), son of Maimun (Rambam from the acronym: Rabbi Moses Ben Maimon; Abu Imran Musa Ibn Maimun, in Arabic), was called Maimonides to remember the great humanist, astronomer, Talmudist, and mathematician Maimun. A fundamental work of Moses ben Maimun is the Guide of the perplexed, in which he tried to reconcile revelation and reason, the Bible and philosophy.[39] It began by demonstrating the existence of God and his attributes. God is the necessary being, who that knows everything, even particular things; he created the world with an act of creative freedom and therefore the world is not eternal but has had a beginning in time. His book was received not only by doctors of the Jewish faith, but also by Muslims and Christians.

He was born in Cordoba, Spain, by Jewish parents, on March 30th, 1138, and was himself a Talmudist, philosopher, astronomer, and physician.[40] From his father he received rabbinical education and was placed at a young age under the guidance of the most illustrious Arab masters. Moses was only 13 when Cordova fell into the hands of fanatical Almohads (rigidly Orthodox, African Arabs). This fact soon put an end to the somewhat liberal rule of the Almoravid Arabs and forced Jews and Christians to choose to embrace the faith of Islam or to leave the Country. Consequently, for 12 years, his entire family led a nomadic life. In 1160 they settled in Fez, Morocco, pretending to be Muslims. Maimonides' reputation was growing steadily, leading the religious authorities to investigate his faith. He was also accused of the crime of abandoning the Islamic faith. They then left Fez and went in 1165 to San Giovanni d'Acri, a Jerusalem suburb and later settled in Fostat (Cairo).

Maimonides suffered from a long illness. Forced to work for self-support, he embraced the medical profession. At the age of 26 he wrote his first medical treatise. His main medical works are a collection known as "Medical Principles" which has been translated into Latin and Hebrew from the original Arabic. At the age of 39, he was appointed as the court doctor to Vizier Alfadhal, regent of Egypt, during the absence of Sultan Saladin the Great, a fighter in the Crusades in Palestine. During this period Richard the Lionheart, also involved in the Crusades, proposed to Maimonides to become his personal doctor, but he did not accept: "I get off my pet, wash my hands, go to my patients and beg them to bring some refreshments for me, the only meal of the day. Then I go to meet my patients and write prescriptions and directions for their ailments. I converse with them, even in a relaxed position from pure fatigue. When night falls, I am so tired that I can hardly speak."

[39] Javanbakht (2010).

[40] Frank (1981), Minkin (1957), and Rosner (2002).

Maimonides and Medicine

Maimonides translated many Arabic books, including the Canon of Avicenna, into Hebrew, Latin and various European languages. He also produced his book, "Regimen Sanitatis," which emphasized a proper diet, personal hygiene, and moderation in the pleasures of life. According to Maimonides, there is a religious duty in offering medical assistance to any sick person in need, regardless of race, age, religious belief, etc., based on the classic Biblical-Talmudic obligation to "return lost objects to their owner": In this case health. Maimonides defined medicine as a basic religious obligation, an important practical means to help others who live in need and to maintain their physical and spiritual well-being. Another important reason for studying medicine and natural sciences is the ideal way to recognize, love and fear God, on the one hand, and to develop adequate attitude and modesty for human beings, on the other. In his halachic-philosophical work "Mishneh Torah" the scientific and philosophical aspects that play a central role are expressly evaluated: Medicine ("imitatio Dei") is the personal guide for a healthy lifestyle and also explains the obligation of each individual toward himself.

While classical medical oaths, such as those of Hippocrates, Asaph, Rabbi Yaakov Zahalon and others, reflect the beliefs of their cultural milieus at the time they were produced, Maimonides' writings are directly rooted in the Jewish tradition and reflect duties and Basic Religious Principles.[41] Between the years 1158 and 1190 Maimonides produced, in addition to numerous minor writings, the work most relevant philosophical "Dalalat al-'a'irin" ("Moreh Nebukim"). The importance of this writing was considerable for the history of philosophy in the Middle Ages. According to Maimonides, there was no contradiction between the truths that God has revealed and those that the human mind has elaborated. All the principles of metaphysics are enshrined in the Bible and the Talmud. Maimonides divided all the positive attributes into five classes and demonstrated with a philosophical principle that God is

> "Intellectus," "intelligens," "intelligibilis"

His Death

Maimonides died in Cairo on December 13, 1204 and was buried in Tiberias, Palestine. His tomb became a place of pilgrimage and the "Moreh" became the "guide" of the enlightened Jews for many generations; his study influenced the thinking of philosophers such as Spinoza, Solomon Maimon, and Moses Mendelssohn. In the thirteenth century some parts of it have been translated into Latin Many Christian scholastics, such as Albert the Great, Duns Scotus, Alexander of Hales, and others, studied its content carefully.

---

[41] Dunn (1998).

After his death, the Jewish community in Egypt built a synagogue bearing his name. Some Jews book an overnight stay in this synagogue, hoping to receive healing through the spirit of this great physician.

Maimonides summed up his theory of knowledge in a letter to the Jews of Marseille in 1194:

> *Know, my Lords, that man must believe only in the following three things:*
> - *first, something that he can clearly grasp through pure and simple reasoning;*
> - *secondly, something that he can perceive with one of his five senses;*
> - *thirdly, what he learns from reliable prophets and wise men of blessed memory.*
>
> *Of one, however, who believes something that does not fit into any of these three categories, it is said, "The fool believes everything".*

His "Oath" concerning the medical vocation and the "Doctor's Prayer" remain to this day.[42]

Both documents, however, may not have been composed by Maimonides himself.

The Prayer appeared printed for the first time in 1783 by the German doctor and pupil of Immanuel Kant, Marcus Herz (see later). The authorship of the entire text is ascribed to this author, as it appears in a letter dated 23/5/1917, from the Chief Rabbi of the British Empire, Joseph M. Hertz, reported later.[43]

The Oath of Maimonides

The eternal providence has appointed me to watch over the life and health of Thy creatures. May the love for my art actuate me at all time; may neither avarice nor miserliness, nor thirst for glory or for a great reputation engage my mind; for the enemies of truth and philanthropy could easily deceive me and make me forgetful of my lofty aim of doing good to Thy children.

May I never see in the patient anything but a fellow creature in pain.

Grant me the strength, time and opportunity always to correct what I have acquired, always to extend its domain; for knowledge is immense and the spirit of man can extend indefinitely to enrich itself daily with new requirements.

Today he can discover his errors of yesterday and tomorrow he can obtain a new light on what he thinks himself sure of today. Oh, God, Thou has appointed me to watch over the life and death of Thy creatures; here am I ready for my vocation and now I turn unto my calling.

---

[42] Bird (1989), pp. 33–34.

[43] Rosner (1998).

The Prayer of Maimonides

Almighty God, Thou has created the human body with infinite wisdom. Ten thousand times ten thousand organs hast Thou combined in it that act unceasingly and harmoniously to preserve the whole in all its beauty the body which is the envelope of the immortal soul. They are ever acting in perfect order, agreement and accord. Yet, when the frailty of matter or the unbridling of passions deranges this order or interrupts this accord, then forces clash and the body crumbles into the primal dust from which it came. Thou sendest to man diseases as beneficent messengers to foretell approaching danger and to urge him to avert it.

Thou has blest Thine earth, Thy rivers and Thy mountains with healing substances; they enable Thy creatures to alleviate their sufferings and to heal their illnesses. Thou hast endowed man with the wisdom to relieve the suffering of his brother, to recognize his disorders, to extract the healing substances, to discover their powers and to prepare and to apply them to suit every ill. In Thine Eternal Providence Thou hast chosen me to watch over the life and health of Thy creatures. I am now about to apply myself to the duties of my profession. Support me, Almighty God, in these great labors that they may benefit mankind, for without Thy help not even the least thing will succeed. Inspire me with love for my art and for Thy creatures. Do not allow thirst for profit, ambition for renown and admiration, to interfere with my profession, for these are the enemies of truth and of love for mankind and they can lead astray in the great task of attending to the welfare of Thy creatures.

Preserve the strength of my body and of my soul that they ever be ready to cheerfully help and support rich and poor, good and bad, enemy as well as friend. power to see what cannot be seen, for delicate and indefinite are the bounds of the great art of caring for the lives and health of Thy creatures. In the sufferer let me see only the human being.

Illumine my mind that it recognize what presents itself and that it may comprehend what is absent or hidden. Let it not fail to see what is visible, but do not permit it to arrogate to itself the Let me never be absent- minded. May no strange thoughts divert my attention at the bedside of the sick, or disturb my mind in its silent labors, for great and sacred are the thoughtful deliberations required to preserve the lives and health of Thy creatures. Grant that my patients have confidence in me and my art and follow my directions and my counsel. Remove from their midst all charlatans and the whole host of ficious relatives and know-all nurses, cruel people who arrogantly frustrate the wisest purposes of our art and often lead Thy creatures to their death. Should those who are wiser than I wish to improve and instruct me, let my soul gratefully follow their guidance; for vast is the extent of our art. Should conceited fools, however, censure me, then let love for my profession steel me against them, so that I remain steadfast without regard for age, for reputation, or for honor, because surrender would bring to Thy creatures sickness and death. Imbue my soul with gentleness and calmness when older colleagues, proud of their age, wish to displace me or to scorn me or disdainfully to teach me. May even this be of advantage to me, for they know many things of which I am ignorant, but let not their arrogance give me pain. For they are old and old age is not master of the passions. I also hope to attain old age upon this earth, before Thee, Almighty God!

Let me be contented in everything except in the great science of my profession. Never allow the thought to arise in me that I have attained to sufficient knowledge, but vouchsafe to me the strength, the leisure and the ambition ever to extend my knowledge. For art is great, but the mind of man is ever expanding.

Almighty God! Thou hast chosen me in Thy mercy to watch over the life and death of Thy creatures.

I now apply myself to my profession. Support me in this great task so that it may benefit mankind, for without Thy help not even the least thing will succeed.

—Translated by Harry Friedenwald, *Bulletin of the Johns Hopkins Hospital* 28: 260–261, (1917)

His Works

Maimonides symbolized the highest spiritual and intellectual achievement of man on this earth, for the Jewish people: "from Moses to Moses, a man similar to Moses was not born, and no one has been since."

Worthy of mention is his famous trilogy: the *Commentary on the Mishnah*, *The Mishneh-Torah,* and The *Guide for the Perplexed*. He also wrote a book on "Logic," a "Book of Commandments," a "Letter to Yemen," a "Treatise on the Resurrection," several commentaries on the Talmud and over 600 "Responsa."

During the last decade of his life as a doctor at the court of the Sultan of Cairo, he wrote some fundamental works in Arabic, including:

- Extracts from Galen
- Commentary on the Aphorisms of Hippocrates
- Medical aphorisms of Moses (Pirke Moshe)
- Treatise on hemorrhoids
- Treaty on coexistence
- Treatise on Poisons and their Antidotes
- Health Regime (Regimen Sanitatis)
- Speech on the explanation of physical adaptation
- Glossary of drug names, in Arabic, Syriac, Greek, Spanish, Persian and Berber.

Rambam's medical works have been translated into English over nearly five decades by Jewish medical ethics experts and later used at Mount Sinai School and Albert Einstein College in New York.

The various chapters deal with multiple aspects of medicine and are very useful, not only for doctors but also for lay people interested in health promotion, Jewish philosophy, and history.

Medical Ethics in Maimonides

"His focus on medicine was rooted in the experience of generations and augmented by his clinical experience; his profound understanding of the psychosomatic and philosophical aspects received due appreciation."

He certainly made mistakes regarding some medical beliefs, but his knowledge and ability to diagnose were amazing, since he was called "one of the greatest physician-theologians-philosophers who ever lived on this earth. May his memory be blessed!"

He recognized that science had not yet reached a certain knowledge of nature and wrote: "The dangers are evident to the wise while the stupid find nothing difficult ... New doubts arise in those who are led to contemplation" and tried to explain the causes of the errors that afflict man. Rambam clearly wrote why health is important to the faith and to the practice of Jewish medicine:

"Since one heads towards the ways of the Lord, when the body is safe and sound, while there is the impossibility of understanding or knowing anything about the Creator when one is sick."

It is therefore mandatory for a man to avoid things that are harmful to the body and look for things that strengthen him "just as a Jew must return a lost object to its owner, doctors must restore the good health of their patients."

Maimonides expounded the ethical doctrine using a series of demonstrative and conceptual elements from Aristotelian philosophy. "True morality is realized in doing good for good without expecting anything else. It is not possible to think of curing a disease of the body without first knowing it."

In the Mishneh-Toah, Maimonides points to 11 precepts, five affirmative, and six negative, as follows:

1. Imitate God's Behavior
2. Join those who know Him
3. Love your neighbor
4. Love proselytes and foreigners
5. Correct the next
6. Don't hate your brothers
7. Don't shame people in public
8. Do not make the poor suffer
9. Don't spread slander
10. Don't take revenge

11. Do not hold a grudge

The importance of the psychological origin of many diseases is a theme taken up numerous times in the discussion, as is the role of the doctor in his relationship with the patient "emotional experiences produce significant changes in the body that are evident and manifest to everyone"; "You must be careful and always consider the movements of the soul."

Marcus Herz

As already stated, Marcus Herz exalted the work of Maimonides.[44]

He was born in Berlin on January 17, 1747 from very poor parents; he was destined for a career in the mercantile field. In 1762 he settled in Königsberg in East Prussia. He soon abandoned his position as a clerk and enrolled at the University. He became a pupil and friend of Immanuel Kant. For lack of means he was forced to interrupt his studies. He was secretary of the rich Russian Ephraim and traveled with him through the Baltic Provinces.

In 1770 he returned to Germany to Halle, where he graduated in Medicine in 1774. He then settled in Berlin where he worked at the Jewish hospital. Beginning in 1777, he held public lectures on medicine and philosophy, aimed at students and the most prominent personalities of the Prussian capital. Some members of the royal family also participated.

He was also a friend and pupil of Moses Mendelssohn and Gotthold Ephraim Lessing. For many years Herz maintained close correspondence with Kant; their letters are considered of great philosophical importance.

He died in Berlin on January 19, 1803.

The earliest known publication of the so-called Doctor's Prayer is found in a German literary journal, Das Deutsches Museum, dated 1783. The initial title attributed was: "The daily prayer of a doctor before visiting his patients, taken from the manuscript of a famous Jewish doctor in Egypt in the twelfth century." A number of versions, abbreviations, or excerpts have been presented in English, German, Hebrew, French, Dutch, and Spanish, and possibly in other languages.

The introduction indicated that the Author of the prayer was Markus Herz and that it was translated at his explicit request. Frequent is the plea addressed to the Almighty to protect the Doctor in facing various obstacles, moral failures, and carelessness. In one of his pleadings, Herz turns to God so that: "Drive away all charlatans, the host of zealous relatives, pedantic nurses, cruel people who arrogantly frustrate the wisest purposes of our profession and often lead Your creatures to death."

Finally, the author invokes divine help to accept instructions from those who are wiser. Many Jewish doctors and some medical schools have also recently used the

[44] Gesundheit and Hadad (2005), Gesundheit (2011), Rosner (1998), Segal (2011), and Siegel-Itzkovich (2013).

"Physician's Prayer" instead of the Hippocratic oath. There is a lively controversy over the identification of the true author of the prayer.

The first Hebrew version of the prayer was published by Isaac Euchel, editor of the Hebrew periodical Ha-Meassef, in 1790. The title indicated that Marcus Herz was its author and that it was translated at his request from German into Hebrew. In 1841, the London newspaper, Voice of Jacob, published the first English interpretation, under the title "A Doctor's Daily Prayer." The writer, using the fictitious name of "Medicus," stated: "The composition of this prayer has been mistakenly attributed to Maimonides, but it is the production of the late Dr. Marcus Herz, a famous doctor from Berlin. It was published by him in the German language, and the Hebrew version is by Itzig Eichel."

In 1914 it was confirmed that Marcus Herz was the true creator of the prayer and in 1935, the Canadian Jewish Chronicle printed a letter from Rabbi Dr. Joseph H. Hertz, answering a question from Sir William Osler and informing that Herz was the true Author. The opinion remained, not completely dissipated, that Herz's writing was in any case the fruit of an impostor.

Arab Medicine, After Maimonides

Maimonides was admired by Christians, Jews, and Arabs of his time. His tomb in Tiberias may still be visited and many Jews make pilgrimages to pay homage to him and remember that his main attention was directed to pharmacology and chemistry. The Arabs themselves have always shown considerable interest in these faculties and have supplied new drugs to Western Europe. To validate their findings they often carried out experiments on animals. The Pharmacopoeia of the Arabs knew a description of over 1,000 products. Among them rhubarb, manna, cloves, senna and many others.

8. In 1770 A.D., *during Persia's Islamic era*, **Mohamad Hosin Aghili** of Shiraz wrote the work Kholasah al Hekmah.[45] *The first chapter of that work contains a list of ethical duties for the physician, which is reported below in condensed form.* He is known also for his comprehensive pharmacology titled "*Ma la Yasa'u al-Tabiba Jahlahu*" (What a physician cannot afford to ignore).

> 1. A physician must not be conceited; he should know that the actual healer is God.
> 2. He should praise his teachers and professor and return thanks to them for their kindnesses.

[45] Bird (1989), pp. 42–43, Kottek et al. (1978), Kottek (1993), Levin (1973), and Rosner (1977–1995).

3. He should never slander another physician. The fault of others should occasion the recognition of his own fault, not be the occasion for pride and conceit.
4. He must speak to patients with civility and good humor and never get angry at the misbehavior and insults of patients.
5. He must protect the patients' secrets and not betray them, especially to those the patients do not want to know.
6. In the case of the transmission of disease, the physician must not turn the second patient against the first.
7. He must be energetic in studying diseases and drugs and earnest in the diagnosis and treatment of a patient or disease.
8. He must never be tenacious in his opinion, and continue in his fault or mistake but, if it is possible, he is to consult with proficient physicians and ascertain the facts.
9. If someone mentions a useless or wrong idea, he must not turn it down definitely but say politely, "Maybe it is true in some cases but, in my opinion, in this case it is more probably such and such."
10. If a prior physician has a better knowledge of a patient or disease, he has to encourage the patient to return to the first physician.
11. If he is not successful in the treatment of a case or if he has found the patient did not have confidence in his work or that the patient would like to refer to another physician, it is better to offer an excuse and ask him to consult another physician.
12. He must not be prejudiced against any method of treatment and never continue any wrong practice.
13. In the treatment of disease, he must begin with simple medicine and not recommend any drug as long as the nature of the disease is resistant to it and it would not be effective.
14. If a patient has several diseases, first of all he has to cure the main disease which may be the cause of complications.
15. He should never recommend any kind of fatal, harmful or enfeebling drugs; he has to know that as a physician he has to do what is conducive to the patient's temperament, and temperament itself is an efficient corrector and protector of the body, not fatal or destructive.
16. He must not be proud of his class or his family and must not regard others with contempt.
17. He must not withhold medical knowledge; he should teach it to everyone in medicine without any discrimination between poor or rich, noble or slave.
18. He must not hold his students or his patients under his obligation.
19. He must be content, grateful, generous and magnanimous, and never be covetous, greedy, ravenous or jealous.

20. He must never covet another's property. If someone offers him a present while he himself is in need of it, he must not accept it.
21. He must never claim that he can cure an impoverished patient who has gone to many physicians, and should not jeopardize his own reputation.
22. He should never be gluttonous and become involved in pleasure-seeking, buffoonery, drinking, and other sins.
23. He must not look upon women with lust but must look at them as he looks at his daughter, sister, or mother.

(Encyclopedia of Bioethics)

The Islamic Perspective

Faced with the disease, a fundamental principle is the emphasis on finding a cure. This comes from a saying of Muhammad:

"There is no disease that God created, for which there is not also its treatment" and furthermore, in another context, he also said: "... seek treatment, because God the Most High did not create a disease for which he has not created a treatment, except for senility."[46]

When a Muslim doctor is making a decision about patient care, that decision should be in the best interest of the patient, both Muslim and non-Muslim. Furthermore, that decision must not be based only on one's own knowledge and experience, but must consider Islamic teaching in this regard, without imposing his religious opinion on the patient.

In relation also to the Adab al-Tabib of Al-Ruhawi who declared: "One must train oneself to use good morals and actions with compassion, mercy, gentleness, chastity, courage, generosity, justice," Islam puts great emphasis on the sanctity of life and the reality of death.

The Koran sets out some principles for which both the Hippocratic Oath and the Doctor's Oath (Geneva Declaration, 1948) were considered unsatisfactory in Muslim circles, because:

- The first refers to a multiplicity of divinities, clearly in contrast with the principle of unity of Islam;
- The second absolutely lacks references to God who is the source of all disease and healing.[47]

[46] Wakim (1944), Reich (1995), and Spinsanti (1985).

[47] Guzzo (2016) and Schacht (1995).

While Islam places importance on saving life (with medical or other treatment), it clarifies that death is a part of the contract (with God) and the final decision (of its term) is God's alone.

In this regard, Muslim jurists have classified the acts according to their morality. Medical interventions may be distinguished:

- mandatory
- desirable and recommended
- permissible and not encouraged, nor discouraged and also those improper, undesirable, illicit, bad by nature.

The Law of God, as such, remains unknown to men and is based on four sources, of which the first three are considered of divine origin: the Koran, the Sunna or Tradition, the Consent of the learned, definitively collected and codified within the nineth century and analogical reasoning (solutions elaborated by medieval jurists). The Koran and the Sunna have no direct references to medicine in the strict sense; however, medieval Islamic scholars who dealt with medicine have tried to deduce a series of hygienic precepts of folk medicine, which are classified under the label of "prophetic medicine."

The Koran is a divine word, "made to descend by God" to the prophet Mohammed between 609–610 and 632 and does not include a term that renders the concept of "ethics." This is confirmed by the use of the expression "ethics of biology" in the Arabic translation. Ethics is not perceived as an independent discipline based on its own principles, but as a "budding of law."

Islamic law gives precedence to the collective need for respect for morality and modesty, considered a guarantee of public order and social stability, with respect to the individual need for care. According to Islamic law, whenever collective and private interests collide, it is the latter that yields; the opposite is true for Western bioethics.

More Critical Remarks

Ethics began to develop in the field of Islamic medicine, with the collection of materials on medical ethics and with the main purpose of increasing help and commitment to the sick, under the aegis of the help and assistance of Allah. Medical ethics was mainly based on the three sources of the Sacred Law, already cited above (The Koran, the Sunnah and the Ijtihad).

Two main virtues have relevance to the field of medicine, both of which constitute two major principles of Islamic ethics, to wit, God-consciousness (*taqwá*) and mercy (*rahmah*).

Sharia (the Law) is evidenced through the following aspects:

- Ethics (akhlāq) and Creed (aqīdah) with the main objectives of protecting (*hifz*) the so-called five necessities, namely religion, life, offspring, intellect, and

wealth. Moreover there are "*commandments*": justice, beneficence, maintaining ties of kinship, keeping promises, honoring trusts, forgiveness, avoiding ignorance, repaying evil with benevolence, fearing only God, patience, gratitude, honesty, and seeking closeness to God through all good deeds; and "*prohibitions*": vice, maleficence, oppression, speaking without knowledge, engaging in fraud and duplicity, corruption, adultery, murder, infanticide, harming others, assaulting animals, committing obscenities, and violating honor.
- Abundant Texts and Expansive Ethical Discussions;
- The Harmony between Ethics and Religion;
- Comprehensive Moral Principles.

God-Consciousness is the Source of Ethics and the objectives of medicine can be summarized as the protection of life, offspring, and intellect, which are three of the objectives of Sharia. However, it must be noted that the protection of these three shared objectives also serves in the protection of religion and wealth.

The following ethical principles serve as a summative outline:

(a) The purpose and mission of medicine should be promotion of the physical, mental, and psychological health of all persons.
(b) The main, essential objectives of medicine intersect with three of the objectives of Sharia; namely, preserving life, preserving offspring, and preserving intellect.
(c) The two ethics, God-consciousness and mercy, are essential ethical principles for those professionals entrusted with the protection of people's lives and with maintaining public and private health for society and individuals.

1. The foundation of Islamic medical ethics is having a "good character," an attitude that historically took shape gradually from the seventh century and was finally established by the eleventh century It was formed from an amalgamation of the teachings of the Koran, the Sunnah of Muhammad as well as the precedents of Islamic jurists (see al-*Shari'a* and *Fiqh*), the pre-Islamic Arab tradition and non-Arab elements (among which Persian and Greek).
2. Chapter 17 of the Koran provides a series of moral provisions (Moral Commandments) which are "among the precepts of wisdom and which are ten in number."

These resemble the ten commandments of the Bible and "represent the most complete statement of the code of conduct that every Muslim must follow":

1. Worship Allah alone (17:22)
2. Be kind, respectful, and humble to your parents (7:23; 17:24)
3. Do not be stingy or wasteful in your shopping (17:26; 17:27; 17:28 and 17:29)
4. Do not engage in "pitiful murders" (17:31)

5. Do not commit adultery (17:32)
6. Do not kill unjustly (17:33)
7. Take care of orphaned children (17:34)
8. Keep your promises (17:34)
9. Be honest and fair in your interactions with others (17:35)
10. Don't be arrogant in your statements or beliefs (17:36; 17:37)

3. The five guiding principles of Islamic Law are:
   - Maintenance of life
   - Protection of an individual's freedom of belief
   - Maintenance of the intellect
   - Preservation of honor and integrity
   - Property protection

Almost all Arab medical books have since then contained a chapter or section relating to medical ethics that subsequently has evolved over time, referring to guidelines regarding ethical or moral problems that concern the life of man. Islamic medical ethics seems to have had considerable influences for the initiation and development of the European one in many aspects, improving moral values. The standards on various topics related to medical ethics, as drawn up in the nineth and eleventh centuries and can be listed as outlined below:

- What your doctor should avoid and what they should guard against
- Visitor behavior
- Treatment of remedies by the doctor
- Dignity of the medical profession
- Examination of doctors
- Removal of corruption among doctors

Among the best achievements of the new Arab culture: The first Islamic jurists introduced a series of concepts that anticipated modern ones: to name a few, moral bodies, brotherhood and social solidarity, human dignity and work, the idea of an ideal law, the condemnation of antisocial behavior, the presumption of innocence, assistance to those in difficulty, care, commercial integrity, freedom from usury, women's rights, privacy, abuse of rights, personal legal status, individual freedom, equality before the law, the supremacy of the law, judicial impartiality, tolerance and democratic participation.

Many of these concepts were later adopted in medieval Europe and effectively benefited Western medicine.[48]

---

[48]Aboukleish (1979), Amine and El Kadi (1988), Bird (1989), pp. 31–32, Cattermole (2006), Filosa (2007), Majeed (2005), Masoud and Masoud (2006), Urquhart (2006), and Peel (2005).

1. The development of efficient hospitals in Baghdad, Cairo, Fez and Damascus, for the care of the sick
2. Medical and surgical information from Muslim doctors.
3. Muslim doctors have placed a lot of emphasis on ethical principles in their practice: a large number of their books have been used for the purpose of medical ethics.
4. Already in the ninth century Abu al-Hasan Ali ibn-e Raban Tabari wrote the first codes of ethics worldwide, regarding the personal characteristics of the doctor, his commitment to patients, to the community and also his obligations towards of his colleagues and his assistants.
5. Rhazes rigorously committed himself to the ethical principles of the physician
6. Ali al-Ruhawi, a Christian who embraced Islam, faced the problems of responsibility and other ethical dilemmas in doctor-patient relationships; what the doctor must avoid and regarding the customs of visitors, medical art for the moral values of the people and harmful habits.
7. The medical recommendations of Ali Ibn Abbas Ahwazi (Haly Abbas), highlighted the ethical recommendations of medicine, particularly in the field of human rights.

Islamic Code of Medical Ethics, 1981

The Doctor's Oath, 2005, Kuwait

The 11 sections of the Code of Islamic medical ethics[49] were indicated in 1981, at the First International Conference on Islamic Medicine in Kuwait. The Islamic Code of medical ethics has been divided into the following chapters:

1. Definition of the medical profession
2. Characteristics of the Doctor
3. The Doctor and his colleagues
4. The doctor and his patient
5. Professional secrecy
6. The role of the doctor in times of war
7. The Sacredness of Human Life
8. Liability and Warranty
9. The doctor and society
10. The physician and modern biomedical advances
11. Doctor's instruction

[49] Avato (1984), Hatout (1983), Islamic Code of Medical Ethics Kuwait Document (2004), and WHO (2005).

A further chapter (12th) concerns the Muslim Physician's Oath:

> I swear to God ... The Great,
> To consider God in the execution of my profession
> To protect human life at all stages and in all circumstances, doing my utmost to save it from death, disease, pain and anxiety
> To maintain people's dignity, cover up their confidences, keep their secrets safe
> To be, always, an instrument of God's mercy, extending my medical assistance near and far, to a virtuous or sinful person, to friend or foe

The hope was agreed that every Muslim physician would "find the guiding light to maintain his professional conduct within the confines of Islamic teachings."[50]

Like other Muslim medical ethics texts, the Code is based on passages from the Koran and demonstrates a explicitly religious, even more so than most contemporary Judeo-Christian Medical Ethics directives. The individual points were resumed and expanded in the USA, in 2017, as follows:

> To fight in the pursuit of knowledge and exploit it for the good but not to the detriment of humanity To revere my teacher, teach my pupil and be fraternal with the members of the medical profession, together with piety and charity
> To live my faith in private and in public, avoiding any malfunction in the eyes of God, his Apostle and my faithful companion.
> And God be a witness to this Oath.[50]

Character of The Doctor

The characteristics of the Islamic doctor must adhere to what is stated by the "International Organization of Islamic Medicine" and are summarized and simplified below for the essential points. The Islamic doctor must have the following characteristics:

- The doctor is truthful whenever he speaks, writes, or testifies. He must be invincible to the dictates of faith, creed, friendship or authority towards pressure to make a statement or testimony that he knows to be false. Witnessing is a grave responsibility in Islam. The Prophet once asked his companions. "Will I tell you about the gravest sins?" When they said yes, he said "Boasting of God's company, wronging one's parents" and, after a short pause, repeatedly said "indeed the gift of bearing false opinions or false testimony".

[50] Code of Ethics Kuwait University (2002).
Filosa (2017), Nanji (1991), and Sonn (1996).

- The physician should have a minimal knowledge of the law, worship and essential elements of Islamic jurisprudence, so that he is allowed to advise patients seeking his guidance on health and body conditions by being aware of the cult rites. Men and women are prone to symptoms, ailments or biological situations such as pregnancy and wish to know the religious ruling regarding prayer, fasting, pilgrimage, family planning, etc.
- Even if "necessity replaces prohibition", the Muslim doctor, however, should spare no effort to avoid resorting to drugs or therapeutic modalities that are surgical, medical or behavioral and which are forbidden by Islam.
- The physician's role is that of a catalyst through which God, the Creator, works to preserve life and health. It is only a tool of God to alleviate people's diseases. To be so designated, the physician must be grateful and always seeking God's help. He must be modest, free from arrogance and pride, and never fall into boasting or glorifying himself, with words, writing or announcements. direct or devious.
- The doctor must strive to keep abreast of scientific progress and innovation. His zeal, complacency and knowledge or ignorance weigh directly on the health and well-being of his patients. Responsibility for others should limit his freedom to waste his time. Since the poor and needy have a recognized right to the money of those who are capable, so patients own a part of the time that the doctor spends studying and following the progress of medicine.
- The doctor must also know that the pursuit of knowledge has a double indication in Islam. Apart from the therapeutic application aspect, the pursuit of knowledge is itself worshiping, according to the guidance of the Koran, "And saying: My Lord, make me progress in knowledge" and "among his worshipers: the educated person fears".
- And "God will make the ranks of those of you who have believed and those of you who have received knowledge grow."[51]

The Patient

(The following text was extracted from the writings of Prof. Mahmoud Abu-Saud, co-founder of the "American Muslim Council" and Dr. Hasan Ghaznawi and Shahid Athar, of Islam-USA)

The condition of man, as regards ethics, is determined by the following principles:

1. man is respected
2. every human being has the right to live; his life is respected and protected
3. equity is considered in religion as an indispensable value
4. doing good is one of the fundamental values prescribed by God
5. no harm must be done.

[51] Code of Ethics Kuwait University (2002) and Filosa (2017).

> Health is a right of every human being, without any discrimination based on race, sex or religion; the assistance provided by the Islamic State begins with the birth and continues with the services of the nursing care to ensure a healthy life into old age; no sick, paralyzed or injured person will be deprived of adequate care.

The Islamic vision of ethics in the medical profession and the publication of the "Code of Ethics in the Medicine and Islamic Health" (see Footnote 51) includes the doctor's ethics, medical obligations toward patients and the community and colleagues, professional secrecy, the institution and the profession, the rights of doctors, social issues toward other patients, transmissible diseases HIV/AIDS, euthanasia, abortion, organ transplantation, violence, advertising and information.

In addition, the international ethical guidelines for the biomedical research involves human subjects and the multiple ethical relationships, according to Islamic morality, following the developments in medicine, such as: human breast milk banks; sex control of the embryo; human, animal and plant cloning; in-vitro children (in vitro fertilization and embryo transfer); surgical sterilization; abortion; visualization of the genitals of the opposite sex for an exam; the beginning of life in man and death; brain death; the inconsistency between regulations and Islamic law; human cadaveric organs, their transport e the transplant; sex change; the minimum and maximum duration of pregnancy; the menstruation and the puerperium; senility and the rights of the elderly; drug and alcohol addiction; infection from HIV/AIDS; prohibitions for impure materials in food and drugs; contemporary medical practices with foods and drinks that can break the fast; reading the human genome and his legal impact; genetic engineering and its impact on humans and nutrition; family genetic education; rights and obligations toward mentally and disabled patients misfits; legal adaptation of medical and life sciences, etc.

The Islamic Oath[52]

The Muslim doctor's oath, taken from the Koran, according to the "Islamic Medical Association" (IMA) of North America, was officially presented and adopted at the IX Annual Convention, at Newark, N.J. in 1977. It was formulated in English and Arabic.

> *Praise to Allah, the Master, the One, Majesty of Heaven, the Exalted, the Glorious, Glory to Him, the Being eternal who created the Universe and all creatures inside and the only Being it contains infinity and eternity. We serve no other God besides you and we consider idolatry asan abominable injustice.*
>
> *Give us sincerity, honesty, modesty and mercy for achieve goals.*

[52] Islamic Medical Association of North America (1977).

Give us the strength to admit our mistakes, to change oursbehaviors according to the tasks assigned to us and to forgive the wrongs of others.Give us the wisdom to bring comfort and advice to all and to preserve peace and harmony.

Make us aware that our sacred profession is concerned with the precious gifts of life and

of the intellect. Therefore safeguard our dignity with honor and piety, in order to dedicate the

our life at the service of humanity; be it poor or rich, wise or illiterate, Muslim or not, black or white.

Give us patience, tolerance, virtue, respect, knowledge and vigilance, with your love in our hearts and compassion for your servants.

We swear this oath in Your name, Creator of all heavens and earth, and we will follow your advice, as you revealed it to the Prophet Mohammed. If you take the life of another human being, it is as if the whole of humanity were killed. If you save a human life, it is as if all humanity be saved.

I undertake to:

- be the instrument of Your Will and Mercy and, in all humility, exercise justice, love and compassion for all of Your creatures;
- extend my hand to the service of all, rich and poor, friends and enemies, regardless of race, religion or color;
- consider human life as a precious and sacred gift, to protect and honor it at all times and in all circumstances in accordance with your law;
- do my best to relieve pain and misery, to comfort and counsel human beings in the resulting illness and worries;
- respect the trust and keep the secrets of all my patients;
- maintain the dignity of health care and honor teachers, students and members of my profession;
- find in the knowledge of your name the good for humanity in support of its dignity;
- have the courage to admit my mistakes and forgive those of others;
- always be aware of my duties towards Allah and His Messenger; and follow their precepts in the public and private sphere;
- Allah grant me strength, patience and dedication to always be faithful to my Oath.

Moreover, each doctor is required to observe the following "Prayer" after taking the oath.

Some highly comparable versions of the Oath have been transcribed.

Below there is another one, quite similar to the previous one and highly significant.

Praise to Allah, the Master, the One, the Majesty of Heaven, the Master, the Glorious, the Glory for Him, the Eternal who created the Universe and all creatures and the only Being who contained the infinity and eternity. We do not serve any god other than You and we consider idolatry as an abominable injustice. Let us equip ourselves with the strength to be truthful, honest, modest, merciful and objective.

Give us the strength of mind to admit our mistakes, change our ways and forgive the sins of others. Give us the wisdom to comfort and advise everyone towards peace and harmony.

Give us the understanding that ours is a sacred profession that deals with your most precious gifts in life and the intellect.

Therefore, make us worthy of this favorable situation with honor, dignity and piety so that we can dedicate our lives to serve humanity, poor or rich, literate or illiterate, Muslim or non-Muslim, in black or white with patience and tolerance with virtue and respect, with knowledge and vigilance, with your love in our hearts and compassion for your servants, your most precious creation.

We take this oath in your name, Creator of all Heaven and earth and follow your advice, as you revealed to the Prophet Mohammed. [Medical oath officially adopted by I.M.A. (Islamic Medical Association) in the United States, 1977]

Turkey (3)

Turkish medicine and its ethics bear the marks of a long history. The ethics of Turkish medicine was formed from Islamic morality, Turkish customs and Hippocratic ideas inherited from Greek medicine. An important milestone was the formulation of the Islamic Code of Medical Ethics (IOMS, 1981), ratified by the First International Conference on Islamic Medicine (Kuwait, 1981) and approved by many Arab and Islamic countries.[53] Despite the differences in the time devoted to teaching, methodology, and course content, Medical Ethics has become a fundamental part of medical education all over the world. In Turkey, education on medical ethics is given both at undergraduate and postgraduate level.[54]

The medical school of the University of Ankara was the first medical school opened after the establishment of the Turkish Republic in 1945.

[53] Medical Ethics, History of the Near and Middle East: III (2004).

[54] Ekmekçi (2016).

The number of medical schools rose from 19 in 1980 to 74 in 2010. In 2010, only 33 of all medical schools could set up a separate department dedicated to Medical Ethics. The increase in the number of medical laboratories has raised concerns about quality and created the need to standardize medical education. Recently, the evolution of the concept of medical ethics has created the need for its teaching. The National Core Education Program refers to medical ethics and states that "one of the objectives of medical university education is to incorporate human and professional values in students and allow them to carry out their profession in line with ethical values."

In Turkish medical schools, medical ethics and medical history studies are brought together in the same Department called "History of Medicine and Ethics."

The course of study includes the following topics:

- Concepts of ethics, bioethics, medical ethics
- Basic ethical theories
- Principles of Medical Ethics
- Paternalism, informed consent and respect for autonomy
- Ethical dilemmas and ethical decision making
- Confidentiality and patient privacy
- Relations with patients

Islamic Bioethics

The medical world would be a much simpler place if a universal bioethics were established through first principles or with only informed consent.[55] Islamic bioethics is closely linked to the general ethical teachings of the Holy Koran and to the tradition of the Prophet Mohammed and therefore to the interpretation of Islamic law.

All Islamic bioethics and the resulting regulations conform to Islamic law and its ethics.

The terms "bioethics" and "medical ethics" are used together with the moral structures surrounding the use and research of medicine and biology. Islamic bioethics emphasizes the importance of preventing disease.

In Islam, human life is considered a priceless gift from God and therefore must be respected and protected.[56]

This is evident in many Koranic verses (or ayat). Within Islamic bioethics there are two fundamental principles that guarantee the preservation of the sanctity of human life:

[55] Weber (2010).

[56] Shomali (2008).

1. Saving a life is mandatory;
2. The unjustified taking of a life is classified as murder and therefore prohibited. Although Muslims recognize and argue that Allah is the ultimate source of life (Koran 2: 258), the Koran illustrates that God instructed them in reason, free will, the ability to distinguish between what is morally acceptable and what is unacceptable (Koran 91: 8) while also providing the provisions of the nature (Koran 45:13).

With these things, Muslims are held accountable for maintaining health and preventing disease. In case the disease does occur, Muslims are obliged to seek medical treatment in an appropriate and Islamic-acceptable manner. The principles of bioethics in the Western world were first developed and described by two American philosophers and bioethics.

[Tom Beauchamp and James F. Childress, in their book Principles of Biomedical Ethics (Already cited. 1995].

These principles have been legitimized by Muslim jurists and have also been supported by Koranic verses.

The fundamental basis of Islamic bioethics is that all decisions and actions must be in accordance with the *Shari'a*.

It does not only concern crimes and penalties (which as such can also include corporal punishment, whipping, amputation or blindness, in addition to the death penalty), but all the behavior of the Muslim.

It is divided into four sectors, covering various moments in life:

1. *Fard* (obligatory), relating to the five prayer breaks during the day, to the pilgrimage to Mecca to be carried out at least once in a lifetime, to alms to the poor, to the Ramadan fasting.
2. *Mustahabb* (recommended) informs about male circumcision.
3. *Makruh* (not recommended) who is not criminally prosecuted, but simply deplored by the community.
4. *Hara-am* (explicitly prohibited): In addition to crimes and offenses, it includes behavioral rules relating to clothing and nutrition.

By evaluating the issues from an ethical and legal point of view, jurists can issue decrees or "*fatwas*" regarding the admissibility of the subject. Any rule that has not been explicitly indicated in religious texts or formulated by jurists is referred to as "*bid'ah*" (innovation) and, if the case, "*haram*" (inadmissible).

The concept of bioethical principles was considered as a purely "Western" innovation, absent in the Islamic health system. The bioethical principles of Autonomy, Benefit, Non-maleficence, and Justice have been legitimized by Muslim jurists as falling within the sphere of Islamic law and have also been supported by verses from the Koran (Koran 3: 104, 16:90 and 17:70). They subsequently became the founding spirit behind the "Muslim Physician's Oath."

References

Aboukleish E. Contributions of Islam to medicine. Islamic medicine. J Islamic Med Assoc North Am. Athar S, editor. 10 (3&4). 1979.

Ahmad W. Medical ethic, Islamic perspective. JIMA. 2005;37:64–6.

Aksoy S. The religious tradition of Ishaq ibn Ali al-Ruhawi: the author of the first medical ethics book in Islamic medicine. JISHIM. 2004;3:9–11.

Amine ARC, El Kadi A. Islamic code of medical professional ethics. JIMA. 1988;20:19.

Amundsen DW. Medicina e religione nella tradizione occidentale, in Enciclopedia delle religioni (IT: Medicine and religion in the Western tradition, in Encyclopedia of religions). Milano; 1996. p. 358.

Amundsen DW, Ferngren GB. Medicine and religion: pre-Christian antiquity. In: Marty ME, Vaux KL, editors. Health/medicine and the faith traditions: an inquiry into religion and medicine. Philadelphia: Fortress; 1982. p. 53–92.

Arawi TA. The Muslim physician and the ethics of medicine. J IMA. 2010;42(3):111–6.

Ardalan M, Khodadoust K, Mostafidi E. A review of Ferdous al-Hekma fil-Tibb by Ali ibn Raban Tabari. J Med Ethics Hist Med. 2015;8:7.

Athar S, Fadel HE. Islamic medical ethics: the IMANA perspective, IMANA Ethics Committee. JIMA. 2005;37:33–42.

Avato FDM. Codice Islamico di Etica Medica (IT. Islamic code of medical ethics). Riv Ital Med Legale: 1177–1191; 1984.

Ben-Tov A. Knowledge and religion in early modern Europe: studies in honour of Michael Heyd. In: Ben-Tov A, editor, vol. 219. University of Erfurt, Yaacov Deutsch, David Yellin College, and Tamar Herzig, Tel Aviv University. Brill; 2013. p. 95–7.

Bird LP. Medical ethics. In: Bird L, Barlow J, editors. Oaths & prayers, an anthology. Richardson, TX: Christian Medical & Dental Society; 1989. p. 1–15.

Castiglioni A. History of medicine. A. Mondadori Ed; 1946. p. 7–11.

Cattermole GN. How Islam changed medicine: Al-Nafis, Servetus, and Colombo. BMJ. 2006;332(7533):120-C.

Code of Ethics Kuwait University. Accredited by the board of the University of Kuwait on 6/18/2002.

Cosmacini G. Medicina e mondo ebraico. Dalla Bibbia al secolo dei ghetti (IT. Medicine and the Jewish world. From the Bible to the century of the ghettos). Laterza ed; 2001. p. 37–41.

Dunn PM. Maimonides (1135–1204) and his philosophy of medicine. Arch Dis Child Fetal Neonatal Ed. 1998;79:F227.

Eisenberg D. Why Jewish medical ethics: an introduction to the system of Jewish law. Aish.com; 2017.

Eiseneberg D. Jewish medical ethics: the role of a physician in Jewish law. Jewish Virtual Library; May 14, 2017.

Ekmekçi PE. Medical ethics education in Turkey; state of play and challenges. Int Online J Educ Teach. 2016;3(1):54–63.

Ferngren GB. The Imago Dei and the sanctity of life; the origins of an idea. In: Euthanasia and the newborn: conflicts regarding saving lives; 1987. p. 23–45.

Filippi L. Lectio Magistralis, Feb…2, 2007 in Trento, by Istituto Trentino di Cultura, all'inaugurazione AA 2006–2007; Corso Superiore di Scienze Religiose; da: Jakobowits I. Ebraismo. In: Spinsanti S, editor. Bioetica e grandi religioni. Milano; 1987. p. 25.

Filosa AM. Rapporto medico-paziente e consenso arabo musulmano. (IT. Doctor-patient relationship and Muslim Arab consent). Diritto e Diritti; 2001. p. 1–8.

Filosa AM. Rapporto medico-paziente e consenso arabo musulmano (IT. Doctor-patient relationship and Muslim Arab consent) OverLex. Portale giuridico. 2007.

Filosa AM. Norme ed Islam, quale integrazione? (IT: Norms and Islam, which integration?) Diritto.it. 2016. (Enciclopedia Treccani on line. Westfalia treaty).

Filosa AM. Atto chirurgico e responsabilità del medico nei confronti del paziente arabo—musulmano, (IT: Surgical act and doctor's responsibility towards the Arab—Muslim patient); 28 Nov 2017.
Frank JB. Moses Maimonides: rabbi of medicine. Yale J Biol Med. 1981;54:79–88.
Freedman B. Duty and healing: foundations of a Jewish bioethic (Introduction). New York: Routledge; 1999. p. 31–44.
Galbi D. Asaph brought professional medicine into ancient Jewish life. Purple Motes. 25 Mar 2012.
Gatrad AR, Sheikh A. Medical ethics and Islam: principles and practice. Arch Dis Child. 2001;84:72–5.
Gesundheit B. Maimonides' appreciation for medicine. Rambam Maimonides Med J. 2011;2(1).
Gesundheit B, Hadad E. Maimonides (1138–1204): rabbi, physician and philosopher. IMAJ. 2005;7:547–53.
Guidi M. Hunain ibn Ishaq. Enciclopedia Italiana Treccani; 1933.
Guzzo LM. Note sui diritti umani nella prospettiva islamica (IT. Notes on human rights from an Islamic perspective). Ordines. 2016;1:72–107.
Haleem MA. Medical ethics in Islam. In: Grubb A, editor. Choices and decisions in health care. Wiley; 1993. p. 1–20.
Halevi HYBB-T, Lavine JB. The thirteen principles of Jewish medical ethics. April 15, 2008.
Halperin M. Milestones in Jewish medical ethics. Medical-Halachic literature in Israel, 1948–1998. ASSIA Jewish Med Ethics. 2004;VI(2):4–19.
Hatout H. Topics in Islamic medicine. Kuwait University; 1983.
Islamic Code of Medical Ethics Kuwait Document. Encyclopedia of bioethics. The Gale Group Inc.; 2004.
Islamic Medical Association of North America. The oath of a Muslim physician. Officially adopted by I.M.A. in 1977.
Jakobovitz I. Sir, Jewish medical ethics—a brief overview. J Med Ethics. 1983;9:109–12.
Javanbakht M. Ali ibn Abbas alMajusi and medical ethics. Tanaffos J. 2010;9(1)
Kinzbrunner BM. Jewish medical ethics and end-of-life care. J Palliat Med. 2004;7(4):558–73.
Kottek SS. Medical prayers and oaths in Jewish lore. Isr J Med Sci. 1993;29(1):75.
Kottek SS, Leibowitz JO, Richler B. A Hebrew paraphrase of the Hippocratic oath. Med Hist. 1978;22:438–45.
Larijani B, Zahedi F. An introductory on medical ethics history in different era in Iran. BARU. 2006;Suppl 1.1:10–6.
Lavine J. Jewish Medicine, Copyright November 29, 2016.
Levey M. Etica Medica dell'Islam medievale con particolare riferimento a "Etica pratica del medico" di Al-Ruhawi. (IT. Medical Ethics of Medieval Islam with particular reference to "Doctor's Practical Ethics by Al-Ruhawi"). Philos Soc. 1967;57(3):1–99.
Levin S. Jewish ethics in relation to medicine. S Afr Med J. 1973;47(21):924–30.
Majeed A. How Islam changed medicine. Medicine and medical ethics in Islamic empire. BMJ. 2005;331(7531):1486–7.
Masoud MT, Masoud F. How Islam changed medicine: Ibn al-Haytham and optics. BMJ. 2006;332(7533):120-a.
McMillan RC, Engelhardt Jr HT, Spicker SF. Dordrecht: Euthanasia and the dignity of dying, University of Navarra Conference, Reidel Edit.; Dordrecht, 1987.
Medical Ethics, History of the Near and Middle East: III. Encyclopedia of bioethics. Turkey: The Gale Group Inc; 2004.
Minkin JS. The world of Moses Maimonides; with selections from his writings. New York: Thomas Yoseloff; 1957.
Muntner S. Hebrew medical ethics and the oath of Asaph. JAMA. 1968;205(13):912–3.
Muntner S. Medicine in ancient Israel. In: Rosner F, editor. Medicine in the Bible & the Talmud. KTAV Publishing House, Inc. Yeshiva University Press; 1995. p. 3–20.
Nanji A. Islamic ethics. In: Singer P, editor. A companion to ethics. Oxford: Blackwell's; 1991. p. 106–18.
Osler W. The evolution of modern medicine; 1913.

Padela A. Islamic medical ethic: a primer. Bioethics. 2007;21(3):169–78.
Peel M. Human rights and medical ethics. J Soc Med. 2005;98(4):171–3.
Pergola R. Ex arabico in latinum: Traduzioni scientifiche e Traduttori nell'occidente medievale. Studi di glottodidattica. 2009;3:74–107.
Pines S. The oath of Asaph the physician and Yohanan Ben Zabda. Its relation to the Hippocratic oath and the Doctrina Duarum Viarum of the Didache. Proc Israel Acad Sci Human. 1975;9:223–64.
Reich WT, editor. Encyclopedia of bioethics, revised edition, vol. 5. New York: Simon & Schuster MacMillan; 1995.
Rispler-Chaim V. Islamic medical ethics in the 20th century. J Med Ethics. 1989;15:203–8.
Rosner F. Medicine in the Bible and in the Talmud. Selections from classical Jewish sources. KTQAV Publishing House, Inc. Yeshiva University Press; 1977–1995. p. 188.
Rosner F. The medical legacy of Moses Maimonides (Chap. 22). KTAV Publishing House Inc. 1998:273–90.
Rosner F. The life of Moses Maimonides, a prominent medieval physician, Einstein. Quart J Biol Med. 2002;19:125–8.
Rosner F, Sussman M. The oath of Asaph. Ann Intern Med. 1965;63(2):317–20.
Rufus Ephesius. Collection des médecins grecs at latins. Paris: Imprimerie nationale; 1879.
Schacht J. Introduzione al diritto musulmano (IT. Introduction to Muslim law), trad. it., Torino; 1995.
Segal E. He didn't have a prayer. On the trails of tradition: explorations of Jewish life and learning paperback. Calgary: Department of Religious Studies, University of Calgary; 2011.
Serour GI. What is it to practice good medical ethics? A Muslim's perspective. J Med Ethics. 2014;41:121–4.
Shomali MA. Islamic bioethics: a general scheme. J Med Ethics Hist Med. 2008;1(1):1–8.
Siegel-Itzkovich J. Maimonides as physician: caring and curing. Jerusalem Post Health Sci. 2013;1:53.
Sonn T. Health and medicine in the Islamic tradition: Fazlur-Rahman's view. JIMA. 1996;28: 189–94.
Spinsanti S. Documenti di Deontologia e Etica Medica. Edizioni Paoline, Cinisello Balsamo; 1985. p. 228(4).
Steinberg A. Medical ethics in an interreligious comparison: Judaism. Ethik in der Medizin. 1998;10:S112–5.
Steinberg A. Jewish medical ethics. Encyclopedia of Jewish medical ethics, English edition, vol. II. Feldheim Pub.; 2003. p. 380–9.
Stokke OMB. The construction of modern Islamic authority: analyzing the medical ethics. Solli, Oslo: Islamic Organization for Medical Sciences, Ed. OK PrintShop; 2014.
Super CW. Ethics as a science. Int J Ethics. 1914;24(3):265–81.
Tabatabai SM. Rhazes's views on medical ethics. J Med Ethics Hist Med. 2008;1(1):10.
Urquhart J. How Islam changed medicine: Ibn sina (Avicenna) saw medicine and surgery as one. BMJ. 2006;332(7533):120-b.
Veatch RM, editor. Cross cultural perspectives in medical ethics. 2nd ed. Boston: Jones and Bartlett Pub.; 2000. p. 240–58.
Wakim KG. Arabic medicine in literature. Bull Med Libr Assoc. 1944;32(1):96–104.
Weber AS. Bioethical reasoning in Islam. Int J Arts Sci. 2010;3(15):607–17.
WHO Islamic code of medical and health ethics. EM/RC52/7 Eastern Mediterranean. September 2005.
Zahedi F. How Islam changed medicine. BMJ. 2005;331:1486.
Zunic L, Karcic E, Masic I. Medical ethics in the medieval Islamic sciences. J Res Pharm Pract. 2014;3(3):75–6.

7 Portugal, Italy, England

Amatus Lusitanus

Sixteenth Century (Portugal)

His real name was João Rodrigues, a marrano (Jew, converted to Christianity), born in Castelo Branco (Portugal) in 1511.[1] He adopted the name of Amatus Lusitanus for religious reasons (Amatus is the Latinization of his surname in Arabic: Chabib). Lusitanus means "from Portugal." He did his preparatory studies for medicine in Salamanca. In local hospitals he also practiced a good surgery. At the age of 18 he was granted a license to practice and was entrusted with the care of patients in two hospitals.

He was a physician, botanist, and multilingual expert and mastered various languages: Portuguese, Latin, Greek, Hebrew, Arabic, Castilian, French, Italian, German, and presumably also English. It seems that he discovered the function of the valves in the bloodstream and the Azigos venous system. He spent the first years of his professional life in Portugal, but fearing to be recognized as a Jew and therefore persecuted, he initially expatriated to the Netherlands and then to Italy, teaching at the University of Ferrara where he also met Francesco Vesalio, brother of the great anatomist Andrew. He mentions his work with him in his *Curationes*, recalling the first time when he saw to dissect a human body. He also exercised his profession in Ancona (1549–1955) and then in Venice, where he looked after Diego Hurtado de Mendoza, the ambassador of Emperor Charles V. In May 1550 he was called to Rome to treat Pope Julius III, with another famous doctor, John Aguilera.

[1] Marrano: An insulting name used by the Spaniards for Muslims and Sephardi Jews in the Iberian peninsula, obliged to adopt the Christian religion, either under coercion as a consequence of the persecution of Jews by the Spanish Inquisition, or for "free" choice, for a question of formality, but they secretly remained faithful to their original religion. Marrano comes from the Spanish (meaning pig) derived from the Arabic ma'ram (forbidden food), like pork.

Schwarz (1925).

R. G. Russo, *Medical Ethics*, https://doi.org/10.1007/978-3-031-42444-1_7

Pope Paul IV, Cardinal Gian Pietro Carafa, the man of the Counter-Reformation and the Inquisition, made his mission a fight against all heresies. He did not tolerate Jews when took up the papal throne. On July 14, 1555 the new pope issues the bull *Cum nimis absurdum* ("Since it is extremely absurd"), in which it places restrictions on the freedoms of Jews and confines them to ghettos. Subsequently, other papal orders reinforced these religious differences and at the end of 1555, Amato moved to Pesaro, and then left Italy in 1556.[2] He settled in the free city-state of the Republic of Ragusa (Dubrovnik) where hygienic and medical practices were well established. In 1559 he joined the local Jewish community in Thessaloniki (Greece).[3] There was a large Jewish community and he could practice Judaism openly and treat Jewish patients.

One of his main books is *Curationum medicium* that was written in Latin and divided into seven "Centuries." Each contains one hundred clinical cases that he has seen. Numbers 6 and 7 report the oath (on God and on the Torah) in which he affirms that all his work is "only to help men." The oath, written after he reverted to Judaism, is one of the most elevated literary documents of medical ethics. At the end of it he recalls and reaffirms the Hippocratic precepts. The Centuries are also a mine of information on medical history of the sixteenth century, on social life and individual biography. He finished his commentary on the work relating to materia medica (medical matters) in 1549 and it was published in Venice in 1553 with the title *In Enarrationes Dioscoridis*. He gave the names of flora and fauna in Greek, Latin, Italian and Arabic, and sometimes in French and German as well; this work is among the first ever published on *materia medica* and earned him an international reputation.

Amatus Lusitanus was struck by the plague that raged in Thessaloniki and died on January 21, 1568.

He may be considered as a precursor of initiation of tolerance in European medical ethics that he anticipated with his "Oath" which includes also other aspects of medical ethics that are completely organic to the very personality of author and distinguish themselves by courage and novelty for its time.

To mention reward of physician for one's labor, difficulties and hardships falling on representatives of medical profession, theme of glorification and exaltation of physician and medical tolerance.

The Oath of Amatus was published in 1561. It owed much to the special conditions existing in Thessaloniki where a new scientific perspective was added to the ethical foundations of medicine. Below is the version of one of his writings, dated 1559,[4] translated (by me) into English.

[2] Leibowitz (1952) and Nardi (1960).

[3] Gershon Lewental (2015) and Durrigl and Fatovic-Ferencic (2002).

[4] Amatus Lusitani (1560) and Friedenwald (1917).

I swear by the immortal God and by his most Holy Ten Commandments, received on Mount Sinai by Moses, after having freed the people from slavery in Egypt, that, in all the things handed down by me to posterity, nothing has ever been real. In some cases, with perseverance and strong will, I refused offers of money; added, or changed, for simple ornament. more eager for the sick to regain their lost health through my work and diligence. This one thing I have always aimed for—to be useful to mortals; in praise as in than to become rich. I have always valued men of any religion the same way—blame, I was not a slave to passions, but always aimed to study the truth; and if I Jews, Christians and Arabs. try to deceive you with such words, God and his minister Raffaele will always be in predicting the course of a disease I have always told the family what I felt in my adversaries. As for the pay given to doctors, I did not want to seem greedy, my soul. always caring for the poor with the same diligence with which I treat the rich. Among pharmacists I favored only those who stood out for their skill in art and goodness of heart.

In prescribing medicines I always took account of the patient's assets. I have never revealed to anyone the secrets entrusted to me nor have I given any harmful drink.

Finally, I never did anything in my work unworthy of a distinguished doctor, having always tried to imitate Hippocrates and Galen, the Fathers, by carefully reading the best writings. suffered the exile, which is not what a philosopher deserves, and I bore it with a strong heart. I had many disciples, to this day; I always treated them like my own children; I taught them conscientiously, exhorting them to follow the best examples. Not from an ambitious spirit was I motivated to publish my writings, which deal with the medical art, but I only had the aim of benefiting men's health in some way.—Thessaloniki, year 5319 (1559)

He was the first to provide new data on gout and gave useful tips for treating kidney stones and other pathologies. His medical works were printed in Venice, Lyon, Paris, Bordeaux, Barcelona, and Frankfurt; the large number of editions attests to the favor with which they were accepted and disseminated.

As for the medical ethics laid out in his oath after his return to Judaism, this was considered one of the most outstanding documents as it emphasizes the philanthropic side of the art of healing and the need to help the poor and needy. It differs (as other Christian oaths also do) from the professional materialism of the Hippocratic Oath. There are 23 different editions of Amatus's works, but still none fully translated into a modern language.[5]

[5] Friedenwald (1944) and Leibowitz (1960).

Jewish Doctors in Italy

The history of the Jews during the diaspora in Italy was the longest and most continuous. Although Jews in Italy have never been very numerous, their history is of particular interest because it covers a period of over 2000 years. They acquired great distinction in the fields of Hebrew letters and the profession of medicine. It is not known when the Jews began to settle in Rome, perhaps as prisoners of war, as slaves and even probably as traders; references to Jewish doctors in the first centuries of the Christian era are very scarce. Closely intertwined with the history of Italy is that of the Roman Catholic Church which has always had a particular attitude toward Jewish doctors as a whole. From the decree of expulsion of Jews who had not been recognized as citizens, dated 139 B.C., one must assume they had already settled in Rome before then. They developed a commercially and politically important community. At the beginning of the reign of Augustus, over 8000 were already counted in Rome. Nero accused them of having set fire to the city, along with the Christians.

The condition of the Jews has undergone frequent changes. They had been banished and then rehabilitated; they had privileges or restrictions at different times, especially with respect to religious observances. The Romans did not encourage the study of medicine among their citizens and their doctors. Few were natives of Rome; they were mostly Greeks or Oriental, Egyptians, and Jews. The Romans had more faith in foreigners than in the natives, Pliny said.

When Christianity became the state religion under Constantine in 312 A.D., Jews were regarded as second-class citizens. St. Basil (330–379) had not hesitated to take a medicine from a Jew, but St. John Chrysostom of Constantinople, who lived in the second half of the fourth century, protested vigorously against those seeking the help of Jewish doctors and advised Christians, of that time, that "it would be better to die." The law of 438 of Theodosius (Code III) forbade the Jews any public office, including that of the official doctor; this marked the beginning of a long series of legal restrictions, which lasted for many centuries.

In 590 Gregory I became pope, and from that moment the Roman Catholic bishops ruled Rome. Gregory had words and actions of sincere favor toward the Jews and their tradition, especially in Sicily.[6] Nevertheless, the condition of the Jews continued to deteriorate. Many restrictions subsequently inhibited them even from showing themselves in public. The first Jewish doctor mentioned was Sabbato ben Abraham Donnolo, in the tenth century. The general condition of the Jews became even worse during the conflict between popes and emperors (1000–1304).

Their story became a story of humiliation and persecution, prohibitions, and restrictions, put into force, evaded, repealed, and reinforced again.

In 1021 a Jewish persecution took place in Rome, due to the alleged desecration of a sacred image, and Pope Benedict VIII sentenced some Jews to death. Later, Pope Nicholas II, in the eleventh century, condemned the persecutions of the Jews.

Pope Innocent III (1198–1216) was the main instigator of many persecutions suffered by Jews in Rome and in all Christian lands. At the Fourth Lateran

[6] Rizzo (2012).

Ecumenical Council, in 1215, he promulgated a law whereby Jews and Muslims had to wear badges of a special shape and were forbidden to work in public offices. In the Council of Beziers in 1246, after repeating the old laws against usury, against the possession of Christian slaves and against them holding certain offices, they were ordered to wear a round badge and Christians were not allowed to hire Jewish doctors. The spiritual suffering due to "forced" conversion to Catholicism was added to the economic hardship. The numerous harsh restrictive measures also affected the Roman economy. Heavy and unjust taxes, demanded in the years between 1604 and 1658, put the entire community in serious difficulty.

Jews were forbidden to use Christian servants and it was also decreed that a Jew should not operate in any science or art (1620). In 1639 a law prohibited the forced baptism of children under the age of seven. The Jewish population of Rome at that time numbered only 4127 souls; economic and subsistence difficulties induced many to resort to calling for support from the "Jewish Community." In the second half of the seventeenth century, harassment of Jewish doctors started again. This is evident in the story of the plague of 1656, described by Jaacov Zahalon[7] a doctor who worked in the Jewish Lazaret (hospital for infectious patients).

Yaacov Zahalon Ben Isaac

Ben Isaac was born in Rome in 1630 and devoted himself to learning Hebrew and to the study of medicine. He was a rabbi and graduate of the Artium ac Medicinae Medicus in Rome, later earning a high reputation. During the plague of 1656–1657 he was one of the doctors who assisted the sick when the health conditions of the community continued to deteriorate. He was then called to the rabbinate of Ferrara in 1680 and held this position until his death in 1693. He was a prolific writer on medicine, homilies, philosophy, and rabbinic commentaries. His most important medical work Ozar ha-ayyim (Treasure of Life) is in thirteen parts. In the introduction he discussed the religious question whether it was lawful and a duty to treat a sick person with medicine and to resort to mutilation if necessary. We read: "We give thanks to God who has provided us with the drugs by which we can be healed of diseases. If life is decreed for me, I will live; if death is decreed, I will die; anyone who takes his own life is guilty."

He also wrote a "Description of the plague in the ghetto of Rome," Where he stated: "No one was allowed to go out into the street, not even the doctors, except at certain hours, to get food. At night no one is allowed to leave their home." Furthermore: "In some cities there are no doctors, but there is a scholar who is able to understand and study this book closely to seek treatment for the sick. This book will benefit the physician who lives far from a city and also the poor who are unable to pay the bills." Ben Yaacov was the author of the first treatise on Jewish ethics, written in Arabic in 1040, Margaret Toboth (Precious Pearls) is divided into thirty chapters, corresponding to the number of days of the month, with prayers for

[7] Ruderman and Veltri (2004).

various occasions (1665). In his preface Jacob lists the following works he left in the manuscript: Morashah Kehillat Ya'akob, on Maimonides; Yeshu'ot Ya'akob, a comment on Isaiah; Titten Emet le-ya'akob, homilies to the Pentateuch; Zahalah u-Rinnah, on the song of Solomon; Kohelet Ya'akob on Ecclesiastes; Derusim 'al-Daniel about Daniel; Oar ha-Shamayim, on theology and philosophy; and Shubu Elai, on the Shema, a prayer in the Jewish liturgy, and the blessings that accompany it.

He was the author of dissertations on the Hebrew and Mohammedan calendars (Venice, 1594–1595), on the figure of Esther in the Bible and on the *qabbalah* in ethics, in particular on repentance, according to Isaac Luria (1595).[8]

He was also the author of "Oar ha-Hayyim," a medical work in 13 parts.

Zahalon Ben Isaac was often consulted on Halachic questions by his contemporaries and was considered one of the three most educated men of his generation. The conditions of the Jewish community continued to decline: it is described in 1682 as totaling 4500 souls, of few of whom were not very poor. Toward the end of the century the community grew again, reaching 10,000 individuals, but their conditions had not improved. During the plague he was obliged to preach from a window open to the street, in via Catalana, while the synagogue was inaccessible. This was life in Rome in the time of Yacoov Zahalon Ben Isaac. Ben Isaac introduced new elements into Jewish deontological texts, such as:

- The social conscience
- The doctor–patient relationship
- The doctor's duty to study constantly
- Scientific research as a doctor's duty
- Teaching as a doctor's duty
- Correctness and loyalty in relations with colleagues

He laid emphasis on the ethical side of medical practice, reporting what he had already said in Olath Shabbatht in order to specify what was expected of a doctor, to gain the patient's trust:[9]

1. He must be a respected person, of good bearing, in order to enjoy the esteem and approval of the whole population; the patient trusts a God-fearing man.
2. He must be familiar with medical science.
3. He must be a man of experience.
4. He must possess the persuasive capacity to allay the patient's worries.

And added: "Before starting his practice, a doctor should be accompanied by another expert during visits to the sick. He must take note of what his teacher prescribes for the appropriate treatments. He must also carefully study the pathologies found during the visits with the Master, in the medical books. If any doubts arise, he should seek the advice of other doctors. Even if the disease is severe, the doctor

[8] Isaac Ben Solomon Luria (1534–1572) (1972).

[9] Friedenwald (1918, 1922) and Jacobs and Broydé (1906).

should address the patient with encouraging and comforting words. He must not belittle the treatments recommended by other authoritative doctors. Once healing is achieved, the doctor need not make any further visits, but should give useful indications for the patient's independent progress, and how to avoid relapses. The doctor must not sell drugs, but prescribe them appropriately; it is the patient who must send the request to the pharmacist. Should the doctor find that the patient is seriously ill, he has the duty to inform his/her relatives, so as not to be slandered if death should occur, and to invite them to assist the patient adequately.

When the doctor visits women, he must always be respectful and must not indulge in lewd thoughts of any nature. He must not accept compensation from the poor, or from relatives or close friends; he must not ask for or accept compensation for services rendered on Saturdays [sabbath] or during holidays. If the patient is a friend of the doctor's and wishes to repay the treatment received or to be received, he must not resort to expensive gifts, but to simple presents. The rabbis admit remuneration for the time required for visits made for religious duties with the same remuneration as for teachers of the Torah."

A doctor must recite the following at least once a week:[10]

The Doctor's Prayer

> Master of the World, you favored me with your grace and filled me with honors and dignity by allowing me knowledge, albeit only a small part, of medical science. You are the Doctor, I am like clay in your hands. If a sick person consults me, whose hour is approaching the end without hope, Thy will be done and make sure that it is not I who hastens that end. May fraternity, peace and friendship reign between me and other doctors. May Your will be to bless my work and the reward that will be bestowed on me for my effort. May I be economically self-sufficient so I will not need to ask poor people for money. If people honor me for my science, let me not brag about it. Strengthen the patient's ability to communicate with me and help me understand his words...

Medical Ethics: John Gregory (Scotland) and Thomas Percival (England)

Eighteenth to Nineteenth Century

Ethics had already been developed in England with the first writings of Thomas Sydenham (1624, 1689) who inaugurated better ethics in medical practice, but its value and influence did not become evident immediately and it was only applied many years later. He was undoubtedly considered the most representative English exponent of medical science in the seventeenth century and was referred to as "the father of English medicine and the English equivalent of Hippocrates," since he stressed the importance of accurate observation and symptoms.

[10] Levin (1973).

Most historians, however, considered the history of medical ethics as though it coincided with the history of medicine.[11]

> Doctor becomes every person who sets out to help others, taking the following four things seriously:
>
> 1. He must one day account to the Supreme Judge for all the lives entrusted to his care;
> 2. all his skill, knowledge and energy, as they were given to him by God, must be exercised for His glory and for the good of humanity, and not for mere gain or ambition;
> 3. There is nothing more beautiful, truly, than reflecting on having cared for a person because, to give an idea of the value and estimate the greatness of the human race, no less than the Son of God became human and with the nobility of his divine dignity died to redeem mankind;
> 4. The doctor himself is mortal and should be diligent and tender in treating his suffering patients, as he himself may one day be sick too.

Historical Period

Hippocrates' ideal was expanded by doctors such as Sir Thomas Browne (1605–1682), one of the first doctors to write on medical ethics and on the care of the whole person. He was the author of Religio Medici in which he said that "attacks" of disease had a "natural" origin but were backed by the devil and by the malevolence of witches. Among the first general practitioners there were religious men and non-believers who, often unconsciously, continued to follow the principles of Christian ethics.[12]

In the seventeenth and eighteenth centuries, simultaneously with British expansionism, medicine in England began to differ from the European model. The College of Doctors, founded by Henry VIII in 1518, promoted formal education in Oxford and Cambridge only for those who had joined the Church of England.

This created a small group of elite doctors who served the Royal Court and the aristocracy, leaving other citizens and the armed forces to seek professionals of lower standing and cheaper. New medical candidates came mainly from the USA and Canada to meet urgent "staff" requirements. The Scottish Enlightenment and its moralism condemned the self-interest that dominated contemporary life and consequently also medicine.

While many changes were taking place in the field of medicine, in Germany Medical Jurisprudence arose, of medical and forensic teaching, as a new area.[13]

[11] Kottek (1993).

[12] Deewhurst (1962), Jonsen (2000), and Joshi and Poojary (2013).

[13] Ryan (1836).

J. Bohn's Dissertationes Medicinae Forensis developed from writings associating Jurisprudence with medicine, and that attitude continued through the century.

John Gregory

This Scottish physician, born in Aberdeen on 3 June 1724, was also a writer and a moralist. After attending King's College and the University of Aberdeen, in 1742 he moved to Edinburgh where he studied medicine. Gregory continued his studies at Leiden in 1745. In 1746, shortly after graduating, he was appointed professor at King's College. He taught mathematics and moral and natural philosophy. He moved again to Edinburgh in 1764 where he began medical practice. He died on 9 February 1773.[14]

Gregory was an active member of the Aberdeen Philosophical Society, First Physician in Scotland under George III and Fellow of the Faculty of Medicine at the University of Edinburgh. With his colleague William Cullen, he gave a series of lectures on the qualifications and duties of a physician, on the theory and practice of medicine (Observations on the Duties and Office of a Physician, Lectures on the Duties and Qualifications of a Physician), and published them in 1772.

That publication helped establish that medicine was a trust-based profession; he discussed conflicts of interest, both in the doctor–patient relationship and in consultations with other doctors, and laid stress on confidentiality toward patients, especially women, and condemned sexual abuse. He wrote that the truth is often a painful duty for doctors, but absolutely necessary, especially with patients in a terminal phase, where there is also collaboration with the clergy. Gregory's writings have been called "the first philosophical and secular medical ethics in English."[15]

His medical ethics is a blend of modern ideas in this science and the ethics of behavior. He described medical morality in the context of private medical practice and patient care at the Royal Infirmary in Edinburgh. He then focused on the crisis of intellectual and moral confidence of the time. The virtues of compassion, firmness, and tenderness (as expressed by Gregory) referred to some women (known to him) of recognized qualities and virtues, thus reflecting the pre-modern idea of "chivalry in the service of the sick."

Gregory also recommended that the doctor must have kindness and adaptability to put up with the contradictions and disappointments of delays in patient care and in applying the suggested treatments. He warned that if instructions to the patient were too strict or too detailed they would not be followed.

He also maintained, however, that the doctor should not be too severe, otherwise he would not be able to grasp the patient's true state. The prudent physician prescribes a regimen which, while not necessarily always the best, may be the best for the patient to follow.

[14] Bastron and McCullough (2007), Gregory (2008), and Haakonssen (1997).

[15] McCullough (1998a, b, 2006, 2007).

The Profession of Medicine

Gregory worried that medicine was not a trade with priority to the doctor's interests rather than the patient's, thanks to scientific and clinically competent treatment. He said that doctors who pursued personal interest at the expense of the patient "have an interest that is distinct and separate from the honor of science" (see Footnote 15).

Doctors should dress formally, but they should not be pretentious or ostentatious "that can scare pediatric patients"; they should not sanction risky self-treatments but they should not complain if their advice is not followed. Gregory lamented the lack of the moral qualities and intellectual knowledge that should have characterized "good medicine." Treatment of affluent patients often led to excessive, sometimes unnecessary and expensive, care, while treatment of the poor in the infirmaries was often scant. He based his ethical beliefs on compassionate in the care of patients. For a long time his work was ignored; he was considered only an Enlightenment physician with a philosophical profile. He started to gain fame in 1970 when he pointed out the close links between philosophy and medicine. He acquired fame as the "Father of medical ethics" fairly recently.

Gregory criticized the mentality of the medical "guild-like mentality," and of many of his colleagues; this dissent was later shared and openly opposed by his successor, Thomas Percival.

- I now speak of the moral qualities particularly required by a doctor.
- The main of these is humanity—the sensitivity that makes us feel the anguish of our fellow men and which, consequently, spurs us to alleviate their sufferings.
- Compassion leads to continuous attention toward the patient; an attention that money can never buy: hence the great comfort of having a friend as a doctor.

> I remember the moral duties of a doctor that spur him to persuade and to recognize and correct his mistakes. A stubborn attachment to an unsuccessful method of treatment is the cause of great presumption; the certainty of infallibility is hardest cure, as it is generated by ignorance.
>
> This can lead to extremes of distrust and lack of humility.

John Gregory published the lectures to his teachers on Duties and Qualifications of a Doctor in 1772, a year before his death. It was in fact only a draft of a Code of Ethics, which discussed issues such as confidentiality and truthfulness (especially if the prognosis was uncertain), considering the needs of patients and not abandoning desperate or near-death cases.

Thomas Percival

Thomas Percival was born in Warrington, England, in 1740. At 17 he enrolled as a student at Warrington Academy for classical and theological studies. In 1761 he moved to Edinburgh where he graduated in medicine in 1765. The Royal Infirmary asked Percival to help settle an internal dispute at the Manchester Hospital. He became interested in the divisions that had grown up between the various branches of the profession: doctors, surgeons, and pharmacists with their different fields of training (university, hospital, and apprenticeship).

In 1794 he drafted a code of conduct toward patients, initially circulated privately as a book on jurisprudence: "Medical Jurisprudence or a Code of Ethics and Institutes, Adapted to the Professions of Physic and Surgery." He published articles on medicine and science in the Royal Society journal "Philosophical Transactions," between 1767 and 1776, which made him one of the leading men of science.

Percival's experience in medical life in Manchester prompted him to write two pamphlets: "Internal Regulation of Hospitals" in 1771 and "Internal Regulation of Hospitals and other Medical Charities" in 1772. He also wrote "Essays, Medical, Philosophical and Experimental" in 1773. In 1775 he published the first of three parts of "A Father's Instruction," which was completed in the late 1800s. He was interested in using mortality statistics for insurance purposes and wrote "Proposals for establishing more accurate and comprehensive bills of mortality in Manchester."[16] He later resumed the work he had begun in 1794. He changed its title to "Medical Ethics" and published it in 1803. Percival's code affirmed the moral authority and independence of doctors in the service of others and laid stress on individual honor. The expression "Medical Ethics," which was not clearly understood for many millennia, was not expressly coined until 1803, when Thomas Percival introduced it in his book entitled "Medical Ethics": describing the professional duties of doctors and surgeons toward their patients, their fellow practitioners, and ordinary people.

Percival may have also documented himself through the work and lectures John Gregory had taught from the chair of medicine in Edinburgh.

The code was written to respond to problems that arose at the Manchester Hospital Infirmary, where conflicts and disputes between medical staff had caused it to close during an epidemic, thereby jeopardizing the care and health of the patients. He therefore maintained that doctors had a duty to put patients' interests before their own; they were expected to gain public trust through adequate service in hospitals and private practice; to maintain collaborative relationships with apothecaries and ensure the necessary services to the health, judicial, and public authorities. He also forecast that his text would be "followed and shared in the years to come." Thomas Percival died in 1804.

Percival is also known for his writings on occupational health.[17]

The expansion of the textile industry in England at the end of the seventeenth to eighteenth centuries was accompanied by numerous medical and social problems. Thomas Percival became involved in these questions on account of his studies of population structure and attempts to eliminate typhus in Lancashire mills. His observations and conclusions greatly influenced Robert Peel (a Tory politician), so much that he introduced a legislative project to eliminate abuses and improve the health and well-being of factory workers. He published several texts illustrating his

[16] Howard (1975).

[17] Percival (1803, 1849, 1965, 1985, 2014a, b, 2015).

interest in public health: "Essays medical and experimental [Vol. II]" on the following subjects:

> *On the orchis root; On the waters of Buxton and Matlock; On the medicinal uses of fixed air; On the antiseptic and sweetening power of varieties of factitious air; On sea salt; On coffee.*

His proposal was not initially adopted by the British Medical Association when it was founded in 1857. The persistent gap between social classes, between doctors and surgeons, and also between university doctors and apprentices meant that in England the new rules of professional conduct were left to individual morality, rather than being formalized in a code of ethics. It was only in 1858 that the General Medical Council regulated the liability of its members and established the power to "disqualify" from the medical register those who transgressed. Practitioners could not benefit from tax and insurance cover without the special license issued by the Medical Council.

Short and concise summary of the Medical Ethics book:

Medical Ethics: or a code of Institutes and precepts, adapted to the professional conduct of Physicians and Surgeons
Contents—Preface
Origin of the work—Suspension of it—Farther progress of it—Addition of supplementary notes and Illustrations
Chapter I Of professional conduct relative to hospital or other medical charities.
Chapter II Of professional conduct in private or general practice.
Chapter III Of the conduct of physicians to apothecaries.
Chapter IV Of professional duties in certain cases which require a knowledge of law.
A Discourse on Hospital Duties, Notes and Illustrations

Extracts from Dr. Percival's "Medical Ethics"

Here are just some of his essential and novel points (see Footnote 17):

I. Doctors and surgeons must assist the patient, respecting the importance required by their functions. They must be modest and combine gentleness with firmness, humility with authority.
II. Each case entrusted to a doctor or surgeon must be treated with attention, firmness and humanity; some reasonable indulgence may be reserved for cases of mental deficiency.
IV. A doctor must not make gloomy predictions, but may possibly advise the patient's friends about the severity of the disease and, if absolutely necessary, tell the patient himself.

V. If surgery is required, this can be communicated to the patient or his family.
VI. When a patient who calls the doctor has already been treated by another, the doctor should propose consulting the colleague. On such occasions, the clinical examination must take place without rivalry or Jealousy.
VII. When these occasions arise the clinical examination should be done without rivalry or jealousy.
VIII. Theoretical discussions during consultations should be avoided, as they cause perplexity and waste of time.
XII. During consultations visiting hours must be respected. The doctor or surgeon who arrives first should wait 5 min for the colleague to arrive before going to see the patient, to avoid unnecessarily repeating questions.
XIII. Visits to the sick must not be too frequent; the doctor would lose some of his professionality, risking an impression of uncertainty in the diagnosis.
XV. Some general rules should be adopted in relation to the fees to be paid by the patients.
XVI. All relatives of doctors must be followed free of charge.
XVIII. Priests must be visited free of charge: this should be a recognized general rule. They can still pay a reasonable fee for the assistance received.
XX. Doctors and surgeons can offer to issue certificates to justify the absence of military and civilians working in the government. These documents, considered public, cannot be issued free of charge.
XXI. The use of drugs prescribed by "charlatans" must be discouraged as it is discouraging for the profession, risky for health and often harmful.
XXII. No doctor or surgeon should disclose a secret remedy, of his own invention or another's property, if proven effective.
XXIV. Diversity of opinions and economic interests can, in medicine, give rise to controversies and disputes; in these situations, the arbitration of other doctors or surgeons should be sought.
XXV. A doctor should not give free advice to wealthy patients as they could be to the detriment colleagues.
XXVII. When a doctor visits a patient, he may see the person has been treated by another professional. The conduct to follow in these situations is to give adequate advice relevant to the circumstances, without interfering with the treatment in progress or, if the case requires it, to initiate a consultation with the doctor who prescribed it.
XXVIII. At the end of each particularly significant case, especially if with a fatal outcome, the doctor must write down all the steps taken in the treatment, in order to extend his own and others' skills.
XXX. The continuity of medical service must be guaranteed regardless of observance of holidays and free time available outside religious duties.
XXXI. An elderly physician, still unaware of any slowing of his faculties, may occasionally be assisted by a younger physician.
XXXII. With advancing age, a doctor must always be fit for his work. Similarly, for a surgeon, this rule is even more necessary if he suffers any defects in sight, touch and steadiness of hand—all essential qualities for operations.

A Few More Points on Medical Ethics

Percival's code of ethics gave physicians a moral mandate for assessing the conduct not only of professional colleagues but of their superiors, employers, or hospital administrators. It was drawn up in response to a particular crisis and to formulate the standard requirements for the modern hospital and proper operation of its infirmaries. Percival knew from personal experience that lay hospital administrators were not always reliable. "Administrators have at times been tempted by gossip or to use poor quality drugs."

Some criteria must be applicable for a professional code of ethics: it must, of course, be an ethical code, applicable to all members of a profession and only to them. This justifies the use of the terms "code," "ethics," and "profession."[18]

Code

A text with these characteristics replaces the documents (statutes and other similar books) that preceded them. Since Percival lacked the authority to adopt the rules that governed all doctors and surgeons in England, Medical Ethics could not be used for that purpose. Before 1803, Medical Ethics had no authoritative formulation. After its publication, there was still no one who dealt with it and, consequently, a code without authority (written or oral) could not be adopted by all medical graduates.

Therefore it could not be considered "the first professional code."

Profession

Several legitimate interpretations can be ascribed to it:

- Synonymous with "vocation" (or "call") and "occupation": any useful activity to which a large part of one's life is dedicated, even without an actual income. It is thus defined as a "discipline" with which its practitioners generally earn their living.
- "Profession" can be used instead, for any legal occupation.
- A philosophical definition that covers "most professions" concerns a certain number of individuals voluntarily organized in the same activity, to earn a living by openly using the same moral ideal in a lawful way. According to this definition, a profession in a specific group of professionals has the consequence of not considering the Hippocratic oath as the first code. To be a professional code, the oath must oblige every member of the profession, taking effect only when

[18] Davis (2003).

"everyone" has sworn and when every new "member" of the same profession takes that oath.
- Ultimately: "A profession is connoted when a certain number of individuals are voluntarily organized in it, to earn a living and openly using a certain moral ideal."

The special standards of conduct will be ethical and will govern the conduct of all group members simply because they are members of that group; they will be morally binding on each member.

Percival's Innovations

Doctors must serve the sick with all the attention due to their important task. They must also study their specialty and combine gentleness with firmness and humility with authority, to inspire gratitude, respect, and trust in their patients. Thomas Percival appears to have been the first person to propose a written code of professional ethics. The duties—some quite detailed—were justified by the main collective responsibility of the profession for caring for the sick. Percival also affirmed this fundamental responsibility in the light of the moral authority and independence of medical professionals; he also stated that even doctors and surgeons had a professional obligation "not to suffer and be held back by considerations of thrift" and to prescribe "drugs" when there were no other alternatives to fatality but the purest charity.

[His code of ethics gave the medical professional a morale mandate to assess the conduct not only of colleagues but also of superiors and employers, hospital administrators, managers and other responsible staff.]

The first code of professional ethics was drafted in response to a particular crisis resulting from a divergence between personal ethics, individual honor, and the requirements of a modern institution, the hospital.

The innovation, the code of ethics, marked out some fundamental elements:

(a) Common standards,
(b) The least possible interpersonal struggle between people dedicated to public welfare, and
(c) The independence of medical professionals from their employers in the service to others.

The American Medical Association (AMA) in 1847 established a Code of Medical Ethics, citing Percival's 1803 work (Medical Ethics in Medicine).[19]

[19] Reiser and Dyck (1977), p. 29 and Veatch (2000), pp. 26–27, 39–41, 53–54.

Some Consequences of These Definitions

Since neither the Hippocratic Oath nor Percival's Medical Ethics can be considered the first true code of professional ethics, the first reasonable candidate is the 1847 American Medical Association (AMA) code. There are at least three reasons. First, it is a code, a systematic statement of rules. Second, it applies to members of the "profession" simply by virtue of membership: all doctors. Third, the code is clearly a code for people who work for a living and whose taxes and expenses are specific for that task.

For some observers and scholars, even this code lends itself to some criticism of priority since it is more a declaration of medical morality not just ethics. The code is explicitly designed to help members of a certain category (in this case doctors) earn a living. Just as a doctor is obliged to give advice or make suggestions for maintaining well-being, so he has the right to be listened to attentively and respectfully. Being obliged to expose his own health and life for the benefit of the community, he has the right, in return, to expect all its members, collectively and individually, to help him provide his services and grant all possible benevolence regarding the prevention of disease.

The public has duties toward the doctor that are necessary so he can respect his, in this "social contract" or "principle of reciprocity." An important distinction can be made between professional morality and professional ethics.

- Professional morality deals with the obligations of professionals including in special circumstances (knowledge, opportunities, expectations, etc.);
- Professional ethics concerns professional codes, as the pivotal documents for implementing professionalism and teaching standards to doctors, nurses, and other health professionals.

The assumption is that there are certain standards (charity, autonomy, and so on) that apply to anyone who works in health care: doctors, nurses, psychologists, administrators, and perhaps even lawyers.

Generally today biomedical ethics today is understood as "biomedical morality."

After Percival's Death

The ethical concept of medicine as a "profession" did not immediately have precise contours and boundaries. Medical ethics certainly derived from the medical philosophy of the Scott Gregory and the Englishman Percival, but others upheld their views and their concepts of the Enlightenment of the science of morality and of the morality of science. Their medical ethics also adapted traditional ideas to the substantial changes in the medical world.

There were many diatribes on medical ethics intended as a code for all those who dedicated themselves to medicine and who had been the forerunners of correct behavior (see Footnote 14).

To better denote the difference in the "new" medical line, the status of the "sick" person was replaced with the new term "patient."

Other Contemporary English Authors

Thomas Gisborne (1758–1846), born in Bridge Gate, Derbyshire, was an Anglican priest and poet. He wrote The Principles of Moral Philosophy in which, referring to the "constitution of civil society," he opposed moral, philosophical, and political principles with a strong evangelical attack, in accordance with the "moral conclusions" of William Paley (1743–1805, an Anglican philosopher, theologian, and pastor), advocating morality as a categorical imperative. Gisborne wrote an "Inquiry into the tasks of men" (1795) and an "Inquiry into the tasks of the female sex" (1797), stressing how much fell under both headings, and the subordination of Man to the social hierarchy, imposed by God.

Gisborne also wrote a volume on the ethics of various professions, including a chapter on medicine (1794). His approach, based on Christian doctrine, provided for "tasks for specific roles," including professional figures such as that of the doctor. He asserted: "... Great doctors like Percival or Gregory can have the wisdom of morality in their professional role. They would not simply have argued, however, that being wise in the field of theoretical medicine also meant being wise in medical practice."[20]

Jukes (De) Styrap (1815–1899), in his "Code of Medical Ethics" of 1878, wrote and published the only important code of medical ethics of Victorian England. He set out some clarifications and explanatory norms for doctors in case of consultations or substitutions between colleagues.[21]

His Code begins with the following address:

"There is probably no social position that offers a more powerful incentive to all that is pure and honorable, selfless and sincere, than the Medical Profession, and none where, in principle, these exalting virtues are better illustrated" and then goes on to list (in 20 pages) the medical responsibilities, as follows:

- The duties of practicing doctors to their patients
- Patients' obligations to their medical advisors
- The duties of practicing physicians in support of professional character and status
- The duties of practicing doctors with regard to professional services and vice versa
- The duties of practicing doctors in consultations
- The duties of practicing doctors when differences arise between them
- The duties of practicing doctors with regard to professional rights
- The obligations of the public toward the profession
- The use and ownership of [medical] prescriptions

[20] Gisborne (1801).

[21] De Styrap (1878, 1995).

After its first publication, the text was revised and expanded in updated editions of 1886, 1890, and 1895. These incorporated consultations with homeopaths, medical etiquette, investigators and how to handle distinguished patients. "To be effective, medical ethics must be based on the principles of religion and morality and incorporate the reciprocal duties and rights of the profession and the public."

In 1882 De Styrap offered his code to the British Medical Association in the hope that[22] it would be adopted as the national ethical standard. The code received no official approval but certainly had considerable influence. In 1986 it was described as the ethical authority accepted by the British Medical Agency, as was demonstrated and made explicit in subsequent editions.

Meanwhile, the new trend of "medical ethics" had moved to the new continent thanks to Doctor Benjamin Rush (1746–1813) who was also a signatory of the United States Declaration of Independence (4 July 1776). He worked in general surgery in the Army and then became a professor of chemistry, medical theory, and clinical practice at the University of Pennsylvania. He was a forerunner of the medical profession, stimulating knowledge and promoting research. In one of his inquiries on the "Influences of physical causes on moral faculty" (Philadelphia 1786) he stressed the need for the doctor to maintain inflexible authority over the patient.[23]

In 1820 it was compiled in the USA and adopted the following year by the Boston Medical Police Standing Committee; the Boston Medical Police[24] deals with the standards of conduct for the profession. Particular attention was paid to Benjamin Rush's conclusions. These issues related to:

- Medical consultations
- Discouraging quackery
- Professional conduct
- Taxes and Exemptions
- Offices competent in the medical field
- Seniority

In the nineteenth century, many codes of conduct began to appear, with the increasing numbers of doctors, hospitals, their specializations and better economic possibilities thanks to new businesses. Medical culture spread, not only in Europe, but in America and Asia too.

While Hippocratic writers warned doctors not to do harm, Gregory and Percival's modern medical ethics, together with other contemporary authors, recognized the need for scientific updates. The real beginning of medical ethics, even if opposed by various wise lawmakers, can still be attributed to Thomas Percival, criticized mainly

[22] Cook (1942), Manzoni (2017), Scovil (1913), and Scovil and Nightingale (1914).

[23] Cosmacini (2007).

[24] Phelps (1820).

for the lack of philosophical foundations. Nevertheless, Percival affirmed the moral authority and independence of doctors at the service of others as well as professional responsibility in the care of the sick and laid stress on the doctor's individual honor. He placed the patient's well-being above any other interest.

For example, Michael Ryan's "Manual of Medical Jurisprudence and State Medicine" (1800–1840) (see Footnote 13) indicated in 1836 the various uses of different professional categories including "Medical Practitioners." Consequently, many doctors in Italy actively picked up the question and produced important treatises.

Here are the Contents of this Manual:

Part I: Medical Ethics
Chap. I Origin of Medicine
Chap. II Hippocrates' Medical Ethics
Chap. III Medical Ethics in the Middle Ages
Chap. IV Ethics of the current age. Dr. Percival's Medical Ethics
Chap. V Medical Ethics in America
Chap. VI Medical Education. Degrees. Diplomas. Appointments. Moral, Physical and Clinical Medicine. Rules in Medicine. Posology or dose adjustment. Action of Medicines on Animals. Pharmacology
Part II: Laws relating to the Medical Profession
Chap. I Laws relating to the Medical Profession in Great Britain and Ireland, with comments
Part III: Medical Jurisprudence
Part IV: Laws for the Preservation of Public Health.

Therefore, if, in the Percival tradition medical ethics was Hippocratic, it was also, according to Gregory's tradition, Socratic. Hippocratic ethics: this establishes the principle of charity that leads doctors and health personnel to apply certain medical practices on their patients, in order to maintain or improve their health.

Socratic ethics: the treatment he proposed had not only a physical or psychological purpose, but aspired to make everyone good and happy.

Conclusion

Ethics: This is a branch of philosophy that deals with the values of human conduct, considering their correctness and incorrectness. The search for what is good for man, for what is right to do or not to do.

Medical Ethics: This is a set of principles and values that govern medical practice, with specific reference to the legitimacy and "rightness" of each medical act.

Etiquette: The rules of decent behavior. In medicine, it means professional conduct toward patients and colleagues.

Florence Nightingale

Nineteenth Century

Florence Nightingale is considered the founder of modern nursing; she was the first to apply the scientific method based on the use of statistics. She was also responsible for the first organization of field hospitals.

Florence Nightingale was born in Florence on 12 May 1820—hence her name, Florence, soon abbreviated to "Flo" 176. She was born into a British upper class family, who owned an estate in Derbyshire and normally resided in Buckinghamshire.[25]

Her father was a pioneer of epidemiology, her maternal grandfather was the abolitionist William Smith who worked hard for the abolition of slave trade, and its subsequent suppression. After receiving a social and cultural education appropriate to her position, she decided to make herself useful to society by looking after sick people. Deeply Christian and inspired by what she considered a "divine call," in 1845 she announced to her family that she wanted to devote herself to the care of sick and destitute people.

She never married, for fear that it would interfere with her vocation. Although she had no medical training, she soon recognized the shortcomings in nursing. The profession was held in scant esteem at the time, and in fact in the army it was equated with maidservants.

In 1847 she met Sidney Herbert, a politician and former defense minister, who helped promote her professional growth. In 1850, she wrote "Suggestions for Thought to Searchers after Religious Truth," a work of theology and feminism that also offers alternatives to atheism.

In the same year she went to Kaiserswerth near Düsseldorf (Germany), where she worked in a hospital run by a group of Lutheran deaconesses who provided high-quality medical care. She returned there in 1851 for a period of training and to prepare the publication "The Institution of Kaiserswerth on the Rhine, for the Practical Training of Deaconesses." From 22 August 1853 to 18 October 1854, Nightingale was superintendent of the Institute for the Care of Sick Gentlewomen in London, where she opened numerous nursing schools and received constant requests for advice to organize nursing work all over the world. Florence offered her collaboration to the British government during the Crimean War and on 21 October 1854, authorized by Sidney Herbert, with 38 volunteer nurses she had trained, she traveled to the military hospital in Scutari, Turkey, a center for veterans and wounded troops from that war. The military hospital, set up in the Selimiye barracks, was in disastrous general conditions but in a few months she managed to transform its organization.

Nightingale and her nurses noted how badly the wounded soldiers were treated and even neglected by the authorities; insufficient medical staff, scarce medicines, neglected hygiene, often fatal mass infections and an under-equipped kitchen made due care difficult. Despite some resistance from the doctors, the nurses thoroughly

[25] Department of Red Cross Nursing (1920), Kopf (1916), Nightingale (1860), and Osborn (1911).

sanitized the hospital and the basic tools. Mortality, however, did not fall: it was only 10% due to injuries, and depended largely on overcrowding, lack of ventilation and deficiencies in the sewage system. Only in March 1855 was a health commission sent from England that solved the last two problems, leading to a drastic reduction in mortality. Her theory of "nursing" centered on the concept of environmental health as fundamental in the treatment of disease. She identified five essential requirements that an environment must possess in order to be healthy:

1. air exchange
2. drinking water
3. efficient sewage system
4. cleaning
5. light

She added other non-essential, but positive, requirements, such as silence, warmth, and diet. While she was still in Turkey, on 29 November 1855, in gratitude for the work done, a "Nightingale Fund" was established, supported by generous donations, for the training of nurses.

Its President was the Duke of Cambridge and Sidney Herbert was honorary secretary.

Probably suffering from a chronic form of brucellosis, Florence returned home, welcomed as a heroine on August 7, 1857, and settled in London at the Burlington Hotel near Piccadilly, where she placed herself in quarantine, forbidding access even to her mother and older sister until she was completely healed.

In response to a specific invitation from Queen Victoria, she played a central role in the establishment of the Royal Commission on the Health of the Army, chaired by Sidney Herbert. To her we owe the Final Report of the Commission, covering more than 1000 pages, with detailed statistics. When the Army Medical College was set up, many hospitals, especially military ones, were organized according to her precious, innovative indications.

In 1858 she became the first female member of the Royal Statistical Society, on the basis of her specific treatises and later was made an honorary member of the American Statistical Association. In the decades that followed she devoted herself to health counseling in England. In 1859 she established and financed the Nightingale Training School at St. Thomas' Hospital in London. This was open to a maximum of 15 students, offered 1-year courses and was marked with strong religious zeal, military-style discipline, and the cultural models of the wealthy families of the time.

In 1860, she published Notes on Nursing, a 136-page booklet that served as a basic text in the nursing school curriculum.[26] The first graduate nurses began working in 1865 at the Liverpool Workhouse infirmary. Florence also raised funds for the new Royal Buckinghamshire Hospital in Aylesbury and in 1869 opened the Women's Medical College. From 1882, her nurses had a growing and influential presence in the profession; they worked in the main hospitals in London, elsewhere in Great

[26] Manzoni (2010), Morgan (1915), and Nutting and Kopf (1921).

Britain and Australia. Nightingale's work inspired the United States Sanitary Commission volunteer corps during the American Civil War.

Florence began collecting statistics on birth rates, mortality, and the causes of death. She was a pioneer in the compilation, analysis, and graphical presentation of data on medical care and public hygiene.

Between 1883 and 1908 she received numerous honors (first woman to receive the Order of Merit). After a long life of work and study and reflection, Florence Nightingale died in London on 13 August 1910. She was buried in East Wellow, Hampshire.

She is remembered in Florence, in Istanbul, in the Selimiye barracks, in the Crimean Memorial, in London and in Buckinghamshire with statues or monuments dedicated to her. Her voice was recorded in 1890 and is kept in the British Library sound archive.

Probably her nursing was largely influenced by the experience of Saint Vincent de Paul (1581–1660), considered the original founder of modern nursing, and by the French daughters of Charity, now nuns.

The Nightingale Pledge, drafted in 1893 by Lystra Gretter, a nurse instructor at the old Harper Hospital in Detroit, Michigan, may seem to be a modified version of the Hippocratic Oath. It is a statement of ethical principles for the nursing profession. It includes a vow to refrain from all that is harmful and malicious and to look after the sick, wherever they are and whenever they need it. In a 1935 revision, the nurses' commitment was expanded to include an oath to become "health missionaries."[27] I solemnly pledge myself before God and in the presence of this assembly to spend my life in purity and to practice my profession faithfully.

I will refrain from all that is deleterious and malicious and will not knowingly take or administer any harmful drugs. I will do everything in my power to maintain and raise the standard of my profession and will keep in safety all personal matters entrusted to my custody and all family matters that I become aware of in the exercise of my profession. I will be true to my work and devoted to the welfare of those assigned to my care.

The Nightingale Commitment

For many years, nurses had no formal code of ethics and used the Nightingale Commitment to guide their practice. Over time it enjoyed alternating appreciation or changes in the various medical institutes that recognized it. It was opposed by traditionalists due to the growing liberalism in some graduate classes. Much of the controversy surrounding Nightingale's commitment is her mention of God. The first formal code for professional nurses was adopted in 1950 and revised in 1960. The current Code of Ethics (2015, ANA (American Nurses Association)) forms a central basis for the profession and guidance of nurses in their decisions and conduct.

[27] Winkelstein (2009).

References

Bastron RD, McCullough LB. What goes around, comes around: John Gregory, MD, and the profession of medicine. Proc (Bayl Univ Med Cent). 2007;20(1):18–21.
Cook SET. The life of Florence. New York: Macmillan Co.; 1942.
Cosmacini G. La religiosità della medicina Dall'antichità a oggi. (IT, The religiosity of medicine from ancient times to today) Laterza Ed.; 2007. p. 15.
Davis M. What can we learn by looking for at? The first code of professional ethics? Theor Med Bioeth. 2003;24(5):433–54.
De Styrap J. Code of medical ethics. London: Ed. J & A Churchill; 1878.
De Styrap J. The codification of medical morality: historical and philosophical studies of the formalization of Western medical morality in the eighteenth and nineteenth centuries, vol. 2: Anglo-American medical ethics and medical jurisprudence in the nineteenth century. In: Baker RB, editor. Dordrecht: Kluwer Academic Publishers; 1995.
Deewhurst K. Thomas Sydenham (1624-1689) Reformer of clinical medicine. Med Hist. 1962;6(2):101–18.
Department of Red Cross Nursing. Am J Nurs. 1920;21(1):38–41.
Durrigl M-A, Fatovic-Ferencic S. The medical practice of Amatus Lusitanus in Dubrovnik (1556-1558): a short reminder on the 445th anniversary of his arrival. Acta Med Port. 2002;15:37–40.
Friedenwald H. The ethics of the practice of medicine from the Jewish point of view. Johns Hopkins Hospital Bulletin No. 318; 1917. p. 256–66.
Friedenwald H. Jacob Zahalon of Rome, medieval rabbi, physician, author and moralist. Bull Med Libr Assoc. 1918;8(1):1–10.
Friedenwald H. Jewish physicians in Italy: their relation to the Papal and Italian States. Am Jewish Hist Soc. 1922;28:133–211.
Friedenwald H. Jews and medicine, vol. 1. Baltimore: Johns Hopkins University Press; 1944. p. 332–80.
Gershon Lewental D. Amatus Lusitanus (Amato Lusitano). Encyclopedia of Jews in the Islamic world. Executive Editor Norman A. Stillman. Brill Online; 2015.
Gisborne T. An enquiry into the duties of the female sex. Publisher T. Cadell, Jun. and W. Davies; 1797. p. 456; New York: Garland Pub.; 1801. p. 495.
Gregory J. Lectures on the duties and qualifications of a physician. John Gregory's writings on medical ethics and philosophy of medicine. In: McCullough LB, Gregory J, Strahan W, Cadell T, editors. (1724–1773), Dictionary of National Biography. London: Oxford University Press; 2004; 2008.
Haakonssen L. Medicine and morals in the enlightenment: John Gregory, Thomas Percival and Benjamin Rush. Amsterdam: Rodopi Ed; 1997.
Howard JK. Dr Thomas Percival and the beginnings of industrial legislation. Occup Med (London). 1975;25(2):58–65.
Isaac Ben Solomon Luria (1534–1572). Revolutionized the study of Jewish mysticism through the Kabbalah. Encyclopedia Judaica "Luria, Isaac Ben Solomon". Jerusalem: Keter Publishing House; 1972.
Jacobs J, Broydé I, Executive Committee of the Editorial Board, Grünhut L, Zahalon; Jewish encyclopedia; 1906.
Jonsen AR. Medical history in India and China in a short history of medical ethics (Chap. 3). Oxford: Oxford University Press; 2000. p. 27–41. (British Medicine in a short history of medical ethics, Chap. 5: 57–62.0.)
Joshi VR, Poojary VB. J Assoc Physicians India. 2013;61(11):860–1.
Kopf EW. Nightingale as statistician. Am Stat Assoc. 1916;15(16):388–401.
Kottek SS. Medical prayers and oaths in Jewish lore. Isr J Med Sci. 1993;29(1):75.
Leibowitz JO. Amatus Lusitanus, Encyclopaedia Judaica. Copyright 1952.
Leibowitz JO. Amatus Lusitanus, Encyclopaedia Judaica, Nardi B. Amato Lusitano, Dizionario Biografico degli Italiani Enciclopedia Treccani-(IT: Amato Lusitano, Biographical Dictionary of Italian Treccani Encyclopedia) Volume 2, 1960.

Levin S. Jewish ethics in relation to medicine. S Afr Med J. 1973;47(21):924–30.
Lusitani A. Curationum Medicinalium, Centuriae Quinta videlicet ac Sexta, (LAT: Medicinal treatments of the fifth and sixth centuries, Venice) Venetiis Ex Officina Valgriliana. p. 196–9; 1560.
Manzoni E. A cent'anni dalla morte di Florence Nightingale: un'eredità che repara il futuro. (IT. A century from the death of Florence Nightingale: an inheritance that prepares the future) In L'infermiere. 2010;1(2):9–11.
Manzoni E. Alle origini del pensiero di Florence Nightingale: le influenze storico-culturali dei secoli [IT. The origins of Florence Nightingales' thought: historical-cultural influences over the centuries]. Grosseto: IPASVI; 2017.
McCullough LB. John Gregory and the invention of professional medical ethics and the profession of medicine. Dordrecht: Springer; 1998a.
McCullough LB, editor. John Gregory's writings on medical ethics and philosophy of medicine. Philosophy and medicine, no. 57; Classics of medical ethics, no. 1. Dordrecht: Kluwer Academic Publishers; 1998b.
McCullough LB. John Gregory's medical ethics and the reform of medical practice in eighteenth century Edinburgh. J R Coll Physicians Edinb. 2006;36(1):86–92.
McCullough LB. John Gregory and the invention of professional medical ethics and the profession of medicine. Springer/Oxford University Press; 2007. Retrieved 24 Jul 2007.
Morgan M. The nurse in literature. Am J Nurs. 1915;15(10):836–8.
Nardi B. Amato Lusitano, Dizionario Biografico degli Italiani Enciclopedia Treccani-(IT: Amato Lusitano, Biographical Dictionary of Italians Encyclopedia Treccani), vol. 2; 1960.
Nightingale F. Notes on nursing: what it is, and what it is not. New York: D. Appleton and Company; 1860.
Nutting MA, Kopf EW. Nightingale centenary. Q Publ Am Stat Assoc. 1921;17(133):650–1.
Osborn HF. Florence Nightingale. Am J Nurs. 1911;11(5):339–41.
Percival T. Medical ethics cited in Ivan Waddington (1975). The development of medical ethics—a sociological analysis. Med Hist. 1803;19:36–51.
Percival T. Percival's medical ethics, or a code of institutes and precepts, adapted to the Professional Conduct of Physicians and Surgeons. 3rd ed. Oxford: John Henry Parker/John Churchill; 1849.
Percival T. (740–1804) Codifier of medical ethics. JAMA. 1965;194(12):1319–20.
Percival T. Surgeons. Birmingham, AL: Classics of Medicine Library; 1985.
Percival T. Medical ethics: or a code of institutes and precepts. Adapted to the Professional Conduct of Physicians and Surgeons; 2014a.
Percival T. Essays medical and experimental: the second edition, revised, and considerably enlarged. To which is added an appendix (Cambridge Library Collection-History of Medicine). Cambridge: Cambridge University Press; 2014b.
Percival T. Percival's medical ethics, or a code of institutes and precepts, adapted to the Professional Conduct of Physicians and Surgeons. Etica Medica,Ovvero un codice di istituzioni e precetti adattati alla condottaProfessionale dei medici e dei chirurghi—a cura di Sara Patuzzo, (IT. Medical Ethics, i.e. a code of institutions and precepts adapted to the professional conduct of doctors and surgeons—curated by Sara Patuzzo, Mimesis Ed. Milano—Udine; 2015.
Phelps S. Boston medical police. Boston: Boston Medical Association; 1820. p. 1–24.
Reiser SJ, Dyck AJ. Ethics in medicine, historical perspectives and contemporary concerns. Reiser et al., editors. M.I.T. Press; 1977. p. 29.
Rizzo R. Papa Gregorio Magno e gli ebrei di Sicilia. (IT. Pope Gregory the Great and the Jews of Sicily). Mediaeval Sophia. Studi e Ricerche sui Saperi Medievali. E-Review semestrale dell'Officina di Studi Medievali. 2012;12: 223–25.
Ruderman DB, Veltri G. Cultural intermediaries Jewish intellectuals in early modern Italy (Chapter 10). University of Pennsylvania Press; 2004.
Ryan M. Manual of medical jurisprudence and state medicine (Introduction). London: Sherwood, Gilbert, Piper Ed; 1836. p. XIII–XL.
Schwarz S. I Marrani del Portogallo. (IT. The Marranos of Portugal). (Israel Monthly Rev) Rassegna mensile di Israele. 1925;1(2):85-0 (Mesuan 5686).

Scovil RE. Florence Nightingale, The American Journal of Nursing. Pub. Lippincott Williams & Wilkins. 1913;14(1):28–33.

Scovil RE, Nightingale F. Florence nightingale and her nurses. Am J Nurs. 1914;15(1):13–8.

Veatch RM, editor. Cross cultural perspectives in medical ethics. 2nd ed. Boston: Jones and Bartlett Pub.; 2000. p. 240–58.

Winkelstein W. Florence Nightingale: founder of modern nursing and hospital epidemiology. Epidemiology. 2009;20:311.

Statement and Initial Development of Medical Ethics in the Nineteenth and Twentieth Centuries

8

Historical Note and Updates to Recent Times

From the 1750s onwards, increasing numbers of professionals were changing their practice of medicine, surgery, and pharmacy to establish a new professional role: the general practitioner. In the period 1750–1850 the traditional tripartite structure of medicine, surgery, and pharmacy was steadily eroded and replaced by the modern structure of medical practice, based on a distinction between general practitioners and hospital consultants.[1]

By 1830, general practitioners were by far the most numerous, probably around 90% of college graduates. In 1791 **Giuseppe Pasta** (1742–1823) from Bergamo issued a brochure entitled Galateo dé Medici (Etiquette for Doctors). The need for guidelines for "Good Practice" was becoming more and more urgent to give citizens comprehensible, broad, correct information from the world of health, alongside a current code of medical ethics, for correct, complete, and understandable ethical information. In the introduction to his Galateo dé Medici Pasta stated: "I do not intend to give new laws for medical creation, but only to recall what is used most among honest professors. Science makes the learned man; such laws make him worthy. Having one without the other only makes us half glorious. We too must have our own code of civilization, our etiquette. I have sketched it out, trying to concentrate the dictates of the great Masters in a few lines. Widespread or Asian—might be boring or forgotten: laconic and aphoristic—perhaps you will like it more and remember it."

It was a modest little book of aphorisms, and dealt with various topics in 32 pages: Personal qualities; The knowledge; The medical examination; The diagnosis, The prognosis; Therapy; Consultation; The fee.

[1] Leake (1927) and Waddington (1975).

R. G. Russo, *Medical Ethics*, https://doi.org/10.1007/978-3-031-42444-1_8

The same introduction was used later (1829) in a publication (in Venice) in conjunction with Dr. **Salvatore Mandruzzato**'s "Galateo degli Ammalati" (Etiquette for sick people). In this work an "Introduction to the sensible reader" specifies: "The dignity and excellence of the ancient art of the Physician requires that no man should approach her to treat her as her minister, with contempt for Religion and severe morality, nor a man poor in judgment, bare of science, rough in morals, and uncouth in manners, and not even a man without compassion and a generous heart."

What today is called "Medical Ethics" reflects, in a small part, all the complex and changing factors that surfaced in the eighteenth century and remained influential thereafter, but are now changing and call for new rules and recommendations.[2]

Doctors are the only appropriate substitutes for doctors, surgeons for surgeons, and pharmacists for pharmacists. This exhortation was initially expressed by John Gregory, from Edinburgh, who presented a very influential volume, "Lectures on the Duties and Qualifications of a Physician" and who helped to find a formal code of medical ethics. The text was brilliant, as fully applicable today as it was more than two centuries ago. Gregory raised the question of whether medicine should be considered an art or a trade. He systematically expounded the qualities that make up a doctor and what education was necessary to prepare a young person for that profession. He emphasized the "humanity" of a doctor, the "sensitivity of the heart and a fundamental compassion through which the patient considers a doctor as a friend."

Another significant figure, as we already know, was Thomas Percival, who had published a book entitled "Medical Ethics." The title of the first chapter is self-explanatory: "Of professional behavior, with respect to hospitals and other medical organizations." The doctor must truly be a man with a great soul, who must not only be worthy and honest but must know his own worth. This is the basis of the spirit of *noblesse oblige* that plays a significant part in medical ethics.

Two distinctive senses are needed: condescension and authority, described as "An aristocratic tradition capable of harming corruption" and "A superior status of the doctor, as such." In the mid-nineteenth century, the medical profession did not have a proper system of professional legitimacy: it was not necessary to attend medical school or pass exams to become a doctor. He (or she) who professed to be a doctor might have graduated from a University, trained through an apprenticeship, or be a total charlatan. While a small medical elite trained university professors or assisted wealthy and fashionable clients, this status was generally achieved through family or social connections.[3]

Thus, apparently, another medical oath was required to certify the "doctor," which would respond more closely to the demands of the medical schools.

The new professional figure of the general practitioner was entrusted with various tasks concerning the community. Health information always had particular moral relevance on account of the serious risks it entailed and the increasing levels

[2] King (1958).

[3] Bird (1989), p. 44 and Starr (1982).

of information both for individuals and the community.[4] Hospitals also developed, acquiring new and more modern characteristics: a new class of doctors began to form. From 1830 onwards, numerous letters from professionals were published in the Lancet, in relation to violations of ethics and etiquette. In 1854 the Association Medical Journal stressed that "The essential requirements in this new class of medical practitioners are extreme vigilance, appropriate for assessing the honesty of an act, and sentiment."

Everything began with the publication of the Galatei[5] which outlined the first steps in the establishment of what would later become "codes of conduct" for doctors. A document very similar to the idea we have of codes was approved in 1897 by the Istrian chamber of doctors: "Professional Code and Tariffs for Medical Services in Private Practice (Tip. L. Bontempo, Pola, 1899)."

Another similar document followed, drawn up by the Chamber of Doctors of Trento: "Professional code established by the Chamber of Doctors in Trento pertinent in the session of July 21, 1900 (Civic Library of Trento): Collection of some laws and health provisions." (Tip. Ed. F.lli Mariotti, Trento 1900).

A few years later it was the turn of the "Code of ethics and medical deontology," approved by the order of medical doctors of Sassari (1903). These two documents, even if published in land ruled by the Habsburgs, were in fact written in Italian by Italians.[6]

As suggested later:[7] "Human rights and medical ethics are parallel mechanisms, the first at the socio-political level and the second more at the level of the doctor-patient relationship ... they are complementary and the use of the two together maximizes the protection available to the patient."

First Activities on Medical Ethics in Various Countries

British Medical Association, 1832[8]

The British Medical Association (BMA) is the union and professional body for doctors in the UK. The principles of ethics also provide essential guidance on legal issues in clinical practice. Mission: concerns doctors. Vision: respected doctors who offer the best health services and: strong representation and expert guidance; response to individual needs and career support in professional development, support from the BMA, inter-connection in a professional community, influence for improvement of health and the profession. The Medical Ethics Committee provides

[4] Corbellini (1994), Premoli De Marchi (2012), Ryan (1836) and Spinsanti (2012).

[5] Patuzzo (2014), pp 31–37.

[6] Patuzzo (2014), pp.49–63

[7] Cohen and Ezer (2013), Gruskin and Dickens (2006) and Peel (2005).

[8] BMA code of conduct. British Medical Association, 7/1/2017.

guidance to the association on current and developing issues in medical ethics and is regarded as one of the leading authorities on ethical issues in the UK and in the international medical world. Issues examined by the Committee include abortion, organ donation and presumed consent, patient confidentiality, and the law on mental capacity. The code of conduct provides guidance on expected behavior and sets standards of conduct that uphold the professional values.

Confederation des Syndicats Médicaux Francais 1845[9]

The principles enshrined in the articles of this Code of Ethics have been supplemented by explanatory notes adopted by the French National Medical Council (CNMF). While these notes may be considered an integral part of the code, they are not the legal rules. These can only be adopted in the course of disciplinary procedures and their legitimacy is subject to judicial review by the French Council of State. In order to reflect ongoing changes in medical practice, the notes will be updated as and when necessary and posted on the CNMF website.

The French Code of Medical Ethics applies to all doctors and to all patients, women and men.

Article 1 (Article R.4127-1 of the CSP) The provisions of this code are mandatory for all physicians conducting a procedure pursuant to article L. 4112-7 of the French public health code or under the terms of an international agreement, as well as medical students acting as a locum or medical assistant. The National Medical Council supervises compliance with the law and any violation, and is responsible for disciplinary proceedings of Medical Association 1847 (AMA).[10]

In USA

Since its foundation, the AMA and the Code of Medical Ethics have set out the values to which doctors commit themselves as members of the profession, together with the principles of medical ethics and the opinions of the AMA Council, on the

---

[9] Kopp et al. (2007).

[10] AMA (2015).

Ethics of the American Medical Association. Philadelphia, T.K. & P.G.Collins Printers. Adopted May 1847.

Proceedings of the National Medical conventions held in New York (May 1846) and in Philadelphia (May 1847). American Medical Association. T.K. & P.G. Collins Printers,1847. AMA Code of Medical Ethics. AMA Principles of Medical Ethics (Revised June 2001). © 2016. AMA Code of Conduct, American Medical Association, Revised August 2016.

AMA Council on Ethical and Judicial Affairs, Code of Medical Ethics of the American Medical Association, Pub. American Medical Association; Riddick (2003). Proceedings of the National Medical Conventions, New York, May 1846 and Philadelphia, May 1847.

D. Introduction to the Code of Medical Ethics. 1847, Code of Medical Ethics. pp. 83–107. T.K. & P.G. Collins, Printers. 1847.

ethical and judicial issues that make up the code, to offer guidance to help physicians respond to the ethical challenges of medical practice. The Code is periodically updated to address the changing situations of medicine.

The latest edition is dated June 2016: the guidelines have been revised, updated, and reorganized.

Preamble "The medical profession has long been enrolled in a body of ethical claims developed primarily for the benefit of the patient." As a member of this profession, a physician must recognize responsibility to patients first and foremost, as well as to society, other health professionals, and himself. The following principles adopted by the American Medical Association are not laws, but standards of conduct that define the essentials of honorable behavior for the doctor.

Principles of Medical Ethics

I. A physician must be dedicated to providing competent care, with compassion and respect for dignity and human rights.
II. A physician must adhere to professional standards, be honest in all professional interactions, and strive to report to the appropriate individuals any physicians lacking character or competence, fraud or deception.
III. A physician must comply with the law and also be responsible for seeking changes in requirements that are contrary to the patient's best interest.
IV. A physician respects the rights of patients, colleagues, and other health care professionals and protects patient confidentiality within the constraints of the law.
V. The physician will continue to study, apply, and advance scientific knowledge, maintaining a commitment to medical education, providing relevant information to patients, colleagues, and the public, obtaining consultations and calling on the talents of other healthcare professionals, when necessary.
VI. A doctor, in providing adequate care to the patient—except in an emergency—will be free to choose who to serve, who to associate with and what is the environment in which to provide medical assistance.
VII. A physician recognizes a responsibility to participate in activities that contribute to the betterment of the community and the improvement of public health.
VIII. While taking care of a patient, the physician must remember his great responsibility for that person.
IX. A doctor must support access to medical care for all people.

—from WMA Principles of Medical Ethics, 2001

The **Declaration of Geneva** is one of the World Medical Association's (WMA) oldest policies adopted by the second General Assembly in Geneva in 1947. It builds on the principles of the Hippocratic Oath, in what is indicated as "The Physician's Pledge" and is now known as its modern version. Further additions and revisions have been adopted and will be discussed and reported in the next chapter in this book. The following is the 1947 version.

The Phisician's Pledge

AS A MEMBER OF THE MEDICAL PROFESSION:
I SOLEMNLY PLEDGE to dedicate my life to the service of humanity;
THE HEALTH AND WELL-BEING OF MY PATIENT will be my first consideration;
I WILL RESPECT the autonomy and dignity of my patient;
I WILL MAINTAIN the utmost respect for human life;
I WILL NOT PERMIT considerations of age, disease or disability, creed, ethnic origin, gender, nationality, political affiliation, race, sexual orientation, social standing or any other factor to intervene between my duty and my patient;
I WILL RESPECT the secrets that are confided in me, even after the patient has died;
I WILL PRACTICE my profession with conscience and dignity and in accordance with good medical practice;
I WILL FOSTER the honor and noble traditions of the medical profession;
I WILL GIVE my teachers, colleagues, and students the respect and gratitude that is due to them;
I WILL SHARE my medical knowledge for the benefit of the patient and the advancement of healthcare;
I WILL ATTEND TO my own health, well-being, and abilities in order to provide care of the highest standard;
I WILL NOT USE my medical knowledge to violate human rights and civil liberties, even under threat;
I MAKE THESE PROMISES solemnly, freely, and upon my honour.

Historical Dates of the AMA'S Activities

An 1845 resolution at the New York Medical Association calling for a national medical convention led to the founding of the American Medical Association (AMA) in 1847. Scientific advancement, standards for medical education, launch of a medical ethics program, improvement of public health: these were the goals of the AMA.

The AMA has revolutionized medicine in the United States. The AMA Code of Medical Ethics was adopted at the meeting of the National Medical Convention in Philadelphia in May 1847 and concerned the definition of standards for professional training and medical conduct worldwide.[11]

- 1873: the judicial council of the AMA is founded to deal with ethical and constitutional medical disputes.
- 1883: the AMA Journal is published
- 1906: AMA publishes the first American medical register listing over 128,000 licensed physicians in the United States and Canada.
- 1910: the Flexner Report is published, calling for new standards for medical schools.
- 1927: the AMA Council publishes the first list of hospitals approved for education.
- 1950: the AMA Foundation for Research and Education is established to help medical schools cover expenses and help medical students.
- 1966: AMA publishes the first edition of Current Procedural Terminology (CPT), a system of standardized terms for medical procedures used to facilitate documentation.
- 1967: the United States Adopted Names (USAN) Council is established to determine nonproprietary design nations for chemical compounds.
- 1990: AMA: Fellowship Residency Electronic Interactive Data Access System (FREIDA) describing residency programs in the United States is available in electronic form.
- 2008: Ronald M. Davis, MD, then the AMA's immediate past-president, apologizes for more than a century of AMA policies that excluded African-Americans from the AMA and also barred them from some state and local medical societies.

AMA promotes the art and science of medicine and the improvement of public health. In the introductory portion, it notes that:

> Medical Ethics is part of general ethics and is based on religion and morality. It includes not only the duties but also the rights of doctors.

The Code is an ever-evolving document like the changes in medicine itself and in the provision of health care. It offers new information on how the core values of the profession apply in daily practice.

Development of the AMA Code

The initial version of the AMA Code of Ethics was revised in the years 1903, 1957, 1980, 2001, and 2016. There was talk of a real revolution in medical ethics.

[11] The American Medical Ethics Revolution. How the AMA's Code of Ethics has transformed physicians' relationships with patients. Baker et al. (1999).

Declaration of Professional Responsibility for Medicine and Social Contract with Humanity

Preamble

Never in the history of human civilization has the well-being of each individual been so inextricably linked to that of everyone else. Plagues and pandemics do not respect national borders in a world of global commerce and tourism. Wars and acts of terrorism recruit innocent people as combatants and view civilians as targets. Advances in medical science and genetics, while promising positive effects, can also do harm. The scale and urgency of these universal challenges require concerted action and a common response from all. Doctors are united by a common goal towards the care of the sick and the suffering.

Over the centuries, individual doctors have met this obligation by applying their skills and knowledge with skill, selflessness and, at times, heroism. Today, our profession must reaffirm its historic commitment to countering natural and man-made attacks on the health and well-being of mankind. Only by acting together and overcoming ideological and geographical divisions can we combat these powerful threats.

In 2008, the Council on Ethical and Judicial Affairs (CEJA) was established, with the aim of maintaining and updating the Code of Medical Ethics and promoting adherence to the professional ethical standards of the Code. For more than 170 years, AMA has been guiding ethics for medical practice with its Code of Ethics. This is a declaration of the values to which doctors individually and collectively commit to adhere; it defines the integrity and establishes the self-regulation of the profession. This Association is dedicated to ensuring that medical activities are sustainable and lead to the best health outcomes for patients. Its strategic plan aims to promote improvements in care and in the doctor/patient relationship.

The three main areas of intervention are:

1. Improve health outcomes.
2. Support and adapt to scientific developments.
3. Achieve appreciable professional results.

Also indicated are the "Duties of Doctors for their Patients" and the "Obligations of Patients for their Doctors."

In Conclusion

The latest edition of the AMA Code, adopted on January 23, 2017, is the result of an 8-year project to review, update, and reorganize the guidelines and to ensure that the code remains a timely, easy-to-use resource. AMA's Ethics Group is responsible for helping to establish policy, the development of educational programs and scientific research into the ethical issues that *physicians encounter* in their training and daily practice.

It has three main components:

1. The Council: analyzes and solves the ethical problems that doctors have to face during their work. The resolutions, approvals, and recommendations formulated in the Council's reports become the official policy of the Association. Violation of these principles constitutes immoral behavior and can justify disciplinary measures, such as censorship, suspension or expulsion from the Medical Society. The CEJA has the following responsibilities:
   (a) Maintain and update the Code of Medical Ethics, in parallel with political developments;
   (b) Promote adherence to professional ethical standards (related to the code) through its judicial function.
2. The Ethical Resource Center: develops practical solutions relevant to all phases of the professional career; it provides students and practicing doctors with the tools to face the new challenges posed by constantly evolving "medicine." It deals with: (a) Guidelines for gifts to doctors; (b) Pocket guides to the Code of Medical Ethics for physicians and medical students; (c) End-of-Life Care; (d) AMA Journal: monthly on-line ethics.
3. The Institute of Medical Ethics: is an academic research and training center. Its staff publishes qualified articles on issues concerning:
   (a) professionalism and responsibility of the doctor
   (b) public health and consequent health care
   (c) respect for privacy in information.

However, the AMA Code of Conduct may be modified at any time.

In Canada

Canadian Medical Association (CMA) 1868

The CMA Code of Ethics, first published in 1868, is probably the most important document produced by the CMA. It has a long and distinguished history of providing ethical guidance to Canada's doctors. Areas of focus include decision making, consent, confidentiality, research, and physician responsibilities. The code is updated every 5–6 years and has a major revision approximately every 20 years. Changes must be approved by the CMA General Council.[12]

[12] CMA Code of Ethics, 2004–2018.

Latest news and developments. February 12, 2020.

The Virtual Care Task Force (VCTF), a collaboration of the Canadian Medical Association (CMA), the Royal College of Physicians and Surgeons of Canada (Royal College), and the College of Family Physicians of Canada (CFPC), has published its recommendations for enable and expand the implementation of virtual assistance in Canada.

The report outlines recommendations for building a pan-Canadian approach to healthcare virtualization.

The task force formed four working groups—interoperability and governance, licensing and quality of care, payment models, and medical education.

Among their key recommendations, the task force calls for:

- national standards for access to patient health information;
- greater support to regulatory bodies to simplify the registration and licensing processes of doctors to allow doctors to provide virtual assistance beyond provincial and territorial borders;
- a framework for regulating the safety and quality of virtual assistance services;
- provincial and territorial governments, in collaboration with key associations, to develop new tariff schemes for in-person and virtual assistance that are neutral with respect to income; and
- the establishment and integration of virtual assistance training in medical schools and continuing training for health professionals.

Sir William Osler

William Osler was a pathologist, educator, great bibliophile, historian, and writer. He was also referred to as the father of modern medicine. He was born in Bond Head (Ontario), southwestern Canada, on July 12, 1849. At 18 he began attending Trinity College in Toronto, then enrolled in the School of Medicine; in 1870 he moved to McGill University in Montreal; he spent a couple of years in Europe, in Oxford and Berlin.

He returned to Montreal in 1874, when he was offered the post of associate professor at McGill University. His work in this university soon became fundamental for the preparation of future doctors.[13]

His capillary researches under the microscope were thorough and particularly appreciated by his students. At the same time he also worked in the "smallpox" department at the Montreal General Hospital. In 1884 he was appointed to the chair of clinical medicine at the University of Pennsylvania, in Philadelphia. Four years later he received an invitation from the newly formed Johns Hopkins University in Baltimore, the first hospital in the Anglo-Saxon world to be divided into specialized

[13] Bensley (1990) and Garrison (1920).

pavilions, according to the criteria established by Florence Nightingale. In December 1891, Osler finished writing his internal medicine text "The Principles and Practice of Medicine." He donated his historical library to McGill University.

In 1893 he founded a new Journal Club, the Johns Hopkins Hospital Bulletin as well as a Society for the study of tuberculosis. In 1905 he was appointed to the Royal Chair of Medicine at Oxford, where he became a member of the Board of Curators of the Bodleian Library. He also proposed the Association of Physicians of Great Britain and Ireland, whose official organ was the Quarterly Journal of Medicine He went to Paris, Rome, Florence, Venice, Verona, Padua, Milan. For his important contributions in the field of modern medicine, Osler was made a Baronet in the Coronation Honors List in 1911.

At the outbreak of the First World War (June 1914), Osler and his wife put all their efforts into health care for wounded soldiers; they set up organized hospitals, shelters, infirmaries, and promoted pharmacological research to combat the most common diseases that afflicted them. He died in Oxford, on December 29, 1919, during the Spanish flu epidemic.[14]

Osler also taught Medical Ethics, bringing his personal ideas to what he considered his "lifestyle": "One, to carry out daily work correctly, without worrying about tomorrow. Two: act according to the Golden Rule, towards professional colleagues and towards patients who are being treated. Three: cultivate a measure of equanimity to allow you to look at success with humility, with the affection of friends, without pride and being ready for the day of pain and suffering, with the courage of a man".[15]

Osler has been claimed by doctors from three different countries (Canada, USA, UK) as "one of them" and his main textbook, "The principles and practice of medicine," has passed 16 editions, has been translated into six languages and was the last major medical text by a single author. Osler gave his name to many diseases and symptoms:

- An Osler sign is the recognition of high systolic blood pressure due to calcification of atherosclerotic arteries.
- Osler's nodules appear on the tips of the fingers or toes. They are characteristic of autoimmune vasculitis caused by subacute bacterial endocarditis.
- Rendu-Osler-Weber disease (also known as hereditary hemorrhagic telangiectasia) is a syndrome of multiple vascular malformations of the skin, nose, oral mucosa, and lungs.
- Osler-Vaquez disease is also known as polycythemia vera.
- Osler-Libman-Sacks syndrome is a warty, non-bacterial, atypical endocarditis. Final stage of lupus erythematosus.
- Osler's row is a parasitic nematode.
- Osler's maneuver: in pseudo-hypertension this consists of palpation of the pulse while measuring with the sphygmomanometer.

[14] Brownell Wheeler (1990).

[15] Millard (2011).

- Osler's syndrome relates to recurrent pain in the form of colic, with typical radiation to the back, chills, and fever.
- Osler's triad: simultaneous presence of pneumonia, endocarditis and meningitis.
- The "Sphryanura osleri" is a trematode worm.

Pickwick's Syndrome" relates to obstructive apnea-hypopnea during sleep.[16]

During his 16 years at Johns Hopkins, he revolutionized the teaching of medicine in the United States and Canada. He led the efforts to bring a scientific approach to patient care. Osler noted: "The practice of medicine is an art based on science." He attached great importance to the clinical environment and argued that the most effective teaching for students was at the patient's bedside. He was among the first to want students to accompany him on his "rounds" of visits to the hospital, providing them with many opportunities to observe and ask questions about each clinical case under consideration. This was his greatest innovation that almost sanctioned an obligation for teachers to their students. The practice is now widespread all over the world.

The transition from a didactic teaching method, focused solely on the textbook, to learning based on practical lessons with a more clinical approach, underlines the importance of medical teaching and training.[16]

He was a keen admirer of the Hippocratic Corps, and no physician has exerted more influence on how physicians should behave than Sir William Osler. From the "Hippocratic Corps" he learned that: The doctor should also be confidential, very chaste, sober. He should have a distinctive look and feel. All behavior must inspire restraint, because these things are beneficial. Be prompt in approaching the patient, not with the head thrown arrogantly backward, but with a lowered gaze and with the head tilted slightly, as art requires, in a humble and uniform way. The hair must not be too smooth, nor the curled beard, as in degenerate youth. He should approach the patient with moderate, not noisy steps, and look calmly at the sick-bed. He should inspire peace and not react to insults from patients: people with "frenetic" disorders often use evil words to doctors. William Osler was not a general practitioner, although he developed encyclopedic experience by devoting himself to pediatrics, hematology, neurology, cardiology, infectious diseases and all aspects of general medicine. He was very sensitive to medicine as practiced at the turn of the twentieth century. He asserted that: "The greatest enemy of the scientific practice of medicine is routine."

In Conclusion

Osler wrote extensively on the new era that he called "scientific medicine," which differed from both homeopathy and allopathy. He lectured on philosophy and the importance of history to inform the choices of his time. The following quote from him is reported:

[16] Christian (1922).

"The practice of medicine is an art, not a profession; a vocation, not a business; a call in which your heart will be stimulated as well as your intellect."

Some aphorisms of his in the medical field are worth noting:

- It is much more important to know the sick patient than to know what disease afflicts him.
- The good doctor treats the disease; the great doctor treats the sick patient.
- Medicine is uncertainty.
- One of the first tasks of the doctor is not to take too many medicines.
- The young doctor uses 20 drugs for each disease and the senior doctor uses only one for 20 diseases.
- There are no real specialties in medicine; to fully understand the most important diseases, a doctor must be familiar with their symptoms in many organs.
- Variability is the law of life; just as no two faces are alike, no two bodies are alike; there are no two individuals who react and behave alike in the abnormal conditions that we recognize as disease.
- The desire to take medicine is perhaps the greatest characteristic that distinguishes humans from animals.

Osler engaged in evidence-based medicine, believing it to be the basis of medical education and traditional medical training. It required all physicians to engage in an ongoing process of education in order to utilize the evidence obtained through research. In addition, evidence-based medicine education had to be integrated with clinical ethics, according to the four classic elements for which doctors work in the best interest of their patients: Autonomy, Justice, Charity, and Non-wickedness.[17]

Sri Lanka Medical Association, 1887[18]

The Medical Association of Sri Lanka (SLMA) brings together doctors of all grades and all sectors of medicine. SLMA is the oldest professional medical association in Asia and Australasia, with a proud history dating back to 1887. It was called the Ceylon Branch of the British Medical Association then later evolved into the Ceylon Medical Association (1951). When Sri Lanka became a Republic in 1972, it became the Sri Lanka Medical Association. Medical Ethics, taught by members of the Department of Forensic Medicine in three of the five medical universities, is an "ethical norm" (normative ethics) based on "traditional" or "classical" ethics. Education includes the teaching of moral principles, illustrated with examples.

Recognizing the importance of incorporating good ethical principles into daily practice, SLMA published its Declaration of Health in 1995.

[17] Osler (2009, 2010), Reid (1931), and Silverman (2012).

[18] Amarasekera (2007) and Karunalathilake (2010).

References

AMA. Evidence-based medicine: a science of uncertainty and an art of probability. Virtual Mentor. 2015;15(1):4–8.
Amarasekera S. Development of ethics and professionalism in Sri Lanka. JMAJ. 2007;50(3):255.
Bensley E.H. Medical luminaries (Osler Library studies in the history of medicine), (1), 1990.
Bird LP. Medical ethics. In: Bird LP, Barlow J, editors. Oaths & prayers, an anthology. Richardson: Christian Medical & Dental Society; 1989.
Brownell Wheeler H. Special report – Shattuck lecture – healing and heroism. New Engl J Med. 1990;322(21):1540–8.
Christian HA. Sir William Osler (1849-1919). Proc Am Acad Arts Sci. 1922;57(18):496–9.
Cohen J, Ezer T. Human rights in patient care: a theoretical and practical framework. Health Hum Rights. 2013;15(2)
Corbellini R. Dall'Etica Medica alla bioetica. (IT. From medical ethics to bioethics). Scienze e tecniche. Oilproject, Pub; 1994.
Garrison FH. Sir William Osler (1849-1919). Science (New Series). 1920;51(1307):1540–8.
Gruskin S, Dickens B. Human rights and ethics in public health. Am J Public Health. 2006;96(11):1903–190.
Karunalathilake I. Sri Lanka Medical Association. JMAJ. 2010;53(6):377–9.
King LS. Development of medical ethics. NEJM. 1958;258(10):480–6.
Kopp N, Réthy M-P, et al. Évolution des structures d' éthique médicale en France. (FR. Changing structures of medical ethics in France). Éthique & Santé. 2007;4(1):12–3.
Leake CD, editor. L'Etica Medica di Percival. Baltimore: Williams & Wilkins; 1927.
Millard MW. Can Osler teach us about 21st-century medical ethics? Proc (Bayl Univ Med Cent). 2011;4(3):227–35.
Osler W. The evolution of modern medicine, ed. Kaplan, chap. VI; 2009. p. 211.
Osler W. L'evoluzione della medicina moderna. (IT: The evolution of modern medicine). Translated by Paolo Fai. EDI Scienze; 2010. 310 p.
Patuzzo S. Storia del Codice Italiano di Deontologia Medica. Dalle origini ai giorni nostri. (IT. History of the Italian Code of Medical Ethics. From its origins to the present day). Ed. Minerva Medica; 2014.
Peel M. Human rights and medical ethics. J Soc Med. 2005;98(4):171–3.
Premoli De Marchi P. Le responsabilità del medico verso la società e verso il paziente. (IT. The responsibilities of the doctor towards society and towards the patient). Accademia University Press; 2012. p. 170–83.
Baker RB, Caplan AL, Emanuel LL, Latham SR, editors. Professionals and society. Baltimore/London: The John Hopkins University Press; 1999.
Reid EG. The great physician. A short life of Sir William Osler. Oxford University Press; 1931.
Riddick FA. The Code of Medical Ethics of The American Medical Association. Ochsner J. 2003;5(2):6–10.
Ryan M. A manual of medical jurisprudence and state medicine. II ed. London: Sherwood, Gilbert and Piper; 1836.
Silverman BD. Physician behavior and bedside manners: the influence of William Osler and The Johns Hopkins School of Medicine. Proc (Bayl Univ Med Cent). 2012;25(1):58–61.
Spinsanti S. Dall'Etica Medica alla bioetica: un cammino accidentato. (IT. From medical ethics to bioethics: a bumpy path). Janus; 2012.
Starr P. The social transformation of American medicine. New York: Basic Books; 1982. p. 89.
Waddington I. The development of medical ethics, sociological analysis. Med Hist. 1975;19(1):36–51.

9 Italy

It is necessary to start again from 1861. After the foundation of the Kingdom of Italy, the most significant pathologies came to light such as (to mention a few) syphilis, tuberculosis, malaria, pellagra, smallpox, and the high rate of infant mortality and neonatal, as well as various pathologies of mothers. The first (spontaneous) health orders born in Milan in 1887, in Naples in 1888, and in Venice in 1889, dedicated themselves to all this and opened up to the possibility of regulating health care.[1]

Sassari (Island of Sardinia)

The first code of Ethics and Deontology for Doctors was published in Sassari, in April 1903.[2]

At the beginning of the twentieth century, it was a highly innovative work, albeit in its incompleteness, as neither professional orders nor any recent provision for a medical self-regulation code existed yet. In about 50 pages the Professional Oath, the Hippocratic Oath and 50 articles were grouped, divided into Titles and Heads. Below are the first three articles, which do not require particular comments due to their modernity and sobriety:

ART. 1. The healthcare professional will be diligent, patient, and benevolent and will always scrupulously keep professional secrecy. He will be affable to the poor, he will not show servile respect to the rich, and he will treat both of them with the same self-denial.

ART. 2. He will also monitor the public health to the extent of its own means.

[1] Belloni et al. (2010) and Patuzzo (2014), pp. 49–63.

[2] Patuzzo (2014), pp. 67–78.
Sassari 2008, YEAR XVIII - N. 2 – May 2008.
Sassari 2014 Supp.n.5 Sassari, Medica, Anno XXIII, Oct 2014.

R. G. Russo, *Medical Ethics*, https://doi.org/10.1007/978-3-031-42444-1_9

ART. 3. When the doctor finds serious conditions in a sick person who is being treated, he must notify the family or whoever takes his/her place in the appropriate way, so that he/she can take those measures that are appropriate.

In the following article, ART. 4, it is stated that the Doctor will not undertake any operational act without first obtaining the consent of the patient or of the persons on whom this depends, if he is a minor or civil incapacitated. Certain cases of urgency, however, authorize derogations from this rule. But in serious circumstances he will ask, if he can, the help of a colleague who takes on some responsibility; this will be done especially when it will be procured an abortion for therapeutic purposes. What will then become part of the mandatory "Informed Consent," anticipated by about 44 years (see Chap. 12); other subsequent information is to better quantify the doctor's mission, still valid and respected today.

ART. 5. In public clinics you should not pay visits, but only place visits to poor patients, recognized as such.[2]

ART. 8. The doctor, in his own interest and in that of his colleagues, must expect a worthy and adequate compensation for his services.

Below is reported the Professional Oath (added only in the 2008 publication).

Being myself aware of the importance and solemnity of the act I perform and the commitment I undertake,

I swear:

- to practice medicine in freedom and independence of judgment and behavior, avoiding any undue influence;
- to pursue the defense of life, the protection of man's physical and mental health and the relief of suffering, to which I will inspire all my professional acts with responsibility and y and promoting the elimination of all forms of discrimination in the health field;
- never to carry out acts capable of deliberately causing the death of a person;
- to refrain from any diagnostic and therapeutic persistence;
- to promote the therapeutic alliance with the patient based on trust and mutual information, respecting and sharing the principles that inspire medical art;
- to stick in my activity to the ethical principles of human solidarity against which, in respect for life and for the person, I will never use my knowledge;
- to make my knowledge available to medical progress;
- to entrust my professional reputation exclusively to my competence and my moral skills;

- to avoid, even outside the professional practice, any act and behavior that could harm the decorum and dignity of the profession;
- to respect colleagues even in the event of conflicting opinions;
- to respect and facilitate the right to free choice of doctor;
- to provide emergency assistance to those in need and to make myself available to the competent authority in the event of a public calamity;
- to observe professional secrecy and to protect the confidentiality of everything that is confided to me, that I see or that I have seen, understood or sensed in the exercise of my profession or because of my state;
- to lend my work, in science and conscience, with diligence, expertise and prudence and according to fairness, observing the ethical rules that govern the practice of medicine and the legal ones that do not conflict with the purposes of my profession.
- YEAR XVIII—N. 2—May 2008—art. 1 paragraph 2, Property Order of the Sassari Doctors

More similar documents were proposed later:[3]

Florence

Code of deontological norms, i.e., medical etiquette, it is extremely important that there are legal bodies which, on the one hand, protect their legitimate professional interests and at the same time ensure the proper exercise of the profession for all those who dedicate themselves to it.

The first codes were elaborated by medical associations born spontaneously following the law n. 455 of July 10, 1910 which formally established the Orders of Doctors.[4]

The original legislation was composed of 11 articles, with which the orders of doctors, pharmacists, and veterinarians were established.

Law 10 July 1910, n. 455, (OJ no. 168 of July 19, 1910) Which Sets Rules for Healthcare Orders. (Published in the Official Gazette No. 168 of 19, 1910)

"Vittorio Emanuele III, by the grace of God and by the will of the nation, King of Italy; the Senate and the Chamber of Deputies approved;

[3] Patuzzo (2014), pp. 79–86.

[4] Flamigni and Mengarelli (2014).
Legge n. 455, July /10/1910 (GU n. 168, July19, 1910).

We have sanctioned and promulgate the following:"

ART. 1. In each Province, the Orders of Surgeons, Veterinarians and Pharmacists registered in the corresponding registers are constituted.

If the number of registered members in a Register does not reach fifteen, the Register itself will be combined with that of the final Province which will be indicated by the Superior Health Council.

Registration in the professional registers managed by the provincial orders thus became obligatory for the exercise of the profession, "in the Kingdom, in the colonies and in the protectorates" (Article 3).

Turin

(1912)—The Turin Medical Association proceeds to publish the Code of Ethics.

(1948)—The Turin Bar Council proceeds to update and revise the Code of Ethics.

(1948)—The FNOM (National Federation of Medical Orders) brings to the attention of all doctors, through the publication in several issues of the "Medical Federation," the Code of Ethics of the Order of Turin, placing it at the basis of a referendum among doctors Italians in view of the drafting of a national Deontological Code.

FNOMCEO

In 1922, during the congress of the Fascist Party, the creation of a trade union association for "intellectual" workers was initiated, with the consequent creation of the National Confederation of Trade Union Corporations, the first fascist medical unions and the Fascist Health Corporation. Later it became evident the need for a professional code valid for all the Italian provinces: such a document was approved only in 1924, inspired by the code in force at the Order of Doctors of the province of Turin, which had been approved in 1910. The latter had given a large space to the relationships of doctors with patients, colleagues, and other health care categories.[5]

The first unified Code of medical ethics, in the Fascist era, was sanctioned when the Orders of Doctors were also established; they gave great importance to the protection of the doctor's dignity, but did not yet consider the patient's consent, as also appears in the documents approved by the Provinces of Genoa, Vicenza, Verona, and Milan. The Code was divided into 37 articles including eight different topics (social duties, medical certificates, professional secrecy, class duty, specialization, duties towards other health professionals, other particular duties).

[5] Patuzzo (2014), pp. 89–98.

The reported norms had no references to patients' rights. There were multiple rules and advice relating to "good and civil conduct" that had to be followed to maintain friendly relations with colleagues.

Law 563 of April 3, 1926 established close subordination to the state.

The 11th Federal Congress of Medical Orders sanctioned the transformation of the FNOM into the National Fascist Federation of Medical Orders (FNFOM) and Royal Decree No. 184 of 5 March 1935 established the new discipline of the medical professions.

Professional orders were abolished:

Article 1 was categorical: "The professional orders of surgeons, veterinarians and pharmacists are abolished."

Discrimination of Jewish doctors appeared following the enactment of the racial laws of 1938.[6]

After World War 2

After the parenthesis of the fascist regime, the Order of Doctors was reconstituted, as well as numerous professional orders and colleges, with D.L.C.P.S. n. 233 of September 13, 1946: "Reconstruction of the Orders of the health professions and discipline of the exercise of the professions themselves" and were attributed to him, in art. 3, the identical functions conferred at the beginning of the century, when the doctors were less than 20,000.

In 1946, Article 1 of the Decree Law 233 of September 13, 1946 stated:

> In each province there are the Orders of surgeons, veterinarians and pharmacists and the Colleges of midwives. The 'Reconstruction of health care orders and professions and discipline of the exercise of the professions themselves' established that the orders of surgeons were established in each province.

The Governing Council of each Order and College had the following powers:

(a) to compile and keep the Register of the Order and the College and to publish it at the beginning of each year;
(b) to supervise the preservation of the dignity and independence of the Order and the College;
(c) to designate the representatives of the Order or College at provincial or municipal commissions, bodies and
(d) organizations;
(e) promote and encourage all initiatives aimed at facilitating the cultural progress of members;

[6] Patuzzo (2014), pp. 99–108.

(f) to contribute to the authorities in the study and implementation of measures that may in any case affect the Order or the College;
(g) exercise disciplinary power over freelance healthcare professionals registered in the Register, except in any case for other disciplinary and punitive provisions contained in the laws and regulations in force;
(h) to intervene, if requested, in disputes between healthcare and healthcare, or between healthcare professionals and persons or entities in favor of which the healthcare professional has provided or lends his professional work, for reasons of expenses, fees and other matters relating to professional practice, providing for the settlement of the dispute and, in case of unsuccessful agreement, giving his opinion on the disputes themselves.

The reconstitution / reconstruction of the Registers, the elections for the executive councils and more must in any case wait for the issuance of the decree of the President of the Republic of April 5, 1950, "Approval of the regulation for the execution of the legislative decree September 13, 1946, n.233, on the reconstitution of the Orders of the health professions and for the discipline of the professions themselves".[7]

Turin

The Order of Doctors of the Province of Turin was established with D.L.C.P.S. of 13 September 1946.

Como

In 1947 the booklet entitled "Doctor's Code" was published.[8] subtitled "Precepts of medical ethics."

The Author presented his writing "TO COLLEAGUES" saying: "… I do not claim, with these precepts, to teach you new things, but simply to remind you of the obligations you have towards God and society. These are duties that require profound piety, Christian virtue, a spirit of sacrifice and self-denial, a lot of diligence, good will, a generous heart and a great spirit of charity …"These advances, alone, represent a strong warning for correct behavior and the text is it then articulates on "The Foundations and the Norms of Christian Morality, for the scientific, professional and didactic exercise of the noble Health Mission." The Code is the work of a Professor of Forensic Medicine at the University of Milan, dedicated to the Bishop of Como and printed in Turin. It therefore lends itself well for a presentation to the medical society of the time.

The subject index includes:

[7] Patuzzo (2014), pp. 117–123.

[8] Judica Cordiglia (1947) and Patuzzo (2014), p. 122

- Duties of the doctor in general
- Doctor's skills
- Need for religious and professional culture
- The doctor in the face of divine laws
- The doctor and the sacraments
- The doctor and professional secrecy
- The doctor in the face of civil laws
- The doctor in front of the customers
- Duties of the doctor in front of colleagues
- Duties of the doctor at the service of the Church

Ultimately, beyond the title, it is a collection of good principles, with a strictly Catholic approach.

Bari

In 1952 the Scheme for a Code of Ethics was published: "The medical profession is the application of Science, the art of thought, the function of conscience."

The text then continues with other notes for professionals, including Relations with the Individual, the Company, and Colleagues. The preliminary texts of the 1910 Turin and Bari codes formed the backbone of the new Code. It was considered mandatory for new graduates who had to commit to its observance and fidelity to the criteria set out therein.

Code of Conduct in Italy

The main stages are listed below:

1953—FNOM appoints a Commission for the drafting of the national Code of Ethics, chaired by Cesare Frugoni, hence the document that will take his name. The Commission takes as its starting point the Code drawn up by the Turin Medical Association.

1954—A study commission is set up within the Roman Society of Forensic Medicine to examine the draft Code of Ethics at the request of the FNOM. The Frugoni Commission concluded its work. The FNOM brings to the attention of Italian doctors, through the full publication in the "Medical Federation", the text of the "Code of Medical Deontology" known as the "Frugoni Code." This Code, in the initial version of 1954 and in the definitive version of 1958, provided the "fundamental" basis for the constitution of the "National Code of Medical Ethics" and of the National Federation of Medical Orders (FNOM) with art. 54.[9]

1972—FNOM establishes a Commission for the revision of the Deontological Code.

[9] Flamigni and Mengarelli (2014) and Patuzzo (2014), pp. 126–131.

1976—FNOM appoints a Select Committee to complete the updating of the Code of Ethics. The Committee, with awork that lasted about a year, draws up the definitive text of the "Code of Medical Ethics" integrating it with the observations of the Italian Society of Health Ethics (SIDeS).
1977—The Committee submits the proposed text to the FNOM Central Committee for approval, which, after some clarifications and changes, is adopted by the Central Committee itself as a text to be presented to the National Council.
1978 (July)—The National Council approves the new "Code of Medical Deontology."
1985 (January)—The Central Committee appoints a Commission for the revision of the Code of Ethics.
1989 (July)—The National Council approves the new "Code of Medical Deontology." It is decided to transform the Study of the Commission into a permanent Commission in order to study any changes that over time will become necessary to bring a constant update of the Code.
1995 (June)—The National Council approves the new "Code of Medical Deontology."
1998 (October)—The Central Committee of FNOMCeO approves the new "Code of Medical Deontology."
2006 (December)—The new Code is approved in Rome by the FNOMCeO National Council.
2014 (May)—Eight years later the new "Code of Medical Ethics" is approved in Turin by the FNOMCeO National Council.
2016 (May 29)—The updated version[10] finally led to the current Code of Medical Ethics (Codex Deontologicus)

—by the National Federation of Orders of Doctors and Dentists (FNOMCeO); version[11] includes the professional oath reported below:

> Being myself aware of the importance and solemnity of the act I perform herein, and of the commitment I undertake, I swear:
> - to practice medicine in autonomy of judgment and responsibility for behavior, counteracting any undue conditioning that limits the freedom and independence of the profession;
> - to pursue the defense of life, the protection of physical and mental health, the treatment of pain and the relief of suffering while respecting

[10] Patuzzo (2014), pp. 135–219. Codice di Deontologia medica del 1978.
Patuzzo (2014), pp. 135–143. Codice di Deontologia medica del 1989.
Patuzzo (2014), pp. 145–153. Codice di Deontologia medica del 1995.
Patuzzo (2014), pp. 155–162. Codice di Deontologia medica del 1998.
Patuzzo (2014), pp. 163–175. Codice di Deontologia medica del 2006.
Patuzzo (2014), pp.177–186. Codice di Deontologia medica del 2014.
Patuzzo (2014), pp. 189–219

[11] FNOMCeO Comunicazione n. 27, Feb./27/2018

the dignity and freedom of the person to whom I will inspire all my professional acts with constant scientific, cultural and social commitment;

- to treat each patient with care and commitment, without any discrimination, promoting the elimination of all forms of inequality in the protection of health;
- never to carry out acts aimed at causing death;
- not to undertake or insist on clinically inappropriate and ethically out of proportion diagnostic procedures and therapeutic interventions, without ever abandoning the care of the patient;
- to pursue a care relationship with the assisted person based on trust and respect for the values and rights of each and on information, prior to consent, understandable and complete;
- to abide by the moral principles of humanity and solidarity as well as the civil principles of respect for the autonomy of the person
- to put my knowledge at the disposal of medical progress, based on the ethical and scientific rigor of research, whose aims are the protection of health and life;
- to entrust my professional reputation to my skills and to compliance with the ethical rules and to avoid, even outside of professional practice, any act and behavior that may harm the decorum and dignity of the profession;
- to inspire the solution of any difference of opinion to mutual respect;
- to provide assistance in urgent cases and to make myself available to the competent authority in the event of a public calamity;
- to respect professional secrecy and to protect the confidentiality of all that is confided to me, that I observe or that I have observed, understood or intuited in my profession or by reason of my state or office;
- to lend my work, in science and conscience, with diligence, expertise and prudence and according to fairness, observing the ethical rules governing the exercise of the profession.

The **"Contents and Purposes"** section is divided into 18 Titles and 79 Articles. The First Article (Definition) is reported:

The Code of medical ethics—hereinafter referred to as the "Code"—identifies the rules, inspired by the principles of medical ethics, which govern the professional practice of the surgeon and dentist—hereinafter referred to as "doctor"—registered in the respective professional registers. The Code, in harmony with the ethical principles of humanity and civil solidarity, to pursue the defense of life, the protection of physical and mental health, the treatment of pain and the relief of suffering while respecting the dignity and freedom of the person to whom I will inspire all my professional acts with constant scientific, cultural and social commitment; commits the doctor to the protection of individual and collective health by monitoring the dignity, dignity, independence and quality of the profession. The Code also regulates behaviors assumed outside the professional practice when deemed relevant and affecting the dignity of the profession.

The "**Final Provision**", as follows:

The Orders of Surgeons and Dentists implement this Code, within the framework of the direction and coordination. The action exercised by the National Federation of Orders of Surgeons and Dentists ensures compliance with it.

The Orders officially deliver the Code, or in any case to make it known to the individual members of the Registers and to carry out training and updating activities on medical ethics and deontology.

The rules of the Code will be subject to constant evaluation by the FNOMCeO in order to ensure that they are updated.

In Conclusion[12]

The Provincial Order of Surgeons and Dentists has specific powers and the following tasks:

- fill in and keep the register of the Order and the College;
- oversee the preservation of the dignity and independence of the Order and the College;
- designate the representatives of the Order or College at provincial or municipal commissions, bodies, and organizations;
- promote and encourage all initiatives aimed at facilitating the cultural progress of members;
- give its contribution to local authorities in the study and implementation of measures that may in any case affect the Order or the College;
- exercise disciplinary power against freelance health professionals registered in the register, except in any case, the other disciplinary and punitive provisions contained in the laws and regulations in force;

[12] Laonigro (2010) and Pepe (2007–08).

- intervene, if requested, in disputes between healthcare and healthcare, or between healthcare professionals and the person or entities in favor of which the healthcare provider has provided or is providing his professional work, for reasons of expenses, fees, and other matters relating to professional practice, providing for the settlement of the dispute and, in the event of an unsuccessful agreement, giving its opinion on the disputes themselves.

Faithful to the values expressed in the Deontological Code, it was later possible to identify a series of positive and negative duties, understood in their legal meaning; they do not express a moral judgment, but the duty to perform or not to perform a given action.

Positive Duties

- Knowledge and observance of the ethical rules: reported in Articles 1 and 2 of the CDM (Code of Medical Deontology) of 2006, as well as the same articles of the CDM of 2014.
- Protection of life, protection of health, relief from suffering: According to the definition offered by the WHO in 1946, health corresponds to a state of complete physical, mental, and social well-being, and not to the simple absence of disease (bio-psycho-social model), is the basis of the assumptions contained in art 4 of the 2006 CDM; CDM of 2014, again in art. 4, takes up the same requests, specifying, however, that the principles of medical action are: freedom, independence, autonomy, and responsibility
- Appropriate use of available resources: In both Codes = Professional and managerial quality. Provision of emergency care: art. 8 of the 2006 CDM is entitled Obligation to intervene; art. 8 of CDM 2014 Duty to intervene. In both cases, the obligation—or the duty—is to provide prompt and effective care to subjects who are in immediate danger of life. Otherwise, in this and similar cases, the subject falls on the cd. Medical fault for omission. The duty of assistance is to be considered of paramount importance, in the context of medical ethics, with respect to the right to conscientious objection, even if legitimate.
- Professional secrecy: Both the 2006 and 2014 Codes report, respectively, in Articles 10 and 11: duty to Confidentiality of personal data.
- Duty to provide clear, complete, and direct information:
- Continuous development of knowledge and skills, or professional updating—Assistance to the incurable patient and respect for the patient's wishes.
- Support in all phases of drug addiction recovery, including the social reintegration of the person involved.
- In case of appointment as medical director, guarantee of compliance with the Code.

Negative Duties

Abstention from:

- therapeutic persistence
- obligations and commitments that you are not able to keep, or from the over-load of work.
- conflict of interest
- comparison and patronage
- intervention on the human genome
- implementation of techniques and methodologies not required by law, or the promotion of practices and therapies lacking scientific evidence.

"**In addition to Italy**, the other member countries of the European Union also have Codes or Guides containing rules of conduct, drawn up by medical organizations, which doctors are required to observe in their clinical practice."

The countries affected by similar laws are: Austria, Belgium, Cyprus, Czech Republic, France, Germany, Greece, Ireland, Luxembourg, Netherlands, Portugal, Romania, Slovenia, Spain, United Kingdom.[13]

References

Belloni G, et al. Per una Storia dell'Ordine dei Medici-Chirurghi e degli Odontoiatri della provincia di Pavia. (IT. For a history of the order of physicians-surgeons and dentists in the province of Pavia). Ed. OMCEO, Industria Grafica Pavese s.a.s.; 2010.

Flamigni C, Mengarelli M. Nelle mani del dottore? Il racconto e il possibile futuro di una relazione difficile. (IT. In doctor's hands ? The story and the possible future of a difficult relationship). Milano: Ed. Franco Angeli; 2014. p. 208.

Judica Cordiglia G. Codice del Medico. Precetti di deontologia medica. (IT. Doctor's Code. Precepts of medical ethics). L.I.C.E. R. Berruti & C. Turin; 1947. 91 pp.

Laonigro P. Le norme deontologiche tra teoria e prassi giurisprudenziale: notazioni sul codice deontologico medico. (IT: The deontological rules between theory and jurisprudential practice: notations on the deontological code doctor). Edition: Amministrazione in Cammino. Rivista elettronica. 2010 May 8. p. 1–34.

Patuzzo S. Storia del Codice Italiano di Deontologia Medica. Dalle origini ai giorni nostri. (IT. History of the Italian Code of Medical Ethics. From its origins to the present day). Ed. Minerva Medica; 2014.

Pepe F. Evoluzione del Codice Deontologico medico in Italia. Tesi di laurea in Medicina Legale. (IT. Evolution of the medical code of ethics in Italy. Thesis in Forensic medicine). Academic Year 2007–08.

[13] Patuzzo (2014), pp. 220–222.

10 Ethics and Professionalism

There are many documents related to the integrity of man and his ethical conduct especially in the field of medicine,[1] from different organizations throughout the world. Students of medical schools often take an oath on graduation, largely based on the Hippocratic Oath, referring to professional responsibility and conduct today. The American Medical Association adopted a Declaration of Responsibility in 2001, covering nine duties and obligations, and future doctors swore that they made these promises freely and on their personal and professional honor. It particularly noted that advances in medical science call for attention and action by the medical profession and in today's "global" world disease respects no frontiers.

More Declarations Followed

(a) **Charter of Medical Professionalism**;[2] born in 2002 from a series of meetings organized by the American Board of Internal Medicine (ABIM), by the European Federation of Internal Medicine (EFIM) and by the American College of Physicians-American Society of Internal Medicine (ACP-ASIM).[3]

It was published almost jointly, with the title "Medical Professionalism in the new millennium: a physician's charter." The Charter consists of a brief introduction, and sets out three fundamental principles and ten commitments, designed to be applicable to different cultures and different political systems.

The practice of medicine in the modern era is faced with many challenges that increase the difficulties on doctor–patient relationships, especially in relation to resources. In fact, while needs are growing, they do not always run parallel with the availability of health care on the market.

[1] Patuzzo (2014), pp. 223–24.

[2] Carta della Professionalità Medica (2002), Medicina e Chirurgia (2015), ABIM Foundation et al. (2002), Medical Professionalism Project (2002), and Familiari and Volpe (2014).

[3] Jotkowitz et al. (2004).

R. G. Russo, *Medical Ethics*, https://doi.org/10.1007/978-3-031-42444-1_10

There are three Fundamental Principles:

- The principle of the centrality of patients' well-being.
- The principle of patients' autonomy.
- The principle of social justice.

and ten Professional Commitments:[4]

1. Professional competence,
2. Honesty with patients,
3. Patients' confidentiality,
4. Maintenance of appropriate relationships with patients,
5. Improvement of the quality of care,
6. Appropriate distribution of limited resources,
7. Scientific knowledge,
8. Maintenance of trust by managing conflicts of interest,
9. Improvement of the quality of services,
10. Professional responsibility.

The commitments to achieve the highest standards of excellence in the practice of medicine underlie and boost the interests and well-being of patients and society itself.[5]

Honor and integrity imply constant respect for the highest standards of behavior and the decision to be fair, sincere, keep one's word, honor commitments, and be simple. Respect for other people (including patients and their families, other doctors and professional colleagues such as nurses, medical students, etc.) is the essence of humanism, at the heart of professionalism and is fundamental for the best collegiality.[6]

Medicine has directed its efforts, together with the "Hippocratic" concepts to professionalism. This term is now interpreted as describing the skills, attitudes, and behaviors expected of individuals during the practice of their profession and covers concepts such as maintaining competence, ethical behavior, integrity, honesty, altruism, service and respect to others, respect of professional codes, justice, self-regulation, etc.[7]

More Notes on Profession and Professionalism

The "Profession" is the form in which medical art presents itself to society, in its task of taking care of a person's health.

"Professionalism" in medicine requires physicians to serve the patient's interests above their personal interest." Medical professionalism implies altruism,

[4] Malliani (2002).

[5] ACGME Project (2004), American Board of Internal Medicine (1999), Mancari (2010), and Nace et al. (2009).

[6] Academic Medicine (2016), Birden et al. (2013), Cruess and Cruess (2008), Wynia et al. (1999), and Wynia (2008).

[7] ACGME (2004), Kirk (2007), and Meakins (2003).

responsibility, excellence, duty, service, integrity, and respect for others, thus already serving as a code of ethics.

The commitments to achieve the highest standards of excellence in the practice of medicine underlie and boost the interests and well-being of patients and society itself (see Footnote 5).

Honor and integrity imply constant respect for the highest standards of behavior and the decision to be fair, sincere, keep one's word, honor commitments, and be simple. Respect for other people (including patients and their families, other doctors and professional colleagues such as nurses, medical students, etc.) is the essence of humanism, at the heart of professionalism and is fundamental for the best collegiality (see Footnote 6).

Professionalism is now interpreted as describing the skills, attitudes, and behaviors expected of individuals during the practice of their profession and covers concepts such as maintaining competence, ethical behavior, integrity, honesty, altruism, service and respect to others, respect of professional codes, justice, self-regulation, etc. (see Footnote 7).

> **A DEFINITION OF MEDICAL PROFESSIONALISM:**[8] from the 2 arguments in the preceding sections, one can appreciate that the key to understanding medical professionalism is not to be found in a simple dictionary definition. Rather, the concept of medical professionalism must account for the nature of the medical profession and must be grounded in what physicians actually do and how they act, individually and collectively. Bearing this in mind, I assert that medical professionalism consists of those behaviors by which we, as physicians, demonstrate that we are worthy of the trust bestowed upon us by our patients and the public, because we are working for the patients' and the public's good. Failure to demonstrate that we deserve that trust will result in its loss, and, hence, loss of medicine's status as a profession.

This concept emerged in the early 1990s in the United States and Canada as a result of the many challenges facing healthcare. In addition to affirming humanistic qualities such as compassion and altruism in the medical world, ethical principles have been strengthened.[9] Ethical priorities are fundamental to medical professionalism, based on improving the well-being and dignity of patients. Honesty and confidentiality are fundamental too, together with other positive professional qualities in the code of ethics.[10]

Some (though not all!) of the values inherent in the Hippocratic Oath are still found in modern professionalism. Some observations, though cited in the Hippocratic Oath (e.g., those relating to abortion and surgical practice), are not in line with current knowledge. An ancient oath cannot encompass all the values of medicine in the twenty-first century. Its meaning lies in the symbolism of an ideal: the safeguarding of human life.[11]

---

[8] Swick (2000).

[9] Academic Medicine (2016), MacKenzie (2007), Mancari (2011), Passi et al. (2010), Premoli De Marchi (2012), Walsh and Abelson (2008), and Wynia et al. (1999).

[10] Cruess and Cruess (2008) and University of Ottawa (2017).

[11] Canadian Evaluation Society (2006).

The ethics related to professionalism also illustrate the expected behavior with other doctors, health professionals, medical students, and tutors. The distinctive signs are competence in a specialized sector, together with the recognition of specific duties and responsibilities towards individuals and society. They are also borne in mind (and evaluated) in the teaching and training given to third parties, and any disciplinary observations concerning lack of competence or non-compliance with the established duties. Medical professionals have a particularly strict obligation to ensure that their decisions and actions serve the well-being of their patients. The various sectors have codes of ethics that specify the obligations arising from this duty.[12]

The definitions of medical professionalism can be summarized in three main points:

1. doctors must master knowledge and skills, in the service of others;
2. doctors will be expected to respect the highest standards of ethical and professional behavior in all their work;
3. the practice of medicine involves trust between doctors and patients.

This relationship between ethics and professionalism indicates that ethical concerns are necessary to address moral issues in medical practice.[13] Some authors, however, have expressed further opinions on professionalism, adding clarification, as in the comments that follow.[14]

Ethics in Professionalism

Medical and professional ethics often establishes positive duties (for instance, what has to be done) to an even greater extent than current law. Understanding medical ethics is based on the principles of charity, non-maleficence and justice. The medical profession is present everywhere, in different national cultures and traditions, and often finds itself confronting complex political, legal, and market forces—occasionally conflicting.[15]

Worldwide Declarations of Professional Responsibility have been declared in a variety of languages, as follows:

> English, Arabic, Brazilian Portuguese, Chinese, Farsi, French, German, Hindi, Indonesian, Italian, Japanese, Korean, Russian, Spanish, Swahili, Urdu.

---

[12] Jonsen et al. (2016) and Professional Ethics and Standards for the Evaluation Community in the Government of Canada (2006).

[13] Dunn (2016).

[14] ABIM, Benson (2017), ACP (American College of Physicians) (2012), AMA (American Medical Association) (2002), Kirk (2007), and MPS (Medical Protection Society Ltd) (2017).

[15] ACP: American College of Physicians AMA: American Medical Association MPS: Medical Protection Society Ltd Ltd? È una società commerciale? (ABIM: American Board of Internal Medicine).

Moreover (Added to Previous Declarations)

Social Contract of Medicine with Humanity

- The priority is the patient's well-being: this principle hinges on altruism, trust, and interest in the patient. The Charter states: "Market forces, social pressures and administrative requirements must not undermine this principle."
- Patients' autonomy. This principle includes honesty with patients and the need to educate and empower them to take part in appropriate medical decisions.
- Social justice. This principle addresses physicians' social contract and distributive justice: that means taking account of the resources available and the needs of all patients, while caring for the patient individually (see Footnote 15).

The Meaning of Medical Professionalism

In 2005 the Royal College of Physicians of London presented a report "Medical professionalism in a constantly evolving world" to redefine the nature and role of medical professionalism in a modern society.

The conclusion it was, briefly, a set of values, behaviors, and relationships to build the trust the public has in doctors. Furthermore, doctors have to commit to observing many professional standards, such as: integrity, compassion, altruism, continuous improvement, excellence, collaboration with other parties in the health-care team.

Professional persons must:

- take pride in doing their job, and pay attention to details;
- take responsibility for their actions and consequences;
- strive constantly to develop and improve their skills;
- not be satisfied with an unsatisfactory result and therefore plan the necessary corrections;
- be ready to recognize mistakes, learn from them and take the appropriate measures to prevent their repetition;
- show respect for those who are consulted in a professional capacity. (MPS) (see Footnote 15)

Not only must doctors reach good decisions for their patients (based on evidence, and the literature), but those decisions must be applied in order to help the patient. "Medical professionals are defined not only by what they must know and do, but, above all, by a deep sense of what a physician must be".[16]

Evaluations and measures of professionalism, based on honesty, altruism, trustworthiness, and respect for others are often interpreted differently, and it is hard to define them fully.

[16] Nichols et al. (2014).

In Conclusion

In almost all cultures and societies today medical practice is concerned with professionalism. Physicians face challenges related to the legitimate needs of patients, the resources available, the dependence of health systems on market forces, and the temptation of physicians to reaffirm their privileged position.

(b) **THE EUROPEAN CHARTER OF PATIENTS' RIGHTS** and the Code of Deontology of the Medical Profession[17] (The Charter of Fundamental Rights of the European Union, in Italy also known as the Charter of Nice), presented on 7 December 2000 in Nice (France) and 12 December 2007 to the European Parliament in Strasbourg.

Principles of European Medical Ethics and Approval of the European Charter of Medical Ethics (Greece)[18]

On 6 January 1987, the then International Conference of Medical Professional Associations and Bodies, with similar remits, established general principles of medical ethics at the European level.[19] The 37 deontological guidelines adopted by CEOM (at that meeting) are reported below.

This text contains the most important principles intended to inspire the professional conduct of doctors, in any field of practice, their contacts with patients, with the society and among colleagues. They also refer to "good medical practice."

The conference recommends that medical professional associations in each Member State of the European Union[20] take the necessary measures to ensure that their respective national requirements relating to the duties and rights of physicians, comply with the principles set out in this text. The associations should take appropriate measures to ensure that the legislation in their country allows for the effective implementation of these principles.

Article 1—The vocation of a doctor consists in protecting the physical and mental health of man and alleviating suffering, while respecting human life and dignity, with no discrimination based on age, race, religion, nationality, social situation, political ideology, or any other reason, in times of war or peace.

---

[17] Principles of European Medical Ethics_C.E.O.M. EJD, Adoption of the CEOM European Charter of Medical Ethics.

[18] Documento di consenso Sanremo (2010), Fondazione Zoé (2011), and Ufficio Stampa FNOMCeO (2011).

Wikipedia.: FNOMCeO.

[19] Carta europea dei diritti del malato (2002).

[20] Carta dei diritti fondamentali dell'Unione Europea (2000).

THE DOCTOR'S COMMITMENT

Article 2—In the practice of his profession, the doctor undertakes to give priority to the patient's health interests. The physician must use his professional knowledge to improve or maintain the health of those who rely on him or his care, at their request; the doctor cannot, in any case, act to their detriment.

Article 3—The doctor is prohibited from imposing personal, philosophical, moral or political opinions on the patient in the exercise of his profession.

INFORMED CONSENT

Article 4—Except in an emergency, doctors must clearly inform a patient of the expected effects and consequences of treatment. They must then obtain the patient's consent, especially if the proposed treatment presents any serious risk. The doctor must not substitute his own concept of quality of life for that of his patient.

MORAL AND TECHNICAL INDEPENDENCE

Article 5—In order to advise and act, doctors must have full professional freedom and technical and moral conditions that allow them to act in complete independence. The patient should be informed if these conditions have not been met.

Article 6—When a doctor acts on behalf of a public or private authority and when the intervention is ordered by a third party or by an institution, s/he must also inform the patient.

PROFESSIONAL CONFIDENTIALITY

Article 7—The doctor is the patient's necessary confidant. Doctors must ensure complete secrecy of all information they collect and discoveries made during contact with the patient. The death of the patient does not release the doctor from medical confidentiality.

Doctors must respect the patient's privacy and take all necessary measures to make it impossible to disclose all the information acquired during the exercise of their profession. If exceptions to medical confidentiality are provided for by national legislation, the doctor can request the prior opinion of an association or professional body with similar competence.

Article 8—Doctors must not collaborate in the creation of electronic databases of medical data that may jeopardize or weaken the patient's right to privacy, security and the protection of their private life.

To comply with medical ethics, any electronic database must be held under the responsibility of a specifically designated doctor. Medical databases cannot be linked in any way to other databases.

COMPETENCE OF THE DOCTOR

Article 9—The physician must refer to all medical resources and apply them appropriately to the patient.

Article 10—Doctors must not claim competence for a competence that they do not have.

Article 11—A doctor must call on a more qualified colleague if any testing or treatment is beyond his or her knowledge.

END OF LIFE CARE

Article 12—In all circumstances, medicine implies constant respect for life, moral autonomy and the patient's free choice. However, in the case of incurable and terminal conditions, doctors can limit themselves to alleviating the physical and moral suffering of the patient by giving adequate treatment and maintaining, as far as possible, the quality of a life that is nearing its end. It is essential to assist a dying person to the end and to act in a way that maintains that person's dignity.

ORGAN TRANSPLANTS

Article 13—When it is impossible to reverse the terminal process of artificially maintained vital function. Physicians must take account of the latest scientific data when certifying the death of a patient. At least two doctors must be responsible for separately drafting a document relating to this situation. They must be independent of the group responsible for the transplant.

Article 14—Doctors responsible for harvesting an organ intended for transplantation can use special treatment to keep the donor organ viable.

Article 15—Doctors who harvest organs must make sure by all possible means that the donor has not expressed a contrary opinion in life, either in writing or through relatives.

REPRODUCTION

Article 16—The doctor must provide the patient or in response to a request, with all useful information regarding re-production and contraception.

Article 17—In compliance with the code of ethics, a doctor may, in the light of his own beliefs, refuse to intervene in the process of reproduction or in the termination of pregnancy or abortion, and should ask the persons concerned to seek advice from other doctors.

EXPERIMENTS ON HUMAN BEINGS

Article 18—The advancement of medicine is based on research that cannot be undertaken without experiments conducted on human beings.

Article 19—The protocol of any planned experiment on a human must be submitted in advance to an ethics committee, independent of the researcher, for advice and opinion.

Article 20—The subject of the experiment must give clear, free consent after having been properly informed of the aims, methods, and expected benefits, as well as of the risks and potential undesirable side effects, of his or her right to refuse participation in the experiment, and withdraw at any time.

Article 21—A doctor may couple biomedical research with medical assistance, in order to acquire new medical knowledge, to the extent that such biomedical research is justified by a potential diagnostic or therapeutic benefit for the patient.

TORTURE AND INHUMAN TREATMENT

Article 22—A doctor must never attend, participate in or accept acts of torture or other forms of cruel, inhuman or de-grading treatment, regardless of the reasons (crime committed, accusation, beliefs) or any other situation, including civil or armed conflict.

Article 23—A doctor must never use his knowledge, skills or abilities to facilitate the use of torture or any other cruel, inhuman or degrading process, for any purpose.

DOCTORS AND SOCIETY

Article 24—To carry out his humanitarian mission, a doctor has the right to legal protection of his professional independence, in times of war and peace.

Article 25—A doctor who acts alone or through a professional organization has a duty to draw the attention of the community to any shortcomings in health care or the independence of professionals.

Article 26—Doctors are required to participate in the development and implementation of collective measures aimed at improving prevention, diagnosis and treatment among patients. In particular, they are required to collaborate, from the medical point of view, in organizing aid, especially in disaster situations.

Article 27—Within the limits of their abilities and possibilities, they must participate in the continuous progress of the quality of health care through research and constant improvements, in order to offer patients treatments that comply with scientific data.

COLLEGIALITY

Article 28—The rules of collegiality have been established in the interests of patients. They aim to prevent patients from being victims of unfair competition; however, doctors can legitimately mention the professional qualities recognized by their peers.

Article 29—A doctor called to take care of a patient already entrusted to one of his colleagues must strive to keep in touch with the latter in the interest of the patient, unless the patient objects to this.

Article 30—It is not a violation of fiduciary duty if a doctor informs the competent professional body of violations of medical ethical rules and professional competence of which he may become aware.

PUBLICATION OF FINDINGS

Article 31—Doctors have a duty to make known in the professional press, first of all, all the discoveries they have made or the conclusions of scientific studies on diagnosis or therapy. They must submit their reports for critical review by their peers, through the appropriate channels, before disclosing anything to the non-medical public.

Article 32—Any description of a medical achievement benefitting only a person, group or school is contrary to the medical code of ethics.

CONTINUITY OF CARE

Article 33—Regardless of the doctor's specialty, s/he must consider it a duty to provide urgent care to a person in immediate danger unless it is certain that another doctor can and is able to provide this care.

Article 34—Any doctor care of a patient undertakes to cooperate with other doctors or colleagues with the appropriate skills, as necessary.

FREE CHOICE

Article 35—The patient's free choice of doctor is a fundamental principle of the patient/doctor relationship. The doctor must respect and guarantee respect for this freedom of choice. A doctor may refuse assistance, except when a patient is in danger.

DOCTORS' STRIKES

Article 36—When a doctor decides to participate in the organized collective refusal to provide assistance, he is not exempted from his ethical obligation towards patients; health care must be guaranteed to patients in need of urgent medical attention and to those already undergoing treatment.

FEES

Article 37—In setting a fee and in the absence of a contract or an individual or collective agreement establishing rates, doctors must take into account the scope of the service provided, any special circumstances, their own skills and the patient's financial situation.

The "Conseil Européen des Ordres des Médecins (CEOM)", of which the Italian FNOMCeO is a member,[21] aims to promote the practice of high quality medicine within the European Union and the European Free Trade Association (EFTA). Its ethical guidelines are related to: Informed consent, Professional secrecy, Doping in sport, Relations with colleagues, Environment and health, Refusal of treatment, Information and advertising, Medical research and therapeutic evidence, Conflict of interest, Appropriate prescription of drugs, Professional updating, Complementary and alternative medicines. On 6 February 1995, besides confirming the previous points, an APPENDIX to the Guidelines was published, establishing the following main points.

Preamble

The previous principles of medical ethics cover the deontological rules on which European medical corporations agree. Developments in the European Union (for example, concerning the basic conditions of free market circulation or EU law on advertising or companies), open up an opportunity for doctors to agree not only on the "ethical basis" of their profession, but also on the

[21] FNOMCeO (2014–2017).

principles of conduct that must be respected in its exercise (for example, how they announce their work or exercise it in companies or associations).

The principles of behavior adopted in the interests of the patient form an appendix to the ethical principles adopted in 1987. They constitute the recommendations addressed to all orders of physicians and related bodies authorized to adopt rules in this area and to doctors themselves.

2. Presentation of medical practice

(a) The practice of a medical profession is neither a trade nor a commercial activity. Whatever type of medicine a doctor practices, whether as an employee or privately, he can make known his titles and qualifications as well as any other indications necessary for information to the patient, in compliance with the provisions in force for professional associations and bodies with similar offices, within the framework of the law. Such information must be clearly distinguishable from any advertising or information which could mislead patients and which could be considered unethical by doctors in all European countries. Also, physicians must not have any such advertising done on their behalf or advertising to be made about them.
(b) A physician practicing in a hospital or other medical center or within the framework of companies or associations must not allow the facility or company manager to specifically advertise his or her knowledge, skills or services to other practitioners.
(c) A doctor can objectively inform other doctors about the medical services he offers. This is particularly applicable to information provided by generalists on specialists. However, it is unacceptable among a doctor's colleagues to specifically highlight his services in relation to those of other doctors.
(d) A doctor exercising working as a medical service provider in a Member State of the EU other than that in which he is domiciled or where he exercises his professional activity and in which he belongs to a medical association (or competent professional organization), must comply with the professional rules of the Member State in which he practices. The same applies if the doctor simply wishes to make his activity known in another Member State; the doctor is authorized to advertise his medical activity on the basis of the ethical and legal rules applicable to professionals of the Member State in which he publishes it.
(e) A doctor can only collaborate with members of other health professions if they work under their supervision or have a well-defined field of expertise corresponding to their qualifications.

Each doctor must be responsible for his medical records and prescriptions.

In 2005, at Sanremo (Italy) (see Footnote 18), the great Project of the European Medicine Charter was launched. Five years later, in March 2010, Sanremo was reconfirmed "Capital of Ethics and Deontology," ratifying a "Consensus Document." On 11 June 2011, 14 delegations from as many European states gathered on the island of Kos to announce and then confirm the European Charter of the Principles of Medical Ethics. The European medical community is committed to respecting the European Charter and the following 16 principles are mandatory.

The president of the FNOMCeO and the other presidents of European Medical Orders have read the Charter which, in addition to taking up the moral bases of the deontological codes of the various countries, follows and stresses the principles of the Hippocratic Oath, in the version updated in 2007.

The expansion and developments of the European Union offer doctors the opportunity to extend their influence, not only on a common ethical basis but also in relation to principles of behavior that must be respected in the practice of their profession, regardless of specialization.

Principle 1: The doctor defends the physical and mental health of man. Relieves pain while respecting the life and dignity of the human person, with no discrimination, in peace as in war.

Principle 2: The doctor undertakes to prioritize the patient's health interests.

Principle 3: The doctor gives the patient, with no discrimination, the most appropriate treatment.

Principle 4: The doctor considers the patient's life and work as determinants of health.

Principle 5: The doctor is the patient's necessary confidant and revealing what they have learned is a betrayal of this trust.

Principle 6: The doctor uses his professional knowledge to improve or maintain the health of those who put their trust in him, at their request; in any case he cannot do anything against them.

Principle 7: The doctor employs all the resources of medical science to be applied appropriately to the patient.

Principle 8: In respect of the autonomy of the person, the doctor acts according to the principle of effectiveness of the treatment, taking into account the fair use of resources.

Principle 9: The practice of medicine involves respect for life, moral autonomy, and the patient's choices.

Principle 10: Health protection is accompanied by constant research to maintain the integrity of the person.

Principle 11: The doctor does never permits torture or other cruel, inhuman or degrading treatment, whatever the situation, including civil or military conflict. He neither assists nor participates in it.

Principle 12: The doctor who intervenes as a simple practitioner with a patient, or as an expert or a member of an institution, ensures full transparency on anything that might appear to be a conflict of interest, and acts independently both morally and technically.

Principle 13: If moral and technical conditions do not allow the doctor to act independently, the doctor informs the patient. The patient's right to care must be guaranteed.

Principle 14: When a doctor decides to participate in a collective refusal to organize treatment, he is not exempted from his ethical obligations towards the patients to whom he guarantees first aid, and any action needed for patients under treatment.

Principle 15: The doctor cannot satisfy requests for treatment that he does not approve.

Principle 16: The doctor exercises his profession with conscience, dignity, and independence.

The European Parliament, the Council, and the Commission solemnly proclaim the following text as the Charter of Fundamental Rights of the European Union.

Presentation

The peoples of Europe in creating ever closer union among themselves have decided to share a peaceful future based on common values. Aware of its spiritual and moral heritage, the Union is founded on the indivisible and universal values of human dignity, freedom, equality, and solidarity; the Union is based on the principles of democracy and the rule of law. It places the person at the center of its action by recognizing Union citizenship and creating an area of freedom, security and justice. These are the first three articles.

Art. 1. Human dignity: human dignity is inviolable. It must be respected and protected.

Art. 2. Right to life:everyone has the right to life. No one can be sentenced to death, or executed.

Art. 3. Right to the integrity of the person. Every person has the right to his or her physical and mental integrity.

In the field of medicine and biology, the following must be respected in particular:

- the free and informed consent of the person involved, according to the procedures established by law,
- the prohibition of eugenic practices, particularly those whose purpose is the selection of persons,
- the prohibition on making the human body and its parts as source of profit,
- the prohibition of the reproductive cloning of human beings.

(c) **CELEX numbers**

The CELEX numbers (Communitatis Europeae Lex) are the unique indicator of each document in the EUR-Lex, prepared in the 24 official languages of the EU. Most documents in EUR-Lex—regardless of the language in which they are written—are assigned a CELEX number, as their unique identifier. Learning how to read these numbers will help you search faster and understand how documents relate to each other.

Documents in EUR-Lex fall into the following 12 areas.

1. Treaties
2. International agreements
3. Legal deeds
4. Complementary legislation
5. Preparatory documents
6. EU jurisprudence
7. National transposition
8. References to national jurisprudence regarding EU legislation
9. Parliamentary questions
10. Consolidated texts
11. Other documents published in the C series of the Official Journal
12. EFTA documents.

(d) **COMMENTARY TO THE FNOMCeO CODE** (see Footnote 21), 75 pages, 2014.

The Code of Ethics—History

- 1912: The Turin Medical Association publishes the Code of Ethics.

1948: The FNOM brings the Code of Ethics of the Order of Turin, basis for a national code of ethics, to the knowledge of all Italian doctors.

1953: The FNOM appoints a Commi for tee to draft the national Code of Ethics.

1954: A study Committee is set up within the Roman Society of Forensic Medicine to examine the draft Code of Ethics.

1954: The Frugoni Committee concludes its work: the FNOM publishes the Code of Medical Ethics in the "Medical Federation."

1972: FNOM revises the Code.

1976: FNOM appoints a select committee to update the Code of Medical Ethics, integrating it with the observations of the Italian Society of Health Ethics (SIDeS).

1977: The proposed text is adopted by the Central Committee itself as a text to be presented to the National Council.

07.01.1978: The National Council approves the new Code of Medical Ethics.

01.20.1985: The Central Committee calls for revision of the Code of Medical Ethics

07.15.1989: The National Council approves the new Code of Medical Ethics.

06.24 and 25, 1995: The National Council approves the revised Code.

07.11.1997: Revision of the Code.

10.02.1998: Observations and proposals of the Provincial Orders. The National Council makes some changes.

03.19.1998: The National Council approves the new Code.

12.16.2006: The National Council approves the revised Code of Medical Ethics reaffirming the role of the doctor as the sole interpreter of a treatment project.
05.18.2014 (Turin): The National Council approves the Code of Medical Ethics by inserting four new articles and restyling duties and vocabulary.

Some changes are made to the text of the Deontological Code on May 19, 2016, November 16, 2016 and December 15, 2017.

Art. 1 Definition

- The Code of Medical Deontology sets out principles and rules that surgeons and dentists registered in the professional Orders of Surgeons and Dentists, hereinafter referred to as "doctors," must observe in the exercise of their profession.

The behavior of the doctor, even outside the exercise of the profession, must be in keeping with its decorum and dignity.

Doctors are required to be aware of the rules of this Code, and ignorance does not exempt them from disciplinary responsibility."

Art. 2 Disciplinary Powers—Sanctions

- Failure to comply with the precepts, obligations, and prohibitions established by this Code of Medical Deontology, and any action or omission, however, unbecoming to the decorum or the correct exercise of the profession, are punishable by the disciplinary sanctions provided for by law. The sanctions must be proportionate to the gravity of the acts.

Object and Scopes of Application

General Duties of the Doctor

The duty of a doctor is the protection of life, the physical and mental health of man, and the relief of suffering with respect for the freedom and dignity of the human person, without discrimination of age, sex, race, religion, nationality, social status, or ideology, in peace as in war, whatever the institutional or social conditions in which they operate. Health is understood in the broadest sense of the term, as a condition of physical and mental well-being of the person.
CHAPTER I—Independence and dignity of the profession
CHAPTER II—Emergency services
CHAPTER III—Special obligations of the doctor
CHAPTER IV—Diagnostic assessments and therapies
CHAPTER V—Professional obligations

Relations with the Citizen

CHAPTER I—General rules of conduct
CHAPTER II—Doctor's duties and citizens' rights
CHAPTER III—Doctor's duties towards minors, the elderly and disabled

CHAPTER IV—Information and consent
CHAPTER V—Care of incurable patients
CHAPTER VI—Transplants
CHAPTER VII—Sexuality and reproduction
CHAPTER VIII—Experimentation
CHAPTER IX—Medical treatment and personal freedom
CHAPTER X—Professional fees
CHAPTER XI—Healthcare advertising and information to the public

Relations with Colleagues

CHAPTER I—Solidarity among doctors
CHAPTER II—Advice and consultation
CHAPTER III—Other relations between doctors
CHAPTER IV—Forensic medicine
CHAPTER V—Relations with the professional associations

Relations with Third Parties

CHAPTER I—Professional work

Relations with the National Health Service and with Public and Private Bodies

CHAPTER I—Deontological obligations of the doctor in employment or contracts and agreements
CHAPTER II—Sports medicine
CHAPTER III—Protection of collective health

FINAL PROVISION: *The Provincial Orders of Surgeons and Dentists are required to distribute the Code of Medical Ethics to individuals on the Register, and to periodically hold refresher and in-depth courses. Doctors and dentists must take the professional oath.*

Professional Oath

Being aware of the importance and solemnity of the work I do and the commitment I undertake, I swear:

- to practice medicine in autonomy of judgment and responsibility for behavior, countering any undue conditioning that limits the freedom and independence of the profession;

- to pursue the defense of life, the protection of physical and mental health, the treatment of pain and the relief of suffering, while respecting the dignity and freedom of the person to whom I will dedicate my professional work, with constant scientific, cultural and social commitment;
- to treat each patient with care and commitment, with no discrimination, promoting the elimination of all forms of inequality in the protection of health;
- never to carry out acts aimed at causing death;
- not to undertake or insist on clinically inappropriate and ethically disproportionate diagnostic procedures and therapeutic interventions, without ever relinquishing the care of the patient;
- to maintain a caring relationship with the patient, based on trust and respect for the values and rights of each, giving understandable and complete information prior to consent.
- to abide by the moral principles of humanity and solidarity as well as the civil principles of respect for the autonomy of the person;
- to put my knowledge at the disposal of medical progress, based on the ethical and scientific rigor of research, whose aims are the protection of health and life;
- to entrust my professional reputation to my skills and to respect of ethical rules and to avoid, even outside professional practice, any action or behavior that could diminish the decorum and dignity of the profession;
- to inspire mutual respect for the solution of any difference of opinion;
- to provide assistance in cases of urgency and to be available to the authorities in the event of a public calamity;
- to respect professional secrecy and to protect the confidentiality of all that is confided to me, that I observe or that I have observed, understood or guessed in my profession or by reason of my state or office;
- to lend my work, in knowledge and conscience, with diligence, expertise, prudence and fairness, observing the deontological rules that regulate the exercise of the profession.

(e) **Charter of CODE OF ETHICS OF THE MARIO NEGRI INSTITUTE FOR PHARMACOLOGICAL RESEARCH—IRCCS**[22]

Milan, 21 December 2016.

The Charter of Values and Code of Ethics promotes the mission of the Mario Negri Institute (Milan, Italy) for Pharmacological Research (hereinafter referred to as the IRFMN) and a system of ethical values and behavioral rules aimed at encouraging employees and third parties involved in the Institute's operations to commit to morally correct conduct as well as compliance with current legislation. The document is divided into two parts:

- Charter of values: The IRFMN requires compliance with certain values. To all people who work in the Institute; to those who finance their research and those who provide support services, the Charter establishes the principles to be fol-

[22] Carta dei Valori e Codice Etico dell'IRCCS Istituto di Ricerche farmacologiche Mario Negri (2015).

lowed and behaviors to be avoided, even when non-observance has substantial consequences only at the level of administrative sanctions (e.g., revocation of authorizations) or has no consequences.
- Ethical code: The Code of Ethics and the Organization and Control Model are drawn to the attention of all recipients by the most suitable methods to ensure timely, appropriate information.

The IRFMN, to ensure full effectiveness of the organizational model, maintains its regular dissemination and continuous monitoring and updating, particularly with regard to the identification and implementation of the most appropriate ways for the prevention of the crimes envisaged under law. The Code of Ethics and the Organization and Control Model are published on the IRFMN website.

References

ABIM, Benson JA. What is medical professionalism? 2017.

ABIM Foundation, ACP-ASIM Foundation, European Federation of Internal Medicine. Medical professionalism in the new millennium: a physicians' charter. Ann Intern Med. 2002;136(3):243–6.

Academic Medicine. Professionalism in medicine and medical education. Volume II. AAMC, 2010-2016. Acad Med. 2016;91(12):163.

ACGME Project. Advancing education in medical professionalism: an educational resource from the ACGME Outcome Project: ©2004 ACGME. A product of the ACGME Outcome Project; 2004.

ACP (American College of Physicians). Physician's charter on professionalism, 5 February 2002. ACP ethics manual. Sixth edition. Ann Intern Med. 2012;156:73–104.

AMA (American Medical Association). Declaration of professional responsibility. Medicine's social contract with humanity, San Francisco, California, December 4, 2001. MoMed. 2002;99(5):195.

American Board of Internal Medicine. Definitions of professionalism; 1999.

Birden H, Glass N, et al. Teaching professionalism in medical education: a best Evidence in Medical Education (BEME) systematic review. Med Teach J. 2013;35(7):e1252–66.

Canadian Evaluation Society. Professional ethics and standards for the evaluation community in the Government of Canada; 2006.

Carta dei diritti fondamentali dell'Unione Europea (IT. Charter of Fundamental Rights of the European Union) (2000/C 364/01), Gazzetta ufficiale delle Comunità europee. 18 Dec 2000.

Carta dei Valori e Codice Etico dell'IRCCS Istituto di Ricerche farmacologiche Mario Negri (IT. Charter of Values and Code of Ethics of the IRCCS Mario Negri Pharmacological Research Institute). 2015.

Carta della Professionalità Medica (IT. Charter of Medical Professionalism)—Version in Italian. 2002.

Carta europea dei diritti del malato (IT. European Charter of Patients' Rights) European Charter of Patient's rights. Brussels. 15 Nov 2002.

Cruess RL, Cruess SR. Expectations and obligations, professionalism and medicines, social contract with society. Perspect Biol Med. 2008;51(4):579–98.

Documento di consenso Sanremo, 2010. (IT. Sanremo consensus document, 2010). http://www.vdanet.it.

Dunn M. On the relationship between medical ethics and medical professionalism. J Med Eth. 2016;42(10):625–6.

Familiari F, Volpe M. Il Medico del Terzo Millennio. Proposta di una "Carta dei valori e delle competenze degli studenti, in un curriculum formativo rinnovato, in Italia (IT. The Physician of the Third Millennium. Proposal for a" Charter of values and skills of students, in a renewed training curriculum, in Italy). Medicina e Chirurgia. 2014;65:2925–30.

FNOMCeO, Commentario al Codice di Deontologia Medica (IT. Commentary on the Code of Medical Ethics). 2014–2017. 75 pages.

Fondazione Zoé. Al via la Carta Europea dell'Etica Medica, (IT. The European Charter of Medical Ethics is underway). 30 Jun 2011.

Jonsen AR, Braddock CH III, Edwards KA. Professionalism, ethics in medicine. University of Washington; 2016.

Jotkowitz AB, Glick S, Porath A. A physician's charter on medical professionalism: a challenge for medical education. Eur J Int Med. 2004;15(1):5–9.

Kirk LM. Professionalism in medicine: definitions and considerations for teaching. Proc (Bayl Univ Med Cent). 2007;20(1):13–6.

MacKenzie CR. Professionalism and medicine. HSSJ. 2007;3:222–7.

Malliani A. Principi e responsabilità della professione medica. (IT. Principles and responsibilities of the medical profession). BIF. 2002;1–2:41–2.

Mancari R. From the Hippocratic Oath to medical professionalism. Congress in Rome, Professionalità: quali valori per la pratica quotidiana? (IT. Congress in Rome, Professionalism: which values for daily practice?). 23–24 Oct 2010.

Mancari R. Professionalità: quali valori per la pratica quotidiana? (IT. Professionalism: what values for daily practice?). HDC Health Dialogue Culture. 24 Aug 2011.

Meakins JL. Medical professionalism in the new millennium. J Am Coll Surg. 2003;196:113–4.

Medical Professionalism Project. Medical professionalism in the new millennium: a physicians' charter. Lancet. 2002;359(9305):520–2.

Medicina e Chirurgia. Carta della Professionalità Medica. (IT. Medicine and Surgery. Charter of Medical Professionalism, Università degli Studi, Milano). 28 May 2015.

MPS (Medical Protection Society Ltd). Medical professionalism—what do we mean? 2017.

Nace MC, Dunlow S, Armstrong AY. Professionalism in medicine: we should set the standard. Mil Med. 2009;174(8):807.

Nichols BG, Nichols LM, et al. Operationalizing professionalism: a meaningful and practical integration for resident education. Laryngoscope. 2014;124:110–5.

Passi V, Doug M, et al. Developing medical professionalism in future doctors: a systematic review. Int J Med Educ. 2010;1:19–29.

Patuzzo S. Storia del Codice Italiano di Deontologia Medica. Dalle origini ai giorni nostri. (IT. History of the Italian Code of Medical Ethics. From its origins to the present day) Ed. Minerva Medica; 2014. p. 31–7.

Premoli De Marchi P. La competenza professionale e le responsabilità del medico verso i colleghi. (IT. Professional competence and doctor's responsibilities towards colleagues). Academia University Press; 2012. p. 84–190.

Professional Ethics and Standards for the Evaluation Community in the Government of Canada. 2006.

Swick HM. Toward a normative definition of medical professionalism. Acad Med. 2000;75(6):612.

Ufficio Stampa FNOMCeO: Approvata a Kos la Carta Europea di Etica Medica, (IT. European Charter of Medical Ethics approved in Kos) Quotidiano Sanità. 13 Jun 2011.

University of Ottawa, Faculty of Medicine. Declaration of professionalism; 2017.

Walsh C, Abelson HT. Medical Professionalism crossing a generational divide. Perspect Biol Med. 2008;51(4):554–64.

Wynia MK. The short history and tenuous future of medical professionalism: the erosion of medicine's social contract. Perspect Biol Med. 2008;51(4):565–78.

Wynia MK, Latham SR, et al. Medical professionalism in society. N Engl J Med. 1999;341:1612–6.

U.S.A. and U.R.S.S.

11

ACP: American College of Physicians (U.S.A.)[1]

2021 ACP Resources for Internists Catalog

The American College of Physicians is the second largest medical specialty organization in the USA. In 2002 the ACP issued a Physician's Charter on Professionalism and in 2012 an Ethics Manual, which ran to several editions.

"The ACP is a diverse community of internists and comprised almost **161,000** internists, subspecialists, residents, fellows, and medical students worldwide." ACP and its members lead the profession in education, standard setting, and knowledge sharing to advance the science and practice of internal medicine, including clinical expertise in the full range of care for adults.

Background[2]

The ACP was founded in 1915 to promote the science and practice of medicine and has since supported internists in their pursuit of excellence. By sharing the latest medical knowledge, offering world-class educational resources and a wide range of additional benefits, ACP has demonstrated its commitment to internal medicine and its practitioners. With its Mission of improving the quality and effectiveness of health care and supporting excellence and professionalism in the practice of medicine, the ACP is accredited as a recognized leader in quality care.

The College's ambitious goals are:

[1] ACP https://www.acponline.org/ ACP About Us ACP Wikipedia

[2] Snyder (2012) and Weinberger (2015).

R. G. Russo, *Medical Ethics*, https://doi.org/10.1007/978-3-031-42444-1_11

I. To establish and promote the highest clinical standards and ethical ideals;
II. To be the primary educational and information resource for all internists;
III. To maintain responsible positions on individual health and public health care policy for the benefit of the public, patients, the medical profession, and ACP members;
IV. To meet the members' professional needs, foster a healthy life for doctors, and promote internal medicine as a career;
V. To promote and conduct research to improve the quality of practice, education and continued training of internists, and to make internal medicine attractive for doctors and the public;
VI. To recognize excellence and distinguished contributions to internal medicine;
VII. To unify the many voices of internal medicine and its subspecialties for the benefit of patients, members, and the profession.

ACP is dedicated to the development and implementation of ethical policies and medical professionalism, offering resources for members and the public. The ACP Ethics Committee oversees the review of reports of unethical behavior regarding College members. The sixth edition of the Manual of Ethics[3] was published in 2012 in the Annals of Internal Medicine and aims to stimulate debate and serve as a reference on ethical issues. The goal is to facilitate decisions in clinical practice, teaching, and research, so as ultimately to boost the quality of care for patients. This edition of the manual examines emerging issues in medical ethics and personal professionalism. It also looks back over old problems that are still relevant. The manual aims to guide doctors in reaching ethical decisions in clinical practice, teaching and medical research, and describes and explains the principles, as well as the doctor's roles in society and with colleagues.[4]

Ethical Issues

The issues addressed include end-of-life care, human rights, medical-industrial relations, research integrity and the protection of research sub-topics, the ethical implications of legislative and regulatory proposals, ethics of technology and health information, relationships with healthcare professionals, family doctors, etc. The following are some of the topics covered in the Manual.

[3] ACP Ethics Manual (2012).

[4] Annals of Internal Medicine: https://annals.org/aim/cmeMOC

Resource management

Physicians have a responsibility to practice effective and efficient healthcare and to use available resources responsibly. Thrifty care, using the most effective means to diagnose and adequately treat the patient, is recommended as a wise and fair thing.

Relations with the medical industry and gifts

Doctors are firmly discouraged from accepting gifts, hospitality, travel, and subsidies of any kind. Even small gifts can influence clinical judgment and increase the perception and/or reality of a conflict of interest

Research on human subjects

All proposed research, regardless of the source of support, must be evaluated by an Ethics Committee to ensure that:

- research plans are sound and reasonable;
- human subjects are adequately protected;
- the benefit-risk ratio is acceptable;
- there is sufficient reason for the proposed research and it is aimed at protecting the subject.
- informed consent and confidentiality are both appropriate and adequate.

Sponsored research

All scientists are bound by obligations of honesty and integrity in their research. Scientists are expected to:

- protect human subjects
- implement applicable research standards
- protect privacy
- objectively record (clinical) tests and results
- submit their work for peer review
- report any conflict of interest.
- When research is sponsored by industry, scientists also need to ensure that they provide the sponsor with the full data.

Physician's Charter on Professionalism[5]

The Physician's Charter on professionalism, developed with the ABIM Foundation, and the European Federation of Internal Medicine are discussed earlier.

About Internal Medicine[6]

> Internal medicine physicians are specialists who apply scientific knowledge and clinical expertise to the diagnosis, treatment, and compassionate care of adults across the spectrum from health to complex illness.

[5] Sox (2002).

[6] ACP American College of Physicians, 2021

Oaths in the U.S.A. (XX Sec.)

The Healer's Oath

The American physician Louis Weinstein (26 February 1908, Bridgeport, Connecticut, March 16, 2000, Newton, Mass.) was a pioneer of infectious disease treatments and a leading medical educator. He received his medical degree in 1943 from Boston University and served as the head of the University for the Treatment of Infectious Diseases from 1947 to 1957. In 1957 he moved to Tufts University School of Medicine, Boston, where he became head of infectious diseases until retirement in 1975. In 1991 he composed the "Oath of the Healer" in which he stressed the need for a preventive approach to mankind's problems, not only of health, but also of malnutrition and poverty[7]. His Oath very elegantly lays down the important rules of moral character and conduct for a doctor, elaborating on the lines of Hippocrates.

He was also responsible for introducing numerous antibiotic treatments and was one of the founders of the modern medical specialty of infectious diseases. His contribution to antibiotic therapy was significant: in the late 1940s, he was already warning about over-use and imminent resistance to these drugs. During the 1950 polio epidemic he rose to prominence as the clinical master of this disease. Bacteria, protozoa, viruses, infected fleas, lice, ticks, mosquitoes, bedbugs, and other agents are always active when neglect, poverty, hunger or war lower defenses, and infection can come from rats, mice, pets or other creatures that fly or crawl, or microorganisms in food and drink and in other areas of our lives.

In May 15, 1991 Weinstein composed the "Oath of the Healer" of which a few fragments, representative for medical ethics, are reported below.

> … I realize that on this day, I become a physician for all eternity. I shall strive to be a person of good will, high moral character, and impeccable conduct. I shall learn to love my fellow man as much as I have learned to love the art of healing…I shall always act in the best interest of my patient and shall never allow personal reward to impact on my judgment. I shall always have the highest respect for human life …
>
> I shall have as a major focus in my life the promoting of a better world in which to live. I shall strive to take a comprehensive approach to understanding all aspects of life. To become the Healer I wish to be, I must expand my thinking…. I am not a God and I cannot perform miracles….

Ethical Oath of the Christian Doctor

The Christian Medical and Dental Association (CMDA) comprises the Christian Medical Association (CMA) and the Christian Dental Association (CDA). The CMDA provides resources, job opportunities, training, and a public voice for Christian health workers and students. CMDA was founded and started work in 1931 at North Western University in Chicago. A new strategy was drafted in 2000.

[7] Weinstein (1991).

The areas of the Association's ministerial activity include evangelization, proselytism, service, dissemination of its principles and procurement of resources. In 2002 it moved to its current location in Bristol, Tennessee, and is now home to more than 80 ministers, representing more than 17,000 medical and dental members all over the world.

The CMDA promotes positions and directs policies on health issues; conducts overseas medical evangelization projects; coordinates a network of Christian health workers for scholarships and professional growth; sponsors medical and dental students. It hosts conferences on marriage and the family; it supplies missionary doctors for the third world with resources for continuing education, and runs university exchange programs abroad.

The CMDA also establishes guidelines for the executive director and staff and offers recommendations on lines of action. Membership is made up of doctors, dentists, and other health professionals. The members come from various political and religious movements and different Christian denominations including Baptists, Anglicans, Lutherans, Catholics, Methodists, Presbyterians, and Orthodox.

The following sentences are from the oath[8] produced by the CMDA House of Delegates on 3 May 1991 in Chicago, Illinois, and amended and updated by the CMDA House of Representatives on 10 June 2000 in Denver, Colorado.

> ....I publicly profess my intent to practice medicine for the glory of God. Humbly I will try to increase my abilities.
>
> ....In turn I will freely impart my knowledge and wisdom to others.
>
> With God's help, I will love those who come to me for healing and comfort.... ...With God's direction, I will respect the sanctity of human life.
>
> I will treat all my patients, rejecting any measures that intentionally destroy or actively end human life, including the unborn, the weak, the vulnerable and the terminally ill.
>
> With the grace of God, I will live in accordance with the standards of my profession.

Oath of the Loma Linda University (LLU)[9]

16 December 1998

The University has been awarded the title of Center for Christian Bioethics. It was founded in 1905 by Seventh Day Adventists, in Loma Linda, California, with the aim of educating future medical professionals and researchers to provide comprehensive and compassionate care for the whole person.

The mission is to continue the teaching and healing ministry of Jesus Christ while educating future medical professionals to excel in their chosen field.

---

[8] CMDA House of Representatives, Christian Physician's Oath Position Statement, Chicago, Illinois. May 3, 1991.

[9] https://home.llu.edu/

The Center offers guidance and information on ethical issues in medicine for health care professionals and families through counseling services, community education, and health policy assessment.

The goal is to improve health care and people's health, encouraging professionalism and decision-making responsibility.

The Center examines ethical issues related to health care in order to improve the health of the community. It also deals with social ethics, to provide society with an adequate framework for the controversial and delicate issues that may arise from poverty, economy, social responsibility, and communication, for the dilemmas arising from the relationship between faith and morals.

The Center for Christian Bioethics, which is based at the School of Religion, is committed to improving education, research, and biomedical ethics and to serving the community by sponsoring events dealing with ethical and social issues from a religious point of view, for people of all faiths, ethnicities, and cultures.

Below the promise that is made:

> I promise the following, before God:
>
> In accepting my sacred call, I will dedicate my life to promoting healing and teaching the ministry of Jesus Christ.
>
> I will give my teachers the respect and gratitude that is due to them. I will impart to those who follow me the knowledge and experience I have acquired….
>
> ….I will maintain the utmost respect for human life. I do not want to use my medical knowledge contrary to the laws of humanity.
>
> I will respect the rights and decisions of my patients.
>
> I will safely keep all the secrets entrusted to me in the practice of my calling.
>
> I will guide my life and practice my art with purity and honor; refraining from immorality: I will not lead others towards immorality with my actions….

In U.S.S.R

Supreme Soviet Oath[10]

The oath of the Soviet doctor

> After having been awarded my degree and authorized to practice medicine, I solemnly swear:
>
> – To devote all my knowledge to the conservation and improvement of human health, to the treatment and prevention of diseases
>
> – To be available in full conscience wherever society calls.

[10] Bird (1989), p. 51, Veatch (1989) and Veatch (2000), pp. 219.

- Always to be ready to provide medical assistance, to relate to the patient and to respect what he confides.
- To constantly improve my medical knowledge and clinical skills to contribute to the development of medical science and practice.
- To refer to the advice and opinions of my colleagues in the interest of my patients.
- To maintain and develop the noble traditions of Soviet medicine, to be guided in all my actions by the principles of communist morality.
- Always to answer the call of a Soviet doctor and keep in mind my responsibility to the people and the State.
- I swear to be faithful to this oath as long as I live.
- Recognizing the danger that nuclear weapons present to humanity, I swear to fight tirelessly for peace and for the prevention of nuclear war.

"The oath of the Soviet doctor" required that doctors be governed by the norms of communist morality and spoke more of their responsibility to the Soviet people and State than to patients. Gradually the flow of literature in the field of ethics increased significantly; it was introduced in the curricula of medical institutes and, despite opposition to Western sources, courses on deontology and medical ethics finally appeared in the early 1990s.

Development of Medical Ethics in Russia

The evolution of medical ethics in Russia was governed by several factors.

First, such Russian concepts as "*obshina*" (community) and "*sobornost*" (spiritual community between people) dictated the supremacy of the collective body over the individual, the State over a person.

Second, Russian medical doctors with university degrees appeared only in the eighteenth century on the heels of the westernization policies of Peter the Great (1672–1725). Medical ethics probably started with Prof. Matvei Mudrov (1776–1831) of Moscow, who followed the Hippocratic credo "to treat not a disease but a patient." He believed that the Hippocratic Oath could serve as the foundation of a code of conduct for Russian doctors as well.[11]

Third, after serfdom had been abolished in 1861 medical care in many rural regions was provided by *zemstva* (local elected councils). Typical patients were illiterate and ignorant peasants who were considered incapable of making reasonable decisions in their own interest and therefore required direction from others.

Medical doctors had idealistic views of self-sacrifice for service to society and the people. In view of the absence of national regulation, some local authorities

[11] Lichterman and Yarovinsky (2005).

adopted their own codes of conduct in medicine and working to enrich oneself was criticized and derided (see, for example, Tolstoy's novels and Chekhov's stories).[11]

In 1901 a Doctor Veresaev (1867–1945) published the first edition of "The Doctor's Notes" which discussed the main ethical issues in work with humans. The main problems of medical ethics in Russian and Soviet settings related to informed consent, human experimentation, abortion, euthanasia, organ and tissue transplantation, abuse of psychiatry, etc. In Soviet ideology, common interests were superior to private ones. Medical confidentiality was considered a "bourgeois" leftover. The diagnosis was not normally revealed to a patient who had an incurable disease (specially cancer). The strong paternalistic traditions of Russian medicine meant that many doctors contested the idea of informed consent. Abortion, euthanasia, transplants on human beings, forensic autopsy and the removal of cadaver organs were legally permitted, though occasionally this was interrupted or canceled. Abortions had been legalized from 1920 to 1936 but then banned until 1955. Active euthanasia was legalized in 1922 for a short period. Human transplantation was adopted only in 1992.

The 1917 Revolution and the subsequent civil war led to a serious decrease in the number of doctors in the country and in the first years after the revolution about 8000 doctors left Russia. Many doctors died from hunger and disease. In 1918 the first "Health Commissioner" was established. For decades, Russian leaders sacrificed health care to financial and human needs for military and space efforts.

Doctors only had access to Soviet medical literature. Information about scientific and clinical advances achieved outside the Soviet Union was not made available by the government to most physicians and the general public. Limited information was available only in restricted areas, in centralized libraries in Moscow and Leningrad (now St. Petersburg). All this, together with environmental pollution, alcoholism, smoking and poor nutrition amounted to a critical public health situation. Soviet health care became disunited, unjust and inadequate, centralized and controlled by the government in all ways. The healthcare system was strictly hierarchical and corruption aimed at obtaining better quality care was rife.

Specific Areas of Ethical Debate and Decisions

Human Rights in the Soviet Union[12]

Here is an overview of the medical ethics issues that have been dealt with, in highly "original" ways, in Russia.[13]

Abortion. Abortions in pre-revolutionary Russia were considered criminal. In 1920 the Soviet government became the first in the world to legalize the termination of a pregnancy at the request of a woman. Then in 1936, seeking ways to improve demographics, abortions were again criminalized. In 1955, with a certain the

[12] Wikipedia: Human rights in the Soviet Union

[13] Cassileth et al. (1995) and Cockerham (1999).

regime, they were again legalized, to reduce the negative consequences of widespread illegal abortions.

Abortion became a common means of birth control. Subsequent laws in 1992 (The Right to Life Society) and in 1993 were established to oppose abortions and were supported by the Russian Orthodox Church.

Confidentiality. The question of doctors' confidentiality was controversial: in the 1920s the People's Health Commissioner announced that it was merely a remnant of bourgeois medicine. The need to keep doctors' secrets was linked to the fear that their elimination would prevent people seeking medical advice and help. The confidentiality requirement only achieved a legal basis in 1970. Until 1993, however, a medical certificate was required to return to work after an illness.

Openness to patients. The subject of disclosure to patients was marked by strong paternalistic tendencies. It was considered unacceptable to inform a terminally ill patient of his diagnosis and prognosis. The practice of informing patients was generally not regulated, so final decisions were left to the discretion of the physician. In 1992, Russian laws on psychiatric treatment and transplantation of human organs and tissues specified rules for informed consent for patients and donors.

The law also established rules regarding the receipt and documentation of informed consent from patients undergoing biomedical experiments. The advent of glasnost (*opening*) in 1985 resulted in public disclosure of information on fatal biomedical experiments conducted on Soviet army soldiers and prisoners under Joseph Stalin (1879–1953) and Lavrenti Pavlovich Beria (1899–1953), and even after them.

Euthanasia. In pre-revolutionary periods there was already opposition to the possibility of euthanasia in certain exceptional circumstances: conscious and insistent requests from the patient; impossibility of reducing suffering with known methods; agreement of a commission of doctors on the impossibility of saving life; preliminary notice of the decision to the heirs.

Most medical ethics specialists, including doctors, jurists and philosophers—with rare exceptions—adopted a fiercely negative opinion about euthanasia, while the public remained more tolerant.

Eugenics and medical genetics. In the first decades of the twentieth century, Russia was among the world leaders in the development of genetics. This interest generated a strong eugenics movement, which flourished in the 1920s. This can be explained by the agreement between eugenics and the central communist ideology of the creation of a "new man" who would be free from the "names" of capitalism. In the 1920s, when ideological control was not yet particularly heavy, the possibilities of creating a new human being were suggested by psychoanalysts and those from other fields of scientific research. In 1994, the Russian Human Genome Project began studying the possible ethical implications of recent developments in human genetics.

Repressive psychiatry. The use of psychiatry as a weapon against political dissidents began under Nikita Khrushchev. The first victim was Zhores Medvedev, who was punished for wanting to publish a book on the elimination of genetics, in 1948. Medvedev was diagnosed by state psychiatrists as mentally retarded and therefore admitted for "treatment."

The widespread use of psychiatry in this way was seen late in Leonid Brezhnev's regime. Hundreds of victims, without any judicial procedure and often without even being physically present, were sentenced for long periods in specific psychiatric hospitals under the jurisdiction not of the Ministry of Health, but of the Ministry of Internal Affairs. The "treatment" ranged from "wall therapy" (keeping patients closed inside four walls) to forced psychotropic injections. The center of expert study and diagnosis of these afflictions was the V. Serbsky Institute for Forensic Psychiatry in Moscow.

Transplants. The adoption in 1992 of a "law on transplantation of human organs and tissues" provided an example of reforms in the Russian health sector. Before the adoption of this law, issues such as the determination of brain death, the rights of donors and recipients, and authorization for the removal of organs and tissues from cadavers were dictated by the in-house instructions of the Ministry of Health—instructions unknown to the population. The government withheld information about scientific and clinical advances produced outside the Soviet Union from most doctors and the general public. Extensive discussion of ethics did not begin until the mid- and late 1960s, when writings on this subject by physicians and philosophers began to appear.

Abuses. Soviets did not protect patients from being used in medical trials without their consent or knowledge. Other abuses occurred too: humans were used in space trials, without their permission, with no explanation or indication of their rights and possibilities of refusing.

On 26 March 1971, the Presidium of the Supreme Soviet approved the Oath and ordered that all doctors and medical students accept it upon graduation, sign a copy and respect it.

Distinctive features of this Oath are: (1) dedication to preventive medicine, (2) commitment to respect the principles of communist morality, (3) responsibility towards the people and the Soviet government.

Although the Hippocratic oath was replaced by the Soviet oath and had no official recognition in Soviet medicine, there was no sense of tension towards the individual patient and the doctor's explicit commitment to the "State." Progress in the ethical foundations had, however, been made, together with the patient's greater participation in medical decisions. However, autonomy and respect for people still do not play the central role that exists in the EU and the USA, though increased awareness of medical ethics has given rise to patients' rights being considered part of individual rights.[14]

On 15 November 1983 the annotation relating to nuclear war was added to the Oath. It can be understood as an example of a call to responsibility in other countries. This was initially ignored. Later, in March 1984, the American Medical Student Association, at its annual convention, passed a resolution calling on students to include in their oath a statement on the physician's duty to work for the

[14]Vlassov (2016).

prevention of nuclear war.[15] The People's Republic of China passed a similar oath in 1988.

The most complete book "Deontology in experimental medicine," from 1988, dealt only with experiments in animals; there was still little public interest in ethical questions of human experimentation. Profound changes came in the 1990s, after the fall of the Soviet regime, in departmental and federal regulations.

For the first time, research with human subjects became part of federal legislation and not just departmental rules. Soviet medical ethics is reflected in the 1991 "Soviet doctor's oath," including the pledge "...to be guided in all my actions by the principles of communist morality, to maintain the high calling of a Soviet doctor and my responsibility to the people and the State." The Soviet doctor's duty was the protection of the State, not the morality expressed by Western medicine in the Hippocratic Oath and the Judeo-Christian tradition. Autonomy and respect for the person did not play the pivotal role it had in Europe and the USA.

The Nuremberg Trials were not reported in the Soviet Union until 1993. Russian doctors actively and individually made efforts to obtain unavailable information and establish contacts with the West. The poor medical care, inadequate diet, environmental pollution, and lack of public health efforts common in Russia only started to be corrected with the fall of the Soviet system. In addition, high mortality and short life expectancy contributed to the decrease in population: in 1993 deaths far exceeded births.[13]

The new 1993 law on patients' rights granted for the first time the right to confidentiality, and to see the results of clinical examinations and medical documents, so as to understand diagnosis and prognosis. It was thus possible to request consultation, be informed of possible experimental treatments, give informed consent or refuse participation. The Russian Constitution finally observed that "no one can be subjected to medical scientific experiments and other experiments without voluntary consent."

In the same year came the most important Russian healthcare law "Fundamentals of the legislation of the Russian Federation for the protection of citizens' health".[16] It introduced new regulations for research on humans. It prohibited research on persons deprived of liberty and laid the groundwork for informed consent, suggesting that participants in clinical trials should be informed about the aims, methods, possible risks and side effects, duration, expected results, and freedom to withdraw.[15]

Article 54 states that only those who have received medical and pharmaceutical training have the right to engage in medical and pharmaceutical activities, attested by the appropriate diplomas. Article 60 specifies that future doctors, upon graduation, take an oath.

In 1994 the first interdisciplinary conference on ethical and legal topics was held in Russia, with the participation of doctors, jurists, philosophers, and theologians. Over the past 15 years, Russia has seen profound changes in all spheres of political, economic, and even medical life.

[15] Cassel et al. (1985)

[16] Lichterman and Yarovinsky (2005) and Yudin (2002).

Brief Notes on Medical Ethics in Recent Russia

Soviet leaders gradually started to maintain acceptable international standards of medical ethics. In 1939 the surgeon and oncologist Nikolai Petrov (1876–1964) published an article, "Questions of Surgical Deontology," in the Bulletin of Surgery; in 1945 he published a booklet with the same title. These publications were the first steps in the rehabilitation of medical ethics.

In 1991 the Russian parliament adopted a law providing medical insurance for Russian citizens: this was an admission of the failure of state medicine. Finally, most people found it hard to accept the idea that health had to be paid for, even though "free medicine" had proved inefficient.[17]

Health care in Russia is mainly governed by Federal Law No. 323 on Healthcare Foundations for Russian Citizens, dated November 21, 2011, and Federal Law No. 326 on Compulsory Insurance in the Russian Federation of November 29, 2010.

Other important legislative provisions include Law no. 61 on the circulation of drugs, dated April 12, 2010.

Universal coverage and healthcare services are guaranteed at no additional cost: primary health care (out-patients and in-patients); emergency services, including specialized medical assistance (e.g., air ambulances) and other specialized medical care for diseases requiring special diagnosis and treatment.

Article 74 of the Law on Healthcare Foundations prohibits doctors and pharmacists from:

(i) accepting gifts, money, paid entertainment, holidays or travel, from companies that produce or distribute medicines or medical equipment;
(ii) entering into written or oral agreements with companies that manufacture or distribute drugs or medical equipment, regarding the prescription or recommendation of certain medicines or equipment to patients;
(iii) accepting samples of medicines or medical equipment from these companies for distribution to patients;
(iv) providing false or incomplete information on the number, type and name of alternative medicines or medical equipment that can substitute for the prescribed medicine or medical device.

The patient (in clinical trials) must not:

- be a minor (under 18 y.o.);
- be a specific case for which the cure of the disease or its improvement uses an advertised product;
- express gratitude for the effect of the advertised product.

The trial must not:

[17]Yudin (1995), Encyclopedia of Bioethics (2017) and Yudin (2002).

- create an impression of the benefits of the advertised product by referring to the results of earlier clinical trials and studies conducted as requirements for registration of the product;
- claim or assume that the target audience of the advertising suffers from certain diseases or health conditions;
- create an impression that a healthy person should use the advertised product;
- imply that it is not necessary to consult a doctor to use the advertised product;
- stress the positive effects of the advertised product, its safety, efficiency and the absence of side effects;
- present a pharmaceutical product as a biological supplement or food supplement or any other non-pharmaceutical product;
- affirm that the natural origin of the advertised product guarantees its safety or efficacy.

Article 74 prohibits pharmaceutical companies sending distributors or representatives to visit medical professionals or doctors treating patients.

Article 75 of the Law on Healthcare Foundations includes a definition of "conflict of interest" whose apparent purpose is to address certain situations not covered by the prohibitions referred to in Article 74. The main rules and principles of cooperation between doctors and pharmaceutical companies are established in the Code of Ethics for Doctors of the Russian Federation, adopted by the medical community in 1997. In particular, the code states that the physician must not accept incentives from pharmaceutical manufacturers or distributors to prescribe their products; the doctor will normally prescribe the medicines on the basis of medical considerations and only in the interest of the patient.

Patient organizations are relatively new in Russia and so far there is no legal or regulatory framework governing their relations with the pharmaceutical industry.[18]

The dissolution of the Soviet Union (1988–1991) involved a process of internal disintegration in the USSR, which began with growing unrest in its various constituent republics, developing into incessant political and legislative conflict between the republics and the central government.

Information about scientific and clinical advances produced outside Russia from physicians and the general public is now available. Young doctors had set up a novel tradition in Russian medicine, which includes the moral bases of the physician's ideology, and has formulated basic values: responsibility, mercy, and compassion as well as purely medical ethics.

References

ACP Ethics Manual. Sixth edition: A comprehensive medical ethics resource. Ann Intern Med. 2012;156(1 Part 2):73–104.

Bird LP. Medical ethics. In: Bird LP, Barlow J, editors. Oaths & prayers, an anthology. Richardson: Christian Medical & Dental Society; 1989.

[18] McDonald and Dementyev (2012).

Cassel CK, Jameton AL, et al. The physician's oath and the prevention of nuclear war. JAMA. 1985;254:652–4.

Cassileth BR, Vlassov VV, Chapman CC. Health care, medical practice, and medical ethics in Russia today. JAMA. 1995;273(20):1569–73.

Cockerham WC. Health and social change in Russia and Eastern Europe. New York/London., Chapter 1: Ed Routledge; 1999.

Encyclopedia of Bioethics. Encyclopedia.com. http://www.encyclopedia.com (17 July 2017).

Lichterman BL, Yarovinsky M. Medical ethics in Russia before the October Revolution (1917). J Int Bioethique. 2005;16(3–4):17–32, 166–7.

McDonald A, Dementyev D. Russia: getting the deal through, life sciences. Salans; 2012.

Snyder L. American College of Physicians Ethics Manual. Ann Intern Med. 2012;156:73–104.

Sox HC. Medical professionalism in the new millennium: a physician's charter on professionalism. Ann Intern Med. 2002;136(3):243–6.

Veatch R. Medical ethics in the Soviet Union. Hastings Center Report; 1989. p. 11–14

Veatch RM, editor. Cross cultural perspectives in medical ethics. 2nd ed. Boston/Toronto/London/Singapore: Jones and Bartlett Pub; 2000.

Vlassov VV. Russian experience and perspectives of quality assurance in healthcare through standards of care. Health Policy Technol. 2016;5:307–12.

Weinberger SE. Challenges for internal medicine as the American College of Physicians celebrates its 100th anniversary. Ann Intern Med. 2015;162(8):585–6.

Weinstein L. The oath of the healer. JAMA. 1991;265(19):2484.

Yudin B. Transl. Schneider R. Medical ethics, history of Europe: contemporary period: IX. Russia; 1995.

Yudin B. Research ethics in Russia. Politeia. 2002;XVIII(67):51–3.

Informed Consent 12

The Nuremberg Code is the most important document in the history of ethics in medical research.[1]

Historical Premises

Historians cite a number of medical guidelines for tracing the history of informed consent in medical practice, providing guidelines for a physician's duty, behavior, and moral responsibility.

In ancient Greece, a patient's participation in decision-making for medical treatment was considered undesirable. It was generally accepted that the physician's primary task was to inspire the patient's confidence in the treatment: this was not to be questioned. The Hippocratic Oath suggested that doctors could withhold most of the information from patients, to give them the best possible care. The rationale was that "the doctor knows better than the patient." Over the centuries, also on the basis of Hippocrate's teachings, doctors exercised the right—and duty—not to reveal anything to the patient. This absolute reserve guaranteed prestige and authority to the medical profession.[2] The *Formula Comitis Archiatrorum*—mentioned earlier—credited to Cassiodorus and possibly among the first writings on medical ethics, required doctors to broaden and deepen their knowledge and the concept of commitment and consultation. A principle that is in accordance with what Hippocrates proposed with the words *επ'ωφελείη καμνόντων* (for the patient's benefit).[3]

Later, in medieval times, medical writing encouraged doctors to use their conversations with patients as an opportunity to offer comfort and hope, emphasizing that they needed to be both manipulative and deceptive. To achieve a cure, it was widely felt that (medical) authority had to be coupled with (the patient's) obedience.

[1] Shuster (1997).

[2] Murray (1990).

[3] Mountokalakis (2014).

R. G. Russo, *Medical Ethics*, https://doi.org/10.1007/978-3-031-42444-1_12

Medical ethics has been preached and expanded over the centuries and even a concept that anticipated "informed consent"—although not yet defined as such—was also formed with other traditional medical ethical guidelines. For example, the Arab doctor Ishaq Ibn Ali Al-Ruhawi wrote *The conduct of a doctor*; then there was Moses Maimonides, a Spanish Jewish philosopher, astronomer, and physician, Thomas Aquinas, an Italian Dominican friar and priest, and others we have already mentioned. However, the Hippocratic oath remained the most enduring guideline for the ethics of doctors in the history of medicine.[4]

There are considerable differences between the prevailing ethics in different societies and cultures (social ethics) and therefore what can be considered right and good for one can be perceived differently for another.

Henri de Mondeville, a fourteenth century French surgeon, wrote about medical practice and outlined his ideas on the Hippocratic oath: "Doctors promise a cure to every patient," hoping for a good outcome. He never talked about obtaining consent, but stressed the need for the patient to trust the doctor.

Benjamin Rush was a US physician in the eighteenth century and was influenced by the "Age of Enlightenment" movement. Because of this, he urged doctors to share as much information as possible with patients. He also recommended that physicians educate the public and respect the patient's informed decision to accept or not refuse a treatment.

There is no evidence that he supported seeking patient consensus and, in a lecture of his entitled "On the Duties of Patients to Their Physicians," he insisted that patients should strictly obey their physician's orders. John Gregory, Rush's teacher, wrote similar views that a doctor might better practice charity by deciding for patients without their consent.

In 1767 a decision by the Anglo-American court (Slater v Baker & Stapleton) judged it reasonable that a patient could know in advance what he would be subjected to and then "courageously" decide whether or not to face medical intervention.

Thomas Percival in 1803 published the book entitled *Medical Ethics*, making no mention of soliciting the patient's consent or respecting their decisions. Patients have a right to the truth, but when the doctor can provide better treatment (for instance, by lying or giving only partial information) he recommended that the doctor do "as he thought best."

When the American Medical Association (AMA) was founded in 1847, it issued a work called "The First Edition of the American Code of Medical Ethics."

A new concept was the idea that doctors should fully disclose all the patient's details when talking to other doctors, but the text did not apply this idea to giving patients information. On the basis of these recommendations Percival's ideas became the guidelines to be observed.

Worthington Hooker, an American physician, followed them in 1849. His book on medical ethics showed an understanding of the AMA guidelines and Percival's philosophy and rejected all directives that a doctor should lie to patients. However, Hooker's ideas were not very influential in those days.

[4] Kumar (2013), Mallardi (2005) and Murray (1990).

In 1850 Hooker wrote: "The great object of the physician should be to cure the patient. This is in his vocation and nothing must be allowed to interfere with it." The physician's moral virtues primarily involved providing assistance through professional commitment, expressed as basic charitable obligations.[5]

In 1891, a Directive of the Prussian Minister of the Interior, addressed to all prisons, stated that tuberculin therapy, used for tuberculosis—at the time still experimental—could not be used against a prisoner's will.

In 1900, the Prussian Ministry for Religious, Educational and Medical Affairs enacted a directive that medical experiments could only be conducted on consenting adults, after adequate explanation of the possible adverse consequences.

In 1914 a sentence in the United States (Schloendorff vs. New York Hospital) stated: "Every adult man capable of understanding and willing has the right to decide what will be done with his body and a surgeon who operates without consent of the patient commits an outrage for which he will be prosecuted for damages."

About a century ago, in 1917, the Polish physician Theodore Heiman unleashed substantial criticism against what he considered the irresponsible experimental practices of his colleagues. In his book *Etyka Lekarska* (Medical Ethics) he strongly criticized the reduction of human beings to experimental material, fostered "consent" and warned against exploiting desperate patients who feared being abandoned by their doctor.[6]

The pre-war German medical association was seen as a progressive and democratic association with substantial public health concerns. For example, compulsory health insurance legislation was in force for German workers.

From the mid-1920s, German doctors were accused by the public and the international medical society of unethical medical practices. The aim was to favor the purity of the Aryan race and therefore to "exterminate those who did not fit their criteria." Racial hygiene extremists merged with National Socialism to promote this criminal goal, a fundamental concept in Nazi ideology.

Doctors were attracted to the scientific ideology and contributed to the establishment of the National League of Socialist Doctors in 1929 with the aim of "purifying the German medical community of Jewish Bolshevism." In response to criticism of unethical human experimentation, the Reich government published "Guidelines for New Therapy and Human Experimentation" in Weimar. The guidelines were based on charity and non-maleficence, but also emphasized the legal doctrine of informed consent, *ante litteram*. In 1931 a Circular from the Minister of the Interior of the Reich identified a draft of the guidelines for new therapies and their experimentation on humans; it referred to the need—in accordance with a legal theory of the time—that these should be implemented only with the consent of the subjects.[7]

The Weimar guidelines were denied by Adolf Hitler. In 1942, more than 38,000 German doctors in the Nazi party helped carry out criminal medical programs, such

[5] Beauchamp (1995).

[6] Heiman (1917).

[7] American College of Obstetricians and Gynecologists (2009), Archives of Internal Medicine (1996) and Encyclopedia of Bioethics (2017).

as obligatory sterilization and others measures, deliberately, and obviously without any consent! A series of trials later accused members of the Nazi party as being responsible for a multitude of war crimes. The contents, developed by two medical consultants of the US court (Andrew Ivy and Leo Alexander), were intended to counter the theses developed by the defense of German doctors. On the basis of normative principles, set out in the American military court's sentence, 23 Nazi doctors were sentenced on August 19–20, 1947 (7 of them to death), for experiments conducted in the concentration camps.

Here is the full text of the Code[8] divided into ten points:

The voluntary consent of the human subject is absolutely essential. This means that the person involved should have legal capacity to give consent; should be so situated as to be able to exercise free power of choice, without the intervention of any element of force, fraud, deceit, duress, over-reaching, or other ulterior form of constraint or coercion; and should have sufficient knowledge and comprehension of the elements of the subject matter involved as to enable him to make an understanding and enlightened decision. This latter element requires that, before the acceptance of an affirmative decision by the experimental subject, there should be made known to him the nature, duration, and purpose of the experiment; the method and means by which it is to be conducted; all inconveniences and hazards reasonably to be expected; and the effects upon his health or person which may possibly come from his participation in the experiment.

1. *The duty and responsibility for ascertaining the quality of the consent rests upon each individual who initiates, directs or engages in the experiment. It is a personal duty and responsibility which may not be delegated to another with impunity*
2. *The duty and responsibility for ascertaining the quality of the consent rests upon each individual who initiates, directs or engages in the experiment. It is a personal duty and responsibility which may not be delegated to another with impunity*

[8] Presented by "Trials of War Criminals before the Nuremberg Military Tribunals under Control Council Law No. 10". Katz (1996).

The Nuremberg Code (1947), BMJ vol. 313(7070):1448, 1996.

Trials of War Criminals before the Nuremberg Military Tribunals under Control Council Law No.10, Vol. 2, pp. 181–182. Washington, D.C.: U.S. Government Printing Office, 1949–1953.

3. *The voluntary consent of the human subject is absolutely essential. This means that the person involved should have legal capacity to give consent; should be so situated as to be able to exercise free power of choice, without the intervention of any element of force, fraud, deceit, duress, over-reaching, or other ulterior form of constraint or coercion; and should have sufficient knowledge and comprehension of the elements of the subject matter involved as to enable him to make an understanding and enlightened decision. This latter element requires that, before the acceptance of an affirmative decision by the experimental subject, there should be made known to him the nature, duration, and purpose of the experiment; the method and means by which it is to be conducted; all inconveniences and hazards reasonably to be expected; and the effects upon his health or person which may possibly come from his participation in the experiment.*
4. *The experiment should be such as to yield fruitful results for the good of society, unprocurable by other methods or means of study, and not random and unnecessary in nature.*
5. *The experiment should be so designed and based on the results of animal experimentation and a knowledge of the natural history of the disease or other problem under study, that the anticipated results will justify the performance of the experiment.*
6. *The experiment should be so conducted as to avoid all unnecessary physical and mental suffering and injury. No experiment should be conducted where there is an a priori reason to believe that death or disabling injury will occur; except, perhaps, in those experiments where the experimental physicians also serve as subjects.*
7. *The degree of risk to be taken should never exceed that determined by the humanitarian importance of the problem to be solved by the experiment. The experiment should be conducted only by scientifically qualified persons. The highest degree of skill and care should be required through all stages of the experiment of those who conduct or engage in the experiment.*
8. *Proper preparations should be made and adequate facilities provided to protect the experimental subject against even remote possibilities of injury, disability, or death.*
9. *During the course of the experiment, the human subject should be at liberty to bring the experiment to an end, if he has reached the physical or mental state where continuation of the experiment seemed to him to be impossible.*
10. *During the course of the experiment, the scientist in charge must be prepared to terminate the experiment at any stage, if he has probable cause to believe, in the exercise of the good faith, superior skill and careful judgment required of him, that a continuation of the experiment is likely to result in injury, disability, or death to the experimental subject.*

Following the Nuremberg Trials, ethics committees, in order to protect the rights, safety, and well-being of subjects participating in a clinical trial, established "Informed Consent."

Article 1. reads:

The voluntary consent of the human subject is absolutely essential

Many of the accused objected that there was no law differentiating legal from illegal experiments. The ten points that defined legitimate medical research constitute the Nuremberg Code, which included principles such as informed consent and the absence of coercion, proper scientific experimentation, and charity towards the participants in the experiment.

The Nuremberg Code was initially ignored, but gained much greater significance some 20 years later. The Ethics Committee set up as a result of those processes set itself the goal of protecting the rights, safety, and well-being of the subjects participating in an experiment.

For the first time in history the concept of "Informed Consent" in the field of bioethics of experimentation on human beings was defined. This implied, in the words of the judges, that "the person involved must have the legal capacity to give consent and must therefore exercise a free power of choice, without the intervention of any element of forcing, fraud, deception, coercion, exaggeration or another further form of obligation or coercion."

Informed consent has been at the heart of medical ethics in the modern era; the purpose of requesting it is to promote the individual's self-determination in the medical decision.[9]

A recurring theme was the relevance of Hippocratic ethics in human experimentation and whether the ideals of Hippocratic morality could serve as an exclusive guide in the ethics of research without any risk to the human rights of the subjects involved.[10]

In Nuremberg, in the person of Nazi doctors, non-traditional medicine was tried, not based on the Hippocratic model and on the medical/patient therapeutic relationship, and therefore the defendants were found guilty, among other things, of having violated medical ethics.[11]

Medical Experiments Permitted

The Code continued to be used (occasionally) in the next half-century, when multiple declarations of international ethics were produced, but not in American or German national codes. However, the Code remains a reference on medical ethics and is one of the most lasting products of the Doctors' Trial. Furthermore, "some

[9] Meisel and Kuczewski (1996).

[10] Annas and Grodin (1995).

[11] Weindling (1996).

medical experiments on humans, if kept within reasonably well-defined limits, comply with the ethics of the medical profession in general. The protagonists of the practice of human experimentation still justify their opinions on the basis that these experiments produce results for the good of society and that they cannot be reconstructed with other methods or alternative tools. However, all agree that some fundamental principles must be respected to satisfy moral, ethical and juridical concepts".[12]

70 Years Later

These concepts have long become an important benchmark for the ethical conduct of medical research. However, in the past there has been considerable debate among scholars regarding the authority, scope, and legal status of the Nuremberg Code, in civilian and military fields.[13] Symbolically, the Code is part of the international democratic system that emerged after the Second World War, with particular attention to respect for human rights, individual autonomy, and informed consent. In the area of human research ethics, the Code was subsequently eclipsed by the Declaration of Helsinki in 1964.

The 1948 Universal Declaration of Human Rights was drafted by the General Assembly of the United Nations, following two world wars. The 1948 code was not adopted by any US government, with the partial exception of the US Department of Defense, in 1953, regarding defense experiments with atomic, biological, and chemical agents.

The question now is whether doctors today can join a profession that truly reflects the definitions and regulations of the Code (of global significance) or whether changes and clarifications are still needed. Is human society ready—or willing—to fully repudiate a phenomenon of which it is ashamed on the one hand, while on the other it still does not seem to be able to do without?

Following the Nuremberg Trials, the concept was proclaimed that "It must never again be allowed that the needs of national security, or any other reason, are used as a justification for the illegal and unethical application on human beings." Many states have actually enacted civil rights laws to complement local laws. In fact, some doctors have been sanctioned for torture and crimes against humanity, in France, Germany, Portugal, Spain, Greece, Turkey, Israel, Iraq, Egypt, Libya, Jordan, USA, and possibly other countries as well. The actions or lack of action of health service providers, sometimes in war, though occasionally regulated by state laws and policies, have resulted in the intentional and unjustifiable inflation of severe physical or mental pain. Such action contrary to international rights is recognized, condemned and fought. That way the Hippocratic commitment not to cause damage or injustice could really be achieved.

[12] Trials of War Criminals, 1949–1953.

[13] Moreno (1997) and Moreno et al. (2017).

Informed Consent

Informed consent has become the primary paradigm for protecting patients' legal rights and guiding the ethical practice of medicine. It can be used for different purposes in different contexts: legal, ethical or administrative. While these purposes overlap, they are not identical, resulting in different standards and criteria for what constitutes "adequate" informed consent. Moreover, this consent is widely accepted as a legal, ethical, and regulatory requirement for most clinical trials relating to research and healthcare.

Not only, however: its principle, aimed at the legitimacy of healthcare, has become the formula for accepting (consent) or refusing (dissent) medical treatment.

Consent presupposes adequate diagnosis, prognosis and the related practicable beneficial interventions, but also risks, foreseeable complications, and possible alternatives.

There are three basic principles:

1. voluntary consent: essential for human participants in research;
2. the human subject must be free to terminate participation if s/he so wishes;
3. the Principal Investigator must terminate the investigation if there is any possible reason that its continuation could result in injury, disability or death.

In particular, the Code provides that subjects "should have the legal capacity to give their consent" without any coercive element (such as fraud, deception, violence, etc.).

Following the Nuremberg Trials and its inevitable legal aftermaths, the United States of America were considered the main supporters and auditors of the informed consent procedure.

The term consent was first used in a medical malpractice court case in the USA in 1957 (Salgo vs. Leland Stanford).[14] In 1960, a Kansas court decision (Natanson vs. Kline) did not allow the physician "to substitute his own judgment for that of the patient through any form of artifice or deception." In 1972, the "Canterbury vs. Spence" ruling established that a patient could freely exercise the right to self-determination only if s/he "possessed such information as to allow a fully informed choice."

In addition, the Patient's Bill of Rights, adopted in 1973 by the American Hospital Association, included the following: "...Ensure appropriate evaluation procedures to ascertain the ability of participants to give informed consent."

Multiple medical teams have gone into the merits and developed and clarified the medico-legal details.[15] Over the course of the twentieth century, the courts extended the doctrine of negligence with regard to EU law in the medical and surgical fields.

---

[14] California Malpractice, vol. 9, Stanford Law Review, p. 731, at pp. 742–43, supra. 1957.

[15] Beauchamp and Childress (1999), Etchells et al. (1999) and Lidz et al. (1988).

When a physician's negligence was accompanied by the violation of duty, the patient's consent was to be considered "incompetent." Currently, a physician's failure to provide adequate information to a patient about treatment is interpreted by the courts as a violation of the physician's duty.

At the beginning of the twenty-first century, there are good reasons to re-assess the ethical significance and practical application of the obligation to seek informed consent. This is especially true with today's numerous medical options, public health concerns, and legal interventions.

Informed consent for medical treatment and participation in medical research is both a legal and an ethical issue. Patients usually receive little training on the question of consent and often have scant understanding of the risks and alternatives of surgical or medical treatments offered. Their decisions are guided more by trust in their doctor or by the information provided by the authority involved.[16]

Over the past 50 years, the informed consent process has been increasingly regulated and standardized; the forms employed are increasingly detailed and complicated, sometimes obscuring important points, and may seem to be designed to serve the interests of institutions and sponsors. Descriptions of the level of risk to participants are kept low and are usually mainly basically informative.

Apps, tablets, videos, interactive computers, robots, personalized digital assistance, mobile phones, and smartphones and other technological innovations can help modernize, modify, and improve informed consent methods. Ethical objectives will guide the informed consent process, in order to make evidence-based practices effective.[17]

Looking at how the concept and the role of consent were born and developed, one must always bear in mind its ancient philosophical origins on the one hand but also the fact that it may have been influenced partly by religion, with moral aspects and the acceleration of deontological progress, often taking parallel paths to needs and progress to take account of new treatments and new biotechnological applications.

This is all relatively new, though not entirely recent. In fact, already at the time of the Egyptian and Greco-Roman civilizations we can find documents showing how the doctor's work had somehow to be preceded by the patient's approval. However, the patient is "ignorant" and does not have the knowledge, the intellectual capacity and the moral authority to oppose the will and decisions of the doctor who, on the other hand, has learned exactly what is best for the patient.

The patient's behavior towards the doctor has always tended towards trust and this attitude is backed by millenary tradition. The suffering patient, always with gratitude and respect, sought treatment but did not ask for explanations, and the doctor was careful not to take the initiative in informing the patient or his family, for two main reasons: (1) to benefit himself and (2) not to be of harm.[18]

---

[16] Grady (2015).

[17] Grady et al. (2017).

[18] Mallardi (2005).

In Conclusion

The whole process of informed consent comprises the following points:

1. to give the participant adequate information about what has been done or is planned;
2. to provide the opportunity for the participant to assess all options, and receive answers to any questions;
3. to make sure the participant understands this information;
4. to obtain the participant's voluntary agreement to participate;
5. to continue providing information as the participant or situation requires.

The informed consent process must give human participants the opportunity, as far as possible, to voluntarily select what will or will not happen to them.

Italy

In Italy, the need for informed consent appeared for the first time in art. 33 of law no. 833 of 23 December 1978 (first law of health reform)[19] which excluded the possibility of carrying out health checks and treatments against the patient's will.

It was only in 1990, when the Court of Assizes of Florence (with sentence no.13, 18 October—later confirmed by the Supreme Court with sentence no. 5639 of 13 May 1992—applied the new law and sentenced a surgeon for the crime of unintentional murder, for having performed an operation (removal of a carcinoma not previously diagnosed, without there being an emergency or immediate danger) on a woman who had given consent only for surgery for the removal of rectal polyps.

The principle of informed consent finds its most important consecration in art. 32 of the Italian Constitution, which reads:

The Republic protects health as a fundamental right of the individual and in the interest of the community and guarantees free medical care to the indigent. Nobody can be obliged to [agree to] a specific health treatment unless obliged by law. The law cannot under any circumstance violate the limits imposed by respect for the human person.

All this is in harmony with the fundamental principle of the inviolability of personal freedom (art.13) which states:

Personal freedom is inviolable. No form of detention, inspection or personal search is allowed, nor any other restriction of personal freedom, except by a reasoned act of the judicial authority and only in the cases and ways provided for by law.

[19] Italian Laws. Update of GU 30/10/2001. Art. 33. Norme per gli accertamenti ed i trattamenti sanitari volontari e obbligatori. [Rules for investigations and voluntary and obligatory health treatments] Oviedo Convention – Council of Europe – 1997.

The Code of Medical Deontology, revised in 2014, establishes the general principle according to which it is forbidden to undertake diagnostic and/or therapeutic measures without first acquiring the patient's informed consent, and the obligation for the doctor to desist if a person capable of understanding and willing expresses documented dissent.

In the Italian Constitution, the Convention for the Protection of Human Rights (confirmed by the Oviedo Convention, 1997, by the European Constitution, 2003), and the various international agreements and national laws that followed and continue to proliferate, the human person must be able to freely give or refuse consent to any intervention on their person. This consent constitutes the basis of the lawfulness of health care, in the absence of which this activity itself amounts to a punishable offense (only in civil law).

Here are some statements regarding informed consent.

Law no. 833, 23 December 1978: Establishment of the National Health Service. "The mandatory health checks and treatments referred to in the previous paragraphs must be accompanied by initiatives aimed at ensuring the consent and participation of those obliged to [receive them]."

Law no. 145, 28 March 2001: Ratification and execution of the Council of Europe Convention for the protection of human rights and human dignity with regard to the application of biology and medicine; and the Convention on Human Rights and Biomedicine, Oviedo, 4 April 1997: "An intervention in the field of health cannot be carried out until the person concerned has given free and informed consent. This person first of all receives adequate information on the purpose and nature of the intervention and its consequences and risks. The subjects may freely withdraw their consent at any time."

Since 1990, there have been numerous interventions on this topic, with consequent measures taken and judgments passed throughout Italy, by courts, the *Preture* (district courts) and Supreme Court.

Here are a few examples from legal decisions, up to 2015:

- Supreme Civil Court, 1994. The doctor is liable for damages resulting from negligence in the duty of complete information.
- Supreme Civil Court, 1997. The doctor cannot act without informed consent which must cover every single phase, the alternatives and the risks.
- Supreme Civil Court, 1997. In a hospital, if consent is lacking the hospital is liable.
- Court of Milan, 2000. Incorrect behavior of the physician in obtaining consent.
- Supreme Criminal Court, 2001. Without informed consent, medical treatment is arbitrary, and criminal.

Doubts have also been expressed about authentic consent.[20] The patient must not be burdened with too much information. Descriptions can be extended

[20] Dworkin (1988).

- Court of Brescia, 2003. Without consent or in the event of improper consent, medical treatment is arbitrary with penal and civil implications.
- Court of Milan, 2005. Responsibility of the healthcare professional for lack of consent even if the intervention was done correctly.
- Court of Milan, 2005. Pre-printed forms are not suitable for informed consent.
- Court of Appeal, Rome 2006. Complete and detailed information for obtaining consent even if the patient is a doctor.
- Civil Court, Paola, 2007. If informed consent is lacking, the patient must be compensated.
- Court of Novara, 2007. Violation of informed consent for different or additional therapies.
- Supreme Criminal Court, United Sections, 2008–2009. In the absence of consent, but the absence of explicit refusal, when the intervention has produced a benefit for the patient's health the doctor has no criminal responsibility (different surgical treatment).
- Supreme Civil Court, 2010. No-one can be tested for HIV without informed consent.
- Supreme Civil Court, 2010. The obligation to inform the patient is not subject to discretionary assessment.
- Supreme Civil Court, 2010. Proof of consent must be given by the doctor.
- Supreme Civil Court, 2010. Professional action (psychological observation) in favor of a minor without the consent of the legal guardian can be sanctioned.
- Supreme Criminal Court, 2010. Without consent, if the outcome is bad there is willful misconduct.
- Supreme Civil Court, 2013. Informed consent cannot be generic and the patient must be informed of the risks of a possible surgical operation.
- Supreme Civil Court, 2014. Cosmetic surgery: informed consent is required.
- Court of Florence, 2015. Plastic Surgery: informed consent is fundamental (on account of foreseeable risks).
- Supreme Civil Court, 2015, Published 2016. In hospitals: The patient must be informed about any shortcomings in the hospital, and the possibility of using more specialized centers; the doctor too must assess any organizational deficit.

indefinitely and there are no limits to specific consensus in clinical research. But how much information does the patient need to be considered "informed"? Perhaps the opinion, the amount and the level of information should be dictated by the individual patient or research subject, not by the doctor. Not all patients can be bothered with all the details, while others want a thorough understanding.

The importance of consent relates to the level of damage that could potentially result from the procedure or from sharing data.

The only exception where the doctor can act without the patient's consent is the state of necessity, to safeguard health (*quoad valetitudinem*) and life (*quoad vitam*).[21] Consent is not required where there is a situation of danger to public health, such as the need to prevent the spread of an epidemic or to isolate the patient.

It is now an established principle that no conscious and capable person can be subjected to any medical treatment against or without his/her will. Therefore today the legitimacy of the doctor's activity is no longer based on the prestige and authority of the professional, but exclusively on the patient's informed consent.

In the information, the following data must be clearly explained to the patient:

- The objective clinical situation
- The description of the medical intervention deemed necessary and the risks arising from failure to do it.
- Any diagnostic and/or therapeutic alternatives
- The techniques and materials to be employed
- The expected benefits
- The presumed risks
- Possible complications
- What the patient must do to avoid complications after the treatment.

Consent to a specific treatment can be expressed by another person only if this person has been clearly delegated by the patient himself. For a minor, the doctor is responsible for the clinical decision after hearing the parents' (or guardians') opinion and, where possible, the will of the subject himself. In the event of urgency and necessity, parental dissent must not affect the medical decision.

If the patient is of age but unable to decide, the designated legal guardian must give or deny the relative consent.

Written consent is mandatory by law:

- when giving or receiving blood
- if you participate in a drug trial
- for serological tests for HIV infection
- for kidney transplantation between living beings
- for the voluntary termination of pregnancy
- for interventions concerning sex change
- for medically assisted procreation

[21] Italian Penal Code, art. 54: "Anyone who has committed the deed having been obliged by the need to save himself or others from a current risk of serious harm to the person, not voluntarily caused by him, nor otherwise avoidable, is not punishable, pro-vided that the fact is proportionate to the danger."

Exceptions to the consent requirement:

- the sick person has explicitly expressed the will not to be informed
- the conditions are so serious and life-threatening that immediate intervention is required (presumed consent)
- a therapeutic trial is already under way, to which the patient had given consent earlier (implied consent)
- the risks concern atypical, exceptional and unpredictable consequences of a surgical intervention
- health treatment is compulsory.

The patient must complete and sign the consent form. This is the last step in an information process that has already begun between doctor and patient.

1. The person involved in a clinical trial must be legally capable of understanding the information provided and giving consent, with no physical or psychological pressure, deception, coercion or any other form of insistence. This responsibility cannot be delegated.
2. Results achieved must be positive, not random or futile and not obtainable by other methods, for the good of the individual and society.
3. The proposal must be backed by findings from animal testing and knowledge of the natural history of the disease or when the expected results justify the experiment.
4. The experiment must be conducted in such a way as to avoid any unnecessary physical or mental suffering or other harm.
5. No experiment should be conducted when death or disabling injury are foreseeable, unless the investigator himself is the subject of the experiment.
6. In the current experiment the risks must never be higher than expected.
7. Adequate support structures must be available for protection of the individual.
8. The experiment must be conducted only by scientifically qualified people.
9. The subject must be free to withdraw from the experiment at any time his/her physical or mental state prevents him/her participating.
10. The investigator must stop the experiment when:
    - s/he considers it risky, in good faith;
    - correct continuation requires skills superior to his/her own;
    - continuation could cause injury, disability or death.

An example of an Informed Consent Form :

THE PATIENT'S DATA
SURNAME AND NAME-------------------------- -------------
DATE OF BIRTH ---------------- PLACE ----------------------
HOSPITAL ----------------- --------------- UNIT---------------
Diagnosis or area for diagnostic orientation

Therapy and/or diagnostic measures and/or rehabilitation

The diagnosis, therapy and/or rehabilitation is carried out on the basis of necessity if the patient is not able to give consent, or there is no-one who can legally give it, so from this point the form need no longer be compiled.

Information has been provided relating to:
1) – The diagnosis or diagnostic orientation
2) – The prognosis and improvement expected of the treatment
3) – The methods for the diagnosis, therapy, and/or rehabilitation
4) – The type of anesthesia (if any)
5) - Any risks or complications (also with reference to any other concomitant pathologies)
6) - Possible diagnostic-therapeutic alternatives to the proposed treatment (including the likelihood of improvement, or risks and complications)
7) - Predictable consequences of failure to carry out the diagnostic and/or therapeutic and/or rehabilitation proposals

In addition (mark the option implemented):
□ The patient, or whoever exercises parental authority, or the legal representative (administrator, guardian, other) has been given information material on the proposed procedure, specifically prepared by the Operative Unit, and a copy signed by the patient is filed in the medical record.
□ In the absence of specific information material, the information transmitted verbally during the interview is summarized in the medical record (or other health documentation), and the patient, or the person exercising parental authority, signs for acknowledgment.
We inform the recipients of the information that should they need further information, they can contact the Operative Unit at the following telephone number .... (a note should be made in the file of any request for further information).
Notes ....
Date ------------- Doctor's signature and stamp...........................

Having verified that the recipient of the information has understood and is aware of the risks and benefits of the proposed diagnosis, therapy and/or rehabilitation, consent is obtained.

EXPRESSION OF CONSENT
I understood what Dr. .... has explained to me.
Therefore I agree:
That the proposed diagnosis, therapy and/or rehabilitation at this Facility will be carried out by:
□ team members □ external consultant
Date --------------
Patient's signature (if adult, capable of understanding, and willing)
....
Signature of parents or guardians (if minor) ....
OR of whoever has this function (having received a copy of the consent document) ....

DISCLAIMER OF CONSENT
I understood what Dr. .... explained to me
But I do not agree
To the proposed diagnosis, therapy and/or rehabilitation at this Facility,

Date -------------------
Signature of the patient (if adult and capable of understanding, and willing) ....
Signature of parents or guardians (if minor) .... or whoever has this function (having received a copy of the consent document)

Doctor's signature and stamp ....

NOTE: withdrawal of consent must be specifically noted in the medical record (or other health documentation) and duly signed by the patient (or parents or legal representative).

SELF-CERTIFICATION FORM FOR PARENTS

Declaration substituting for the sworn statement (Article 47 of Presidential Decree no.445, 18/12/2000)

Date --------------------

Signature of the patient (if adult and capable of understanding, and willing)

....

Signature of parents or guardians (if minor) .... or whoever has this function (having received a copy of the consent document)

Doctor's signature and stamp ....

NOTE: withdrawal of consent must be specifically noted in the medical record (or other health documentation) and duly signed by the patient (or parents or legal representative).

Declaration substituting for the sworn statement (Article 47 no. 445 of Presidential Decree 18/12/2000). I, the undersigned ....
born in ....
on .... resident in town............... street and no..................
Aware of the responsibilities and penalties set out in Article 76 regarding false declarations or certifications:
- declare that I am the parent of the minor ....
- have been informed of the provisions governing consent for minors
- that my marital status is as follows
□ am married □ widowed □ separated □ divorced in a situation of
□ joint custody □ custodial parent...... □ other............
Place and date.................

The declarant (legible full signature) ....
This self-certification was:
□ signed by the party concerned in the presence of the employee in charge
□ presented together with an unauthenticated photocopy of an identity document.
PLEASE NOTE:
An information sheet is always attached to the Form, referring to the articles of the Civil Code regarding the exercise of parental authority.

Informed Consent forms vary depending on the medical and/or surgical specialties involved, for example:

1. Medical Area and its multiple and structured subspecialties, in the specific operative units;
2. Surgical Area and its multiple and structured subspecialties, in the specific operative units;
3. Area of Diagnostic Medicine and Services;

4. Dentistry Area,
5. Public Health Area.

There are some limits to the application of the consent rules:[22]

1. Autonomy: there are many distinct conceptions of individual autonomy and their ethical importance can differ in the light of local legislation and/ or traditional laws.
2. Age and health: Informed consent should not be sought for the very young or very ill, mentally impaired, demented or unconscious, or simply frail or confused. Often people cannot give informed consent to emergency treatment.
3. Informed consent procedures in medicine are sometimes useless for certain health policies.
4. The medical treatment of individuals employs personal information about third parties that may be disclosed without their consent.
5. Some people with adequate competence for consent are under duress and therefore less able to refuse the requests of others: for example, prisoners and soldiers

In Conclusion

Informed consent cannot obviously be relevant for all doctors' decisions, because it cannot be provided by patients who are incompetent, it cannot be used in the choice of public health policies, it cannot be guaranteed for the disclosure of third party information, and cannot be obtained from those who are vulnerable or dependent. However, informed consent is important for the ethically acceptable treatment of individual patients who are competent and free, i.e., in cases where no third party information is needed.

Listed here are a few of the topics that have appeared historically to be most connected with informed consent. Some are discussed elsewhere in this book.

Medical Ethics, Hippocratic Oath, Jewish Medical Ethics, FNOMCEO Code 1916 and 1924, European Charter of Medical Ethics, Principles of European Medical Ethics, ACP American College of Physicians, Oath of the Soviet Union, Loma Linda, AMA American Medical Association, Informed Consent, WMA World Medical Association, Geneva Declaration, Universal Declaration of Human Rights, Helsinki Declaration, Belmont Report, CIOMS, Good Clinical Practice.

Other topics might be covered in a future publication, for instance on civil rights, human experimentation in some specific conditions, human rights in general, research on human subjects, medical torture, universal declaration of human rights, etc.

---

[22] O'Neill (2003) and McLean (2007).

References

American College of Obstetricians and Gynecologists. Informed consent. ACOG Committee Opinion N°. 439. Obstet Gynecol. 2009;114:401–8.

Annas GJ, Grodin MA, editors. The Nazi doctors and the Nuremberg Code. Human rights in human experimentation. Boston University; 1995. 400 pag. 12

Archives of Internal Medicine. Informed consent. 1996;156(22):2521–6.

Beauchamp TL. Worthington Hooker on ethics in clinical medicine. In: Baker R, editor. The codification of medical morality. Philosophy and medicine, vol. 49. Dordrecht: Springer; 1995.

Beauchamp TL, Childress JF. Principi di etica biomedica (IT. Principles of medical ethics) 1944, (1a ed. 1979), Italian translation by S. Buonazia, Le Lettere, Firenze; 1999.

Dworkin G. The theory and practice of autonomy. Cambridge: Cambridge Univ. Press; 1988. p. 6.

Encyclopedia of Bioethics. Informed consent: I. History of informed consent. Encyclopedia.com. http://www.encyclopedia.com (22 June 2017).

Etchells E, Sharpe G, et al. Bioethics for clinicians: 3. Capacity. CMAY. 1999;155(6):657–61.

Grady C. Enduring and emerging challenges of informed consent. NEJM. 2015;72(9):55–862.

Grady C, Cummings SR, Rowbotham MC, et al. The changing face of clinical trials. Informed consent. NEJM. 2017;376(9):856–67.

Heiman T. (POL. Etika Lekarska = Medical Ethics): L'Etica Medica e le funzioni del medico [IT. Medical ethics and the doctor's functions]. Warsaw; 1917.

Katz J. The Nuremberg Code and the Nuremberg Trial. A reappraisal. JAMA. 1996;76(20):1662–6.

Kumar NK. Informed consent: past and present. Perspect Clin Res. 2013;4(1):21–5.

Lidz CW, Appelbaum PS, Meisel A. Two models of implementing informed consent. Arch Intern Med. 1988;148:1385–9.

Mallardi V. Le origini del consenso informato [IT. The origins of informed consent]. Acta Otorhinolaringol Ital. 2005;25:312–27.

McLean SAM. What and who are clinical ethics committees for? J Med Ethics. 2007;33(9):497–500.

Meisel A, Kuczewski M. Legal and ethical myths about informed consent. Arch Intern Med. 1996;156(22):2521–6.

Moreno JD. Reassessing the influence of the Nuremberg Code on American medical ethics. J Contemp Health Law Policy. 1997;13:347–60.

Moreno JD, Schmidt U, Joffe S. The Nuremberg Code 70 years later. JAMA. Published online 17 August 2017.

Mountokalakis TD. Modern medical ethics and the legacy of Hippocrates. Hospital Chronicles. 2014;9(4):229–31.

Murray PM. The history of informed consent. Iowa Orthop J. 1990;10:104–9.

O'Neill O. Some limits of informed consent. J Med Ethics. 2003;29:4–7.

Shuster E. Fifty years later: the significance of the Nuremberg Code. NEJM. 1997;337(20):1436, 1449.

Weindling P. Human guinea pigs and the ethics of experimentation: the BMJ's correspondent at the Nuremberg medical trial. BMJ. 1996;313:1467–70.

Medical Ethics in the World 13

Ethics, also known as moral philosophy, is the branch of philosophy that involves the organization, defense, and recommendation of the concepts of right and wrong conduct. Many individuals tend to compare ethics with their own feelings, even if being moral is not unequivocally a matter of dealing only with one's feelings. Ethics deals with guidelines relating to right or wrong action, good, and evil, as a rule for rights, commitments, advantages for society, decency or particular ideals. Today's medical ethics directly addresses life: it is considered important for behavior in a clinical trial and in the wider fields of medicine, from the search for a correct diagnosis to the treatment phase and beyond, during the last moments of life, and in relation to possible transplants and related practices.

This chapter refers to some events or episodes in the twentieth century that greatly influenced the definition and implementation of medical ethics, at the international level. Here is a brief list:

1. World Medical Association (WMA),
2. Geneva Declaration,
3. International Code of Medical ethics,
4. Universal Declaration of Human Rights,
5. Declarations of Helsinki and Taipei,
6. Other meetings organized and sponsored by the WMA,
7. World Health Organization (WHO).

WMA

The World Medical Association was founded shortly after the end of World War II, in Paris, September 18, 1947: the inauguration of this new international organization had the goal of establishing and promoting the highest standards of ethical behavior and care. Its current headquarters are in Ferney-Voltaire, France. The

R. G. Russo, *Medical Ethics*, https://doi.org/10.1007/978-3-031-42444-1_13

WMA works with academic institutions, global organizations, and individual experts; it has adopted numerous qualified policies and has issued statements on a number of ethical questions connected with medical professionalism, human care and research, and public health. The WMA Board and its standing committees regularly review and update existing policies and develop new policies on emerging ethical issues.[1] The WMA is an organization in constant evolution, in defense of the interests of patients and a defender of the medical profession. When it was founded physicians from 27 different countries met at the First General Assembly. In 2007 the Association counted representatives of 84 medical associations with a membership of about 8 million doctors.[2] The Current Number of Constituent Members, in 2021, is 115.

The Official Journal of the WMA is the Medical World Journal, published since 1954 by the Latvian Medical Association, in Riga, Latvia, and available online. Since its official launch in January 2005, the WMA Medical Ethics Manual has been distributed to medical journals and medical schools throughout the world.

Every year the WMA General Assembly (GA) reviews some existing policies and/or adopts new ones. The WMA Executive Committee (ExCo) at its latest meeting, on July 22, decided not to hold the GA as a traditional in-person assembly, on account of the COVID-19 pandemic. And scheduled the GA, Council and Committee Sessions as virtual meetings. The COVID-19 pandemic meant it was still not feasible to plan a hybrid (in-person/online) WMA Scientific Session on October 23, 2020 in Cordoba. Jointly with their Spanish colleagues, therefore, the WMA Executive Committee postponed the Scientific Session. The new date will be published as soon as possible.

The ethical projects currently under way are:

- Medical education,
- Human resource planning in the medical field,
- Patient safety
- Leadership and career development,
- Defense of doctors' rights,
- Medicine and safety at work,
- Strengthening democracy in medical associations,
- Policies related to public health issues,
- Tobacco consumption and vaccination control projects,
- Medicine in prisons,
- Update on tuberculosis,
- Antibiotic resistance.

---

[1] WMA: WhatWeDo, Medical Ethics.

[2] Wikipedia Associazione Medica Mondiale. (IT. World Medical Assembly).
Bird (1989), pp. 47–48, Guraya (2014) and World Medical Association (1949–2006).

There are also these:

(a) The Handbook of WMA Policies: Topics important for human health.
(b) Medical Ethics Manual: A manual distributed to medical journals and medical schools around the world
(c) WMA Oath
(d) WMA White Paper on Social Media and Medicine: Role of social media in health care provision.

The Handbook of WMA Policies

Various topics relating to human health are continuously debated, with particular focus on medical ethics. The main task is to develop guidelines for human research. The Policies Handbook is published as a WMA position document, covering multiple ethical and social issues. The questions raised for discussion are generally relevant to doctors around the world.

At the III General Assembly in London, in 1949, the International Code of Medical Ethics was produced, and later amended by the XXII World Medical Assembly, in Sydney, August 1968, by the XXXV Medical World Assembly, in Venice, October 1983 and by the LVII Medical World Assembly, Pilanesberg, South Africa, in October 2006.[3]

Medical Ethics Manual

After World War II medical leaders in many countries saw the need to restore the reputation of the profession in response to the extensive violations of medical ethics perpetrated in Nazi Germany and elsewhere. The first task of the new Association was reformulation of the Hippocratic Oath. This new oath was named the "Geneva Declaration." The next task was to adapt and update the principles in line with developments of medicine and society.

Medical Ethics Manual, third edition, 2015, WMA, Ferney-Voltaire Cedex, France, related to: publication

1. Bioethics
2. Doctor–Patient–Ethics Relationships
3. Doctor's Role
4. Research Ethics
5. Professional Relations
6. Education, medical ethics
7. Clinical Case Reports
8. Manuals.

[3] WHO-Who we are, WMA-Who we are.

WMA Oath: 1948[4]

"The WMA DOCTOR'S OATH" was adopted by the WMA General Assembly in Geneva in September 1948 and modified **at** the 22nd World Assembly in Sydney in August 1968. It was further renovated and modified in 1983 and 2005 to take account of Hippocrates' Oath in modern times (2006).

At entry as a member of the profession, "new" doctors must agree to the following:

I solemnly undertake to consecrate my life to the service of humanity: I will reserve the respect and gratitude due to my teachers and I will practice my profession with conscience and dignity.
My patient's health will be my first concern; I will keep the honor and noble traditions of the medical profession.
My colleagues will be my brothers.
I will not allow differences in religion, nationality, race, political party or social status to affect me and my patient.
I will maintain the utmost respect for human life from its conception.
I do not want my medical knowledge to conflict with the laws of humanity, even under threat.
I make these promises solemnly, freely and on my honor.

WMA: White Paper on Social Media and Medicine

Social media has become a practical reality for millions of people around the world including doctors, medical students, and patients. Social media generally involve different platforms and applications that allow user-generated content to be created and shared electronically. This proposed policy had the following aims:

- To examine the professional and ethical challenges relating to the increasing use of social media by doctors, medical students, and patients.
- To establish and maintain high professional and ethical standards.

Geneva Declaration, 1948[5]

The Geneva Declaration was adopted by the WMA General Assembly, and amended in 1968, 1984, 1994, 2005, and 2006. It was drafted by doctors, with a view to laying greater stress on the humanity of medicine—closer to the Hippocratic

[4] WMA International Code of Medical Ethics 2006.
WMA Policy © 2018 The World Medical Association.
[5] https://it.wikipedia.prg/wiki/Declaration_medical_world-cite_note-1.

oath—especially after the crimes committed in previous years. The final version of the Doctor's Oath, after revisions and amendments, is shown above.

The Geneva Conventions now constitute a body of international law, also known as "Geneva law." The four Geneva Conventions of 1949, the two Additional Protocols of 1977 and that of 2005 are the basis of international humanitarian law. Since 1949 those on both sides in wars have committed themselves to protecting the sick, the wounded, the shipwrecked, medical personnel, ambulances and hospitals; prisoners must be treated and cared for. There are detailed rules on the treatment of prisoners of war and protection from acts of violence and arbitrariness, especially for civilians.

A further task was to develop guidelines for human research. In 1964 these were adopted in the Declaration of Helsinki.[6] This document was periodically reviewed, until it was replaced by "Good Clinical Practice" (ICHGCP) in 2008.

Every year the WMA GA reviews some existing policies and/or adopts new ones. Their acceptance requires 75% of voters to reach consent, even if some doctors hold positions contrary to the local ones of governments, health system administrators, and/or commercial enterprises. At the May 1997 WMA Council meeting, decisions were taken regarding: Human Cloning; Tobacco products; the Geneva Declaration; Palliative Care; The Doctor's Imbalance; The rights of hospitalized children; The rights of the unborn child; Suspension of doctors' licenses for serious criminal offenses; Doctors involved in torture.

Comments

The amendments to the Declaration have been criticized by some Catholic doctors, as they may run counter to the inviolability of human life; for example, the original text specified "health and life," which later became only "health"—"health will be my first concern." The "conception of life," "from the moment of its conception" had to be eliminated from a code of ethics that rejects all ideologies, politics, ethnicities, religions, etc. and is a supporter of a right to equality and broad citizenship.

The Geneva Declaration constitutes a modern affirmation of doctors' commitment to the humanitarian principles of medicine. Conceived as a modern Hippocratic oath, it is considered one of the fundamental documents of medical ethics and is intended to be sworn by doctors upon admission to the medical profession.

Also considered was the extent to which the Geneva Declaration is disseminated and used as an oath by physicians entering the medical profession; this varies widely from country to country. The Declaration does not include any reference to

[6] Bird (1989), pp. 61–63.
WMA Helsinki 1964, WMA Taipei 2016. Declaration of Helsinki.
Millum (2013).
Ndebele (2013).
WMA Helsinki.

acceptance of the patient's self-determination, which has since been established as one of the most important principles of medical ethics and is explicitly mentioned in other WMA documents.

Proposed Changes

1. An amendment to the principle of professional autonomy: "I will take up my profession with conscience and dignity and in accordance with good medical practice";
2. The addition of the following to improve consistency with other relevant literature: "My health and my well-being depend on the well-being of my patient: this will be my first consideration";
3. The addition of a clause to highlight the importance of respecting the patient's autonomy;
4. The addition of a clause that reflects the doctor's obligation to share medical knowledge for the benefit of the patient and the advancement of health care;
5. The addition of a clause expressing the need for doctors to look after their own health (i.e., the doctor's well-being) so as to be available to provide the best possible care.

International Code of Medical Ethics, 1949

After approval of the Geneva Declaration, the II WMA General Assembly analyzed a report on War Crimes and Medicine. This prompted the WMA Council to appoint a study committee to prepare an International Code of Medical Ethics, which was adopted in London in October 1949.

A number of amendments were made by various countries in 1968 (Sydney), 1983 (Venice), and 2006 (Pilanesberg).

WMA has organized and run the following courses:

1. Ethics—Fundamentals of Medical Ethics and Objectives;
2. Doctors working in prisons.

WMA International Code of Medical Ethics

Doctors' Obligations in General

A physician:

- must always exercise his or her independent professional judgment and maintain the highest standards of professional conduct
- must respect the right of a competent patient to accept or refuse treatment
- must not allow his judgment to be influenced by personal gain or unfair discrimination

- must be dedicated to providing competent medical service in full professional and moral independence, with compassion and respect for human dignity
- must treat patients and colleagues honestly and report to the authorities any physicians who practice unethically or incompetently or engage in fraud or deception
- must exercise his profession without being influenced by profit motives.
- must not accept any financial benefits or other incentives solely for referring patients or for prescribing specific products
- must respect the rights and preferences of patients, colleagues, and other healthcare professionals
- must recognize his important role in educating the public, but should use due caution in disclosing or spreading information on discoveries or new techniques or treatments through non-professional channels
- has only to certify what he has personally verified
- must strive to use healthcare resources in the best possible way to help patients and their community
- must seek appropriate care and attention if he suffers any mental or physical illness
- must abide by local and national codes of ethics
- must provide emergency care as a humanitarian duty, unless he is sure that others are willing and able to provide it
- must be present in situations where he acts on behalf of third parties and must ensure that the patient has full knowledge of this situation
- must not enter into any sexual or other abusive or exploitative relationship with a current patient.

Doctors' Obligations Towards All Patients

A physician

- must always keep in mind the obligation to preserve human life from its conception. Therapeutic abortion is only permissible if the doctor's conscience and national laws permit it
- owes his patient complete fidelity and all the resources of his science. Whenever an examination or treatment is beyond his/her capacity s/he must call in another doctor who has the necessary skills
- must keep absolute secrecy about everything s/he knows about the patient because of the trust placed in him/her
- must provide emergency care as a humanitarian duty, unless he is sure that others are willing and able to provide it.

Doctors' Obligations Towards Colleagues

A physician

- behaves towards colleagues as s/he would have them behave towards him/her
- does not compromise the patient–doctor relationship of colleagues in order to attract patients. When medically necessary, a doctor communicates with colleagues who are involved in the care of the same patient. This contact must respect patient confidentiality and be limited to the information indispensable.
- must not ensnare patients from his colleagues
- must abide by the principles of the Geneva Declaration approved by the World Medical Association

A few steps are considered unethical:

- any personal advertising unless explicitly authorized by the national code of medical ethics;
- collaboration in any medical service in which the doctor does not have full professional independence;
- receipt of any money, other than a fair professional rate, in connection with services rendered to a patient, even with the patient's knowledge;
- any action or advice that could lessen a person's physical or mental strength.

To Summarize

The physician must abide by the principles of the Geneva Declaration approved by the World Medical Association.

Universal Declaration of Human Rights, 1948[7]

This document on individual rights was signed in Paris on 10 December 1948, and was promoted as a draft by the United Nations, for application in all Member States.

Preamble

Considering that the foundation of freedom, justice, and peace in the world recognizes the dignity of all members of the human family and their equal and inalienable rights; whereas the disregard and contempt for human rights have led to acts of barbarism that offend the conscience of humanity; and that the advent of a world in

[7] Loewy (2007).

which human beings enjoy freedom of speech and belief and freedom from fear and need has been proclaimed as the highest aspiration of man; it is imperative that human rights be protected by legal norms, if you want to avoid man being obliged to turn, as a last resort, to rebellion against tyranny and oppression; it is essential to promote the development of friendly relations between nations; the Members of the United Nations have reaffirmed in the Charter their faith in fundamental human rights, in the dignity and worth of the human person, in the equality of rights of men and women, and have resolved to promote social progress and a better standard of living in greater freedom; the peoples of the Member States have undertaken to pursue, in cooperation with the United Nations, universal respect and observance of human rights and fundamental freedoms; a common understanding of these rights and freedoms is of the utmost importance for the full realization of these commitments.

The General Assembly

Proclaims this universal Declaration of Human Rights as a common ideal to be achieved by all peoples and all nations, in order that every individual and every organ of society, having this Declaration constantly in mind, endeavors to promote, by teaching and education, respect for these rights and freedoms and to guarantee, through progressive measures of a national and international character, the universal and effective recognition and respect both among the peoples of the Member States themselves and among those of the territories subject to their jurisdiction.

> ***The recognition of the inherent dignity of all members of the human family and of their rights, equal and inalienable, constitutes the foundation of freedom, justice and peace in the world.***

The main articles of the Universal Declaration, related to medical ethics, are set out below:

Art. 1—All human beings are born free and equal in dignity and rights and must in conscience act towards one another in a spirit of brotherhood.

Art. 2—(a) Everyone is entitled to all the rights and freedoms set forth in this Declaration, without distinction of race, color, sex, language, religion, political opinion, nationality, wealth and birth.

(b) Furthermore, no distinction will be established on the basis of the political, juridical or international status of the country or territory to which a person belongs, whether they are independent, subject to trust, not autonomous or any other limitation of sovereignty.

Art. 3—Everyone has the right to life, liberty and security of his person.

Art. 4—No individual may be held in a state of slavery or servitude; slavery and the slave trade will be prohibited in any form.
Art. 5—No individual shall be subjected to cruel, inhuman or degrading treatment or punishment.
Art. 6—Everyone everywhere has the right to recognition of his or her legal personality.
Art. 7—All are equal before the law and are entitled, without any discrimination, to adequate protection.
Art. 18—Everyone has the right to freedom of thought, conscience and religion; this right includes the freedom to change religion or belief and the freedom to manifest, in public or private, one's religion or belief, in practices, worship and observance of rites.
Art. 19—Everyone has the right to freedom of opinion and expression, including not being pestered about their opinion, and also has the right to seek, receive and disseminate information and ideas through any medium and regardless of borders.
Art. 20—(a) Everyone has the right to freedom of peaceful assembly and association.
(b) Nobody can be obliged to be part of an association.
Art. 26—(a) Everyone has the right to education. Elementary education must be compulsory. Education must be free at least in the elementary and fundamental classes. Technical and vocational education must be made available to all and higher education must be equally accessible to all on the basis of merit.
(b) Education must be aimed at the full development of the human personality and the strengthening of respect for human rights and fundamental freedoms. It must promote understanding, tolerance, friendship between all nations, racial and religious groups, and must favor the work of the United Nations for the maintenance of peace.
(c) Parents have the right of priority in choosing the education for their children.
Art. 30—Nothing in this Declaration can be interpreted as a right by any State, Group or Person for the purpose of exercising activities or actions aimed at the cancellation of the rights and freedoms set forth herein.

Helsinki + Taipei, 1964[8]

In 1964 the guidelines were adopted together with Helsinki Declaration (HD). The WMA HD of 1964–2014 was considered the "Evolution of ethics in medical research." The HD is in fact the best known political declaration of the WMA. The

[8] World Medical Association (2013).

first version was adopted in 1964 and it has been modified seven times. The most recent version (2013) is the only official one: all previous versions have been replaced and should not be used or cited except for historical purposes. Since 2016, the Taipei Declaration (TD) on ethical considerations relating to health databases has completed the HD, taking account of the need for an ethical approach to human research involving new therapies, new medicines, and new bio-medical instruments.

The HD was perceived as a set of precepts for the guidance and protection of human rights in experimentation. It is a basic document in the history of ethics and scientific research which, until then, did not apply any Code to regulate its ethical aspects. The HD developed the first ten principles indicated in the Nuremberg Code and later reported them in the WMA Geneva Declaration (1948).

The HD addresses the following issues:

- Human research must be based on the results of laboratory and animal experimentation
- Research protocols must be reviewed by an independent committee before the start of a study or trial
- Informed consent from research participants is essential
- Research must be validated by scientifically qualified people in the medical field
- The risks must not outweigh the benefits.

Basic Principles of Clinical Research, According to the HD

- respect for the individual
- the right of self-determination after adequate explanation for participation in the research
- the researcher's duty to safeguard the health of the patient or volunteer
- the need for research must always be stressed
- the individual's well-being has precedence over the interests of society
- ethical considerations must always take priority over current laws or regulations
- continuous vigilance must be exercised on the growing vulnerability of the individual
- when the subject participating in research is physically or mentally unable to join, or is a minor, permission should be based on the consent of another person acting on behalf of the subject.

Doctors are not relieved of criminal, civil, and ethical responsibilities under national laws related to medical ethics.

The DH comprises 37 articles. (Here we look at those focusing mainly on medical ethics.)

1. The WMA drafted the HD as an expression of ethical principles for bio-medical research, including the use of biological samples of human origin and other identifiable data.

4. It is the physician's duty to safeguard and protect the health, well-being, and rights of patients. Science and conscience must be held at the service of this mission.
10. Doctors are required to comply with national regulations on the subject, as well as ethical, legal, and international regulatory standards.
12. Bio-medical research involving human beings must be carried out only by experienced, qualified personnel with adequate ethical and scientific knowledge. Research on patients or healthy volunteers must be supervised by a competent, qualified physician or other professional.
22. The design and conduct of each study must be clearly described and explained in a research protocol. The protocol must set out the ethical considerations in each case and their relevance to the principles of this Declaration. It must include all information relating to sponsors, institutional affiliations, financial aspects, potential conflicts of interest, incentives for the subjects involved, and provisions for the treatment and/or compensation of subjects harmed as a result of participation.
23. Before the start of the study, the protocol must be submitted to the relevant Ethics Committee for examination, comments, suggestions or obligations, approval and subsequent monitoring. No amendment to the protocol can be made without review and further approval. The results of the study and its conclusions must be reported to the Ethics Committee.
25. Informed consent must be given voluntarily, preferably in writing. If consent cannot be obtained in writing, it must be formally documented and witnessed.
26. Every patient has the right to refuse participation in the study and withdraw at any time and without any consequence.
36. Researchers, investigators, sponsors, and publishing houses have ethical obligations regarding the publication and dissemination of research results. Negative and inconclusive findings must be publicly available in the same way as positive results.

Representatives of the OECD[9] met in Helsinki on 5–9 July 2015 to assess developments in ethics and the security of cooperation; they proposed innovative resolutions adhering to the dictates of the Declaration.

The Taipei Declaration (TD)

The TD set out to strike a balance between the rights of individuals providing their products or data and other purposes based on confidentiality and privacy. The main risk scenarios involve not so much science as the commercial, administrative or political use of data. The risk from outside the field of medicine may involve the

[9] The OECD, Organization for Economic Development and Cooperation, established on 14 December 1960 is an international organization that works to build better policies for better lives. Today 37 countries are members, including Italy, and there are 70 non-members.

abuse of marketing, cost reductions, and politics. Therefore, the TD addresses any use of health databases and is not limited to research.

As doctors are the primary custodians of confidential health information, they have an obligation to their patients, but also to others to whom they entrust their data and samples (e.g., blood or tissue).

While there is a strong possibility of finding cures and remedies for many medical problems, diseases, and suffering, the main challenge lies in the considerable risk of abuse and misuse of health databases and bio-banks.

Meetings Indicated and Sponsored by the WMA in the Twentieth and Twenty-First Centuries[10]

The WMA has designed and held various meetings at different times. Here are some of the main ones, with brief descriptions of the topics covered and any comments or provisions that may touch ethics.

[10] WMA Chicago.
WMA Copenhagen 2007.
WMA Divonne-les-Bains 2003 WHA Ferney Voltaire 2001.
WMA International Code of Medical Ethics WMA Ginevra 1948.
WMA Helsinki 1964 WMA Helsinki Declaration WMA Sydney 1968.
WMA Lisbon 1981.
WMA Manual of Medical Ethics 2005 WMA Montevideo 2011.
WMA Moscow 2015.
WMA Oslo 1970.
WMA Ottawa 1988.
WMA Pilanesberg 2006.
WMA Seoul 2008.
WMA St Julian 1991.
WMA Stockholm 1994.
WMA Sydney 1968.
WMA Taipei 2016.
WMA TelAviv 1988.
WMA Tokyo 1975.
WMA Venice 1983.
WMA Washington 2002.
WPA Hawaii 1977.
Bird (1989), pp. 61–63.
Helsinki. Bird (1989), p. 64. Sydney.
Bird (1989), p. 65. Oslo.
Bird (1989), pp. 66–68. Hawaii.
Declaration of Geneva (1948). Adopted by the General Assembly of the World Medical Association in Geneva, Switzerland, September 1948.
WMA Manual of Medical Ethics 2005.
Millum (2013).
Ndebele (2013).

Sidney Declaration, Australia (1968)

The 1968 Sidney Declaration (revised in 1983) relates to *human death and organ transplantation*. Among other things, it states that "the clinical interest lies not only in the state of conservation of isolated cells, but in the fate of a person." In the case of transplantation, there is a rule requiring the simultaneous presence of two doctors who endorse the removal of one or more organs taken from a deceased person, whose death must be confirmed by the certainty that it had become irreversible despite any resuscitation technique that may have been used. In most countries, establishing the time of death is the legal responsibility of the physician and must remain so.

Oslo Declaration, Norway (1970)

This Declaration relates to *abortion*.

The main conclusions are:

(a) The first moral principle for the physician is respect for human life, as expressed in the Geneva Declaration.
(b) The life of the unborn child is a matter of individual conviction and conscience that must be respected.
(c) Therapeutic abortion can only be practiced when it complies with national legislative requirements and if the following principles are approved:
(d) Abortion must be done only as a therapeutic measure.
(e) The decision to terminate a pregnancy must be approved in writing by at least two doctors selected for their competence and professionalism.
(f) The procedure must be done by a competent physician in places deemed suitable.
(g) If the doctor believes that his/her beliefs do not permit him to advise or perform an abortion, he can refuse the task, but at the same time must ensure the availability of a qualified colleague.

Tokyo Declaration, Japan (1975)

The Declaration relates to *torture*.

Torture is defined as the intentional, systematic or arbitrary infliction of physical or mental suffering with the aim of forcing another person to provide information, make a confession, or for any other reason.

Doctors are unequivocally prohibited from tolerating, participating in or condoning the practice of torture or any other forms of cruel, inhuman or degrading coercion. It also bans force-feeding during a hunger strike by mentally healthy people.

Here are some of the main points:

- Doctors must ensure the confidentiality of all personal medical information concerning the patient.

- The doctor must refuse to be present when torture or any other form of cruel, inhuman or degrading treatment is used or threatened.
- WMA must back up international communities, national medical associations, colleagues, and their families who receive threats or retaliation for not participating in similar practices.

Hawaii Statement (1977)

The Declaration concerns the minimum ethical standards of the *psychiatric profession.*

Even if the conduct is based on the individual psychiatrist's personal conscience, guidelines approved by the World Psychiatric Association are needed to clarify the ethical implications of this profession. The wide cultural differences and the different legal, social, and economic conditions in various countries around the world have also to be considered.

Some relevant points are summarized here:

- The purpose of psychiatry is to treat mental illness and promote health.
- Every psychiatrist must offer the patient the best available therapy.
- When there is a need, or requested by the patient himself, the psychiatrist must call on a colleague.
- Confidentiality, trust, cooperation, and mutual responsibility are required.
- No procedure or any treatment should be given against or independently of the patient's wishes.
- If a patient or others request action contrary to scientific knowledge or ethical principles, the psychiatrist must refuse to cooperate.
- Informed consent is essential.

Lisbon Declaration, Portugal (1981)

The Declaration concerns the *rights of the patient.* Some relevant points are listed here:

- Right to the best medical care available and with no discrimination whatsoever.
- Every patient has the right to be treated by a doctor who is free to make clinical and ethical judgments, with no external interference.
- The patient has the right to continuity of health care.
- The patient has the right to freely choose and change doctor and hospital or other health care institution, public or private.
- The patient has the right to consult various doctors.
- The patient has the right to decide freely and to be informed about the possible consequences of this choice.
- An adult patient has the right to consent to or refuse any diagnostic or therapeutic procedure or to participate in clinical research.

- The patient is considered legally incompetent if s/he is a minor or otherwise legally incapable, or unconscious. In such cases, the consent of a legal representative is required.
- If an appointed representative is not available but medical intervention is urgent, the patient's consent can be assumed.
- Doctors must always do their utmost to save a patient's life after a suicide attempt.

Declaration of Venice, Italy (1983)

The Declaration reaffirms that the *doctor's duty is to heal*, where possible, to alleviate suffering and to protect the interests of their patients. There can be no exception to this principle even in the case of incurable or end-stage disease.

The patient's consent is always required; if they are unable to express their will, consent be sought from the family members.

The doctor must not prolong the agony of the dying, in response to their request (if the patient is conscious) or the request of his relatives.

A few relevant points:

- The WMA condemns both euthanasia and assisted suicide, deeming them immoral practices, even if they are requested by the patient himself or his relatives.
- When caring for a dying patient the physician's primary responsibility is to permit the patient a dignified death.
- Doctors should inform relatives of any possible adverse effects of palliative care.
- The patient's decision-making autonomy must be respected even in the terminal phase of life.
- The doctor must not use therapeutic means that bring no benefit

Declaration of St. Julians, Malta (1991)

The Declaration concerns a *hunger strike*.

Hunger strikes occur in various settings, but especially when people are detained (prisons, immigration centers, etc.). They are often a form of protest from people who have no other way of making their requests known.

- Doctors must try to prevent coercion or mistreatment of detainees and must disagree when it occurs.
- Doctors must respect the individual's autonomy. Forced feeding is unjustifiable but artificial feeding (i.v. drip) is ethically acceptable.
- Doctors must make objective evaluations and must not allow others to influence their judgment. They must not violate ethical principles, such as carrying out medical interventions for non-clinical reasons.

Stockholm Declaration, Sweden (1994)

The Declaration relates to the state of *disaster*.

The definition of a disaster in this document focuses on the medical aspects. A disaster is the sudden occurrence of an event, usually violent, with consequent heavy material damage and numerous victims. This causes an acute and unexpected imbalance in the skills and resources of the medical profession. The treatment of survivors must be in accordance with basic ethical principles and not influenced by other reasons.

- The physician should consider only the state of health and should ignore considerations based on any other criteria
- All survivors have the right to identical respect and the most appropriate treatment.
- The same ethical principles must be guaranteed by anyone involved, including other paramedics.

Ottawa Declaration, Canada (1998)

This Declaration *concerns child health*. It aims at improving the health care rights of children around the world.

Donations or financial donations are solicited to address this problem.

Tel Aviv Declaration, Israel (1999)

This is a universal appeal to *medical ethics and human rights*. In many nations—but not all—ethics and human rights are fully respected.

Medical ethics, based on a social contract stipulated between the health professions and human society, establishes a set of principles to adequately evaluate new treatments or new clinical interventions before their application. Failures of individual doctors to recognize their ethical obligations to patients and communities can damage their reputation.

- WMA requires medical schools to guarantee the teaching of research in the field of ethics and human rights.
- WMA hopes that medical ethics and human rights will be taught at all stages of postgraduate medical education.

Ferney-Voltaire Declaration, France (2001)

This Declaration *concerns placebo-controlled clinical trials*. The new guideline provides for the prudent use of a placebo in clinical research, with the warning that it should be employed only in cases where there is no proven therapy.

Washington Declaration, U.S.A. 2002

This statement is about *biological weapons*.

The growing threat of biological weapons that could be used to cause devastating epidemics internationally is recognized.

The release of organisms that cause smallpox, plague, anthrax, or other diseases produced by new microbial agents, could prove catastrophic. The WMA believes that medical associations and all those involved in health care must have a responsibility to condemn the research, development or use of such weapons as morally and ethically unacceptable.

- It is essential that doctors monitor the occurrence of cases or groups of unknown infectious diseases and contact specialists in the diagnosis of infectious diseases, promptly reporting cases to health authorities.
- Legally recognized bio-medical research must be promoted, and the work of unscrupulous scientists who have the evil aim of producing more dangerous biological weapons must be countered.
- The WMA and the associations of doctors and health professionals around the world must promote a rule that condemns the development, production or use of toxins and biological agents that have no justification for peaceful prophylactic, protective or other purposes.
- An international consortium, shared with the World Health Organization, the United Nations and other such bodies, must be established to monitor the threat of the use of biological weapons, to prevent their proliferation and to develop a coordinated plan to monitor the onset of infectious diseases.

Declaration of Divonne-les-Bains, France (2003)

This is a resolution of the WMA Council on the relationship between *law and ethics*.

Ethical values and legal principles are closely related. In some cases, the law requires unethical behavior. If a doctor has operated solely in accordance with legal provisions, he may not have respected the ethical principles he is expected to hold to in the exercise of the profession. In such cases, when the law conflicts with ethics, doctors must take steps to have the law changed.

Manual of Medical Ethics, U.S.A. (2005)

The *WMA Ethics Manual* was presented in January 2005; the second edition, dated 2009, was distributed to medical journals and schools around the world. The following translations are available: French, Spanish, Macedonian, Albanian, Chinese, Korean, Indonesian, German, Arabic, Turkish, Russian, Bulgarian, Japanese, Estonian, Georgian, Slovak, Lithuanian, Latvian, Persian, Ukrainian, Polish and Slovenian. A text in Italian has not yet been published.

In 2015, a third edition was issued, which is currently used by all medical associations and organizations worldwide as a reference and in-depth text.

Its contents are as follows:

Chapter One—Main features of medical ethics
Chapter Two—Doctors and patients
Chapter Three—Doctors and Society
Chapter Four—Doctors and Colleagues
Chapter Five—Medical Research
Chapter Six—Conclusions
Appendix A: Glossary
Appendix B: Medical Ethics Resources on the Internet
Appendix C: Inclusion of medical ethics and human rights in the curriculum of medical schools

> This manual can only provide a basic introduction to medical ethics and some of its central themes.
>
> It is intended to give an assessment of the need for continual reflection on the ethical dimension of medicine and in particular on how to deal with the ethical issues encountered in one's practice.

Resolution of Pilanesberg, South Africa (2006)

The proposed resolutions have clear ethical relevance:

- Professional accountability for *standards of medical care*
- HIV/AIDS and the medical profession
- Fight against HIV/AIDS
- Disease in the terminal phase
- Human organ donation and transplantation
- Ethical issues related to patients with mental illness
- Determination of death and organ recovery
- Therapeutic abortion
- Assisted reproduction techniques
- Animals in bio-medical research
- Medical ethics in case of disaster
- Abuse and neglect of minors
- Patient defense and confidentiality
- International Code of Medical Ethics
- Hunger strikes

Copenhagen Declaration, Denmark (2007)

This Declaration relates to ethics in *telemedicine*. Telemedicine is the practice of medicine for which diagnostic and therapeutic interventions, decisions, and recommendations are transmitted by computer. Telemedicine is particularly useful when a doctor cannot be physically present within a reasonable time. The doctor–patient relationship must therefore be based on mutual trust and respect.

Seoul Declaration, South Korea (2008)

The Seoul relates to *professional autonomy and clinical independence*. It affirms the following principles:

6. The central element of professional autonomy and clinical independence is the guarantee that individual doctors have the freedom to exercise their professional judgment in the care and treatment of their patients, without undue influence from external subjects or individuals.

General Assembly, Montevideo, Uruguay (2011)

Among the *various topics* discussed in Uruguay, and the subject of future statements, were:

- Independence of medical associations: No government should interfere with the independent functioning of national medical associations. Tobacco and child protection: It was stated at the meeting that about 700 million children breathe air polluted by tobacco smoke, especially in their homes. This has led to concerted action to protect them from the effects of smoking.
- Disaster preparedness: WMA must become a key communication channel for national medical associations in the event of a disaster.
- Doctors with double loyalties: development of a new reporting system for cases of doctors enslaved by governments, using torture. Doctors can be pressured into and have to violate their professional ethics.
- Leprosy: Doctors must fight the prejudice and discrimination against people suffering from this disease.
- Tuberculosis in prisons: The increase in its incidence in prisons and other places of detention must boost the vigilance of the medical facilities in charge, in order to avoid contagion and the spread of the disease.

General Assembly, Moscow, Russia (2015)

Among the *various topics* discussed were:

- Mobile Health: new regulations have been adopted to protect patients who use mobile health devices (pacemakers, wheelchairs, mobile phones, monitoring devices, etc.)
- Well-being of doctors: attention is needed to prevent and deal with stress and illness among doctors; the severity of their mental and physical illnesses must be reduced and the incidence of suicides reduced.

- Alcohol Statement: New legal measures have been proposed to combat the problem of alcohol-related harm, including strengthening health systems, raising the price, banning minors, marketing rules, and limiting use in industrial policies.
- Nuclear weapons: declaration of condemnation for the development, testing, production, storage, transfer, distribution, threat, and use of nuclear weapons.

All governments are required to work towards their reduction: there are currently more than 16,000 nuclear warheads in nine countries.

7. Street boys; Riot control agents
8. Medical schools and study curricula must always be focused on ethical dictates and human rights. Individual doctors can fail when they lack knowledge of ethical obligations, and this can harm patients and the community, or the reputation of doctors themselves.

General Assembly, Chicago, U.S.A. (2017)

The WMA recognizes the need to protect the *privacy* of the identifiable personal information it collects when the user uses the WMA site.

General Assembly, Harpa, Reykjavik, Iceland (2018)

The WMA, before the Icelandic General Assembly, initiated the "WMA *medical ethics conference*" summarizing the ethical issues faced over the years. The WMA has been working for the past 70 years on how to foster medical ethics as a physician's mission. Their findings indicate that ethical issues still need to be investigated further to improve the WMA overall assessment.

Adopted by the 70th WMA General Assembly, Tbilisi, Georgia (October 2019)

1. The WMA reiterates its strong commitment to the *principles of medical ethics* and stresses that the utmost respect for human life must be maintained. Therefore, the WMA is firmly opposed to euthanasia and physician-assisted suicide.
2. For the purpose of this Declaration, euthanasia is defined as a physician deliberately administering a lethal substance or carrying out an intervention to cause the death of a patient with decision-making capacity at the patient's own voluntary request. Physician-assisted suicide refers to cases in which, at the voluntary request of a patient with decision-making capacity, a physician deliberately enables a patient to end his or her own life by prescribing or providing medical substances intended to cause death.
3. No physician should be obliged to participate in euthanasia or assisted suicide, nor should any physician be obliged to make referral decisions to this end.

4. Separately, the physician who respects the patient's basic right to refuse medical treatment does not act unethically in forgoing or withholding unwanted care, even if respecting such a wish results in the death of the patient.

WMA General Assembly, Cordoba (Spain) (2020)

The *COVID-19 pandemic* meant we could not plan a hybrid (in-person/online) WMA Scientific Session on 23 October 2020. Jointly with our Spanish colleagues the WMA Executive Committee therefore decided to postpone the Scientific Session. The new date will be circulated later.

(October 26, 2021)

Globally, the numbers of weekly COVID-19 cases and deaths increased slightly during the past week, with over 2.9 million cases and over 49,000 new deaths, a 4% and 5% increase, respectively. With the exception of the European region, which continues for the fourth consecutive week to reported an increase in new COVID-19 cases (18% increase as compared with the previous week), other regions reported a decline. The largest decrease in new weekly cases was reported from the African Region (21%), followed by the Western Pacific Region (17%). The European and South-East Asia regions reported an increase in new weekly COVID-19 deaths, 14% and 13%, respectively, as compared with the previous week. The largest decline in new weekly deaths was reported from the Western Pacific region showing a 13% decrease as compared to the previous week. As of October 24, over 243 million confirmed cases and over 4.9 million deaths have been reported since the start of the pandemic. In this edition, three special focus updates are provided on:

- WHO COVID-19 global rapid risk assessment
- Age and sex distribution from WHO COVID-19 global surveillance
- SARS-CoV-2 Variants of Concern (VOCs) including an update on geographic prevalence and a focus on the Delta lineage AY.4.2 is also provided

World Health Organization (WHO)

The World Medical Association (WMA) is often confused with the World Health Organization (WHO). Both deal with international health problems, but the WHO is a United Nations agency funded by governments, which by their very nature are political in perspective: therefore the WHO is inevitably subject to political influence. The WMA, on the other hand, is funded by voluntary national medical associations.

"It is apolitical, embracing a wide range of members with a diversity of languages, cultures and healthcare systems, and all share the same ideals and respond to those who save their patients".[11]

[11] United Nations. Universal Declaration of Human Rights.

Doctor's duties

- *Practice the profession independently and maintain the highest standards of conduct*
- *Respect a patient's right, properly informing him/her they can accept or refuse treatment*
- *Do not allow your judgment to be influenced by personal gain or unfair discrimination*
- *Provide a competent service in full professional and moral independence, with compassion and respect for human dignity*
- *Behave honestly with patients and colleagues and report those who engage in fraud or deception to the appropriate authorities*
- *Do not derive any financial benefit or receive other incentives for prescribing specific products*
- *Respect patients' rights and preferences, as well as those of your colleagues and other healthcare professionals*
- *Recognize one's role towards the public; use due caution in disseminating discoveries, new techniques and treatments through non-professional channels*
- *Certify only what has been personally verified*
- *Utilize healthcare resources for patients' and the community's greatest benefit*
- *Seek adequate care and attention for mental or physical illnesses*
- *Comply with local and national ethics regulations*

WHO: Ethical Principles

The main goal at WHO is to build a better and healthier future for people around the world. Working in more than 150 countries, WHO Secretariat staff work side-by-side with governments and other partners to ensure the highest possible level of health for all people.

As a specialized agency of the United Nations, WHO is firmly committed to the following ethical principles:

- *Integrity*: behaving in accordance with ethical principles and acting in good faith, intellectual honesty and fairness.
- *Accountability*: Taking responsibility for one's actions, decisions and consequences.
- *Independence and impartiality*: behaving only in the interests of the WHO and ensuring that personal opinions and beliefs do not compromise the ethical principles, official duties or interests of the WHO.
- *Respect*: respecting the dignity, value, equality, diversity and privacy of all people.
- *Professional commitment*: a high level of professionalism and loyalty towards the Organization, its mandate and its objectives.

Offenses

These are situations that involve a significant risk for WHO, but are not limited only to:

- fraud
- corruption
- waste of resources
- sabotage
- substantial and specific danger to public health or safety
- sexual exploitation and abuse.

The WHO information policy is also rooted in the following approach:

- staff members are required to report irregularities;
- the Organization has a duty to protect whistleblowers from retaliation;
- the Organization has a duty to resolve a problem by adopting remedies and taking disciplinary action, as appropriate;
- retaliation, however, constitutes incorrect conduct.

Non-employee personnel are encouraged to report any suspected wrongdoing to WHO. The informant's identity is protected.

Exploitation and Prevention of Sexual Abuse

- WHO prohibits sexual exploitation and sexual abuse and considers such acts as serious conduct, which can constitute grounds for disciplinary sanctions, including summary dismissal and criminal prosecution.
- WHO prohibits any act of sexual abuse or sexual violence and prohibits the exchange of money, work, goods, assistance or services for sex, including sexual favors or other forms of humiliating, degrading or exploitative behavior towards beneficiary populations in countries that are members of the WHO.
- WHO strictly prohibits sexual activity with children.
- Staff have a duty not only to refrain from sexual relations with the people who receive their services, but also to report any cases in which signs of sexual exploitation and abuse may be suspected or detected.

Responsible Search Code of Conduct

Research in the WHO is a fundamental tool for the progress and achievement of health and the Organization is committed to respecting the highest standards of scientific quality and ethical integrity.

The Code of Ethics of Professional Conduct is applicable to all staff members involved in research, as well as to WHO collaborators.

The responsibility of the WHO is:

- to ensure that partner institutions have codes of conduct that uphold the principles in line with the WHO code;
- to seek advice and assistance, as appropriate, from the normal channels, the Office of Compliance, Risk Management and Ethics (CRE), the Ethics Review Committee (ERC) and the Office of the Legal Adviser (LEG), where applicable;
- to report any suspicion of non-adherence to the Code to the supervisors for action or the integrity hotline, where applicable;
- to take action to address suspected wrongdoing, including collaborators and partner institutions: for example, terminating contractual commitments or withdrawing from publication projects.

Conflicts of Interest

A conflict of interest arises when a secondary interest interferes with the primary interest of the WHO and its staff. The scope of the conflict of interest goes beyond financial interest.

Statements for Staff

WHO has strict ethical principles of integrity, independence, and impartiality. WHO staff members are required to disclose on an annual basis any interests that may conflict with their duties as international civil servants.

Declarations for Experts

Each year WHO scientists and other technical experts contribute to the solution of global health-related problems by participating in expert committees, advisory groups, conferences, study, and scientific groups and other activities.

To be effective, the work of the WHO and the contributions of its experts must be objective and independent, in reality, not only apparently.

References

Bird LP. Medical ethics. In: Bird LP, Barlow J, editors. Oaths & prayers, an anthology. Richardson: Christian Medical & Dental Society; 1989.

Guraya SY. Ethics in medical research. J Microsc Ultrastruct. 2014;2(3):121–6.

Loewy EH. Oaths for physicians – necessary protection or elaborate hoax? MedGenMed. 2007;9(1):7.

Millum J, Wendler D, Emanuel EJ. The 50th anniversary of the Declaration of Helsinki: progress but many remaining challenges. JAMA. 2013;310(20):2143–4.

Ndebele P. The Declaration of Helsinki, 50 years later. JAMA. 2013;310(20):2145–6.

World Medical Association. International Code of Medical Ethics. World Med Assoc Bull. 1949–2006;1(3):109–11.

World Medical Association. Dichiarazione di Helsinki della World Medical Association. Principi etici per la ricerca biomedica che coinvolge gli esseri umani. [IT. Ethical principles for biomedical research in humans]. Evidence. 2013;5(10):1–5.

14 The Catholic Doctor's Prayers: Vatican City

Historical Background

Every form of ethical declaration implies a moral imperative, both by the individual and by an entire organization, by a religious community or by a government body.

Many Christian physicians' prayers have existed since ancient times, and the most modern sometimes reflect more heterogeneous and multifaceted perspectives.

In the ancient world, doctors often expressed their ethical commitments in the form of oaths, which were an integral part of their initiation ceremony. Like many medical "prayers," ancient oaths reflected the belief that success in the healing profession required an alliance with divinity for the effective treatment of disease. Ancient oaths often asked the deity to inspire physicians to fulfill their moral obligations and those who honored their sacred trust were rewarded and those who violated it were punished.

A series of medical oaths have already been indicated and set out in detail in this book. Certainly, further clarifications and changes will be made; we cannot imagine what the changes will be, but most likely they will be based on cultural, ethnic and perhaps social grounds. Many other factors will probably be involved and it is inappropriate to limit them to our current knowledge. Some of the changes already appear and will also be discussed in later chapters.

> Future success in using codes to control medical practice may depend heavily on ethical norms in society.[1]

Prayers can be assimilated to real oaths, as they attest to an end and certify one's devotion to that end.

[1] Angelo (2009).

R. G. Russo, *Medical Ethics*, https://doi.org/10.1007/978-3-031-42444-1_14

1. The promise (or even the purpose) is a commitment to behave in a certain way that we will follow, with God.
2. The vow, on the other hand, is made not only to strengthen the commitment, but also to transform action or life into an act of praise for the Lord. The essence of the vow consists in transforming the person's actions or even whole life, by dedicating it exclusively to the greater glory of God, to his worship. The vow undoubtedly has greater weight than the promise and it is therefore logical to take a vow when you know that you can be faithful to it.
3. The oath is different from the vow: it is a call to God to witness what one says or promises to do.[2] St. John Paul II, in his long pontificate, also had the opportunity to write a prayer for doctors.

José Maria Simón Castellví (President of the International Federation of Catholic Medical Associations) recalled this on June 29, 2000 and then again on January 22, 2011 in the Vatican newspaper *Osservatore Romano.* This "ethical press review" came as a surprise, as the Hippocratic oath was also mentioned, defined as "A document known not only in the field of medicine and which, in some universities, is solemnly read when the degree is awarded."

This suggestion—almost a warning—was circulated throughout the Catholic world and had immediate weight, as evidenced by the almost immediate translation into all languages and diffusion on all continents.

In practice, the act of prayer unites many faiths and beliefs even very distant from each other. From the earliest times, religious formulas have made the contract placed under divine protection "valid, inviolable and sacred".[3]

The prayer reported on June 26, 2000 is repeated in other similar invocations, in the Christian-Catholic tradition.

The Doctor's Prayer (Saint John Paul II)

Lord Jesus, Divine Physician,

who in your earthly life have favored those who suffer and have entrusted the ministry of healing to your disciples, make us always ready to alleviate the pains of our brothers. Make each of us, aware of the great mission entrusted to us, strive to be always, in your daily service, an instrument of your merciful love.

Enlighten our minds, guide our hands, make our hearts attentive and compassionate. Grant that in every patient we see the features of Your divine Face.

You, who are the Way, grant us the ability to imitate you every day as doctors not only of the body but of the whole person, helping those who are sick to walk their earthly path with confidence, up to the moment of Meeting You.

[2] Monteleone (2004).

[3] Medical Codes and Oaths: I. History, II. Ethical Analysis. Encyclopedia of Bioethics. Encyclopedia.com. 17-18/9/2017 http://www.encyclopedia.com.

You, who are the Truth, give us wisdom and science, to penetrate the mystery of man and his transcendent destiny, while we approach You to discover the causes of evil and find the appropriate remedies.

You, who are Life, grant us to proclaim and bear witness to the "Gospel of life" in our profession, committing ourselves always to defend life, from conception to its natural end, and to respect the dignity of every human being, especially the weakest and most needy.

Make us, O Lord, good Samaritans, ready to welcome, care for and console those we meet in our work.

Following the example of the Sainted Doctors who preceded us, help us make a generous contribution to constantly update and renew the tools for health care.

Bless our studies and our profession, enlighten our research and our teaching.

Finally, grant us that, having constantly loved and served You through our suffering brothers, at the end of our earthly pilgrimage we may contemplate Your Glorious Face and experience the joy of encountering You, in Your Kingdom of infinite Joy and Peace. Amen

Another Doctor's Prayer

Lord, let my mind always be clear and enlightened at the patient's bed, let no extraneous thoughts distract me.

May erudition and experience always guide me and ensure I always work serenely. Because great and noble is this scientific knowledge, aimed at maintaining the health and life of Your creatures.

Remove from me the idea that I can know everything.

Give me the strength, the desire, and the opportunity to constantly expand my knowledge. Today I can discover things that yesterday I would not even have suspected because this art is great and the human mind never tires of learning. It ensures that in the patient he sees only the man. You, O Generous, have chosen me to watch over the life and death of Your creatures.

Now I am preparing for my visit. Stay close to me in this arduous task, so it can turn out well. Because without your help, man cannot even manage small things.

The Sick Person's Prayer

O Lord, sickness knocked on the door of my life, uprooted me from my work and transplanted me to another world, the world of the sick. A tough experience, O Lord, a reality it is hard to accept.

Yet Lord, I thank you for what I have learned and am learning from this disease; I have touched the frailty and precariousness of life firsthand, I have freed myself from many illusions.

Now I look at everything with different eyes: what I have and what I am does not belong to me, it is your gift; I have discovered what it means: "to depend," needing everything and everyone, not being able to do anything alone: I felt loneliness, anguish, loss, but also affection, love, and the friendship of many people.

Lord Jesus, even if I find it difficult, I will say: Your will be done!

I offer you my sufferings and unite them with yours.

Help the doctors, nurses, relatives, friends, and all those who, day and night, sacrifice themselves for me.

Give each one a big, patient, generous heart.

Support me in my sufferings, give me confidence, patience, courage, and if it is what you want, give healing to me and to others.

More Prayers from the Doctor

1. My God, fill my soul with love for my art and for all creatures.

   Do not let the thirst for gain and the pursuit of glory influence the practice of my art, distancing me from the noble duty of doing good to all creatures.

   Grant that in him who suffers I see nothing but a man.

   Make my mind clear at the sick bed, so I can remember what the intellect and science have taught me.

   Grant, O Lord, that my patients have faith in me and in my art. Make them follow my prescriptions and my advice. Remove from their bed the charlatans, the crowds of relatives always generous with advice and the wives who believe they know everything about everything, since they are dangerous people who often manage, with their vanity and presumption, to make even the best treatments fail, and often lead the patient to death. If the ignorant criticize me and make fun of me, let the love for my art be stronger than their ridicule so that I can persevere in justice regardless of the prestige, research, and age of my enemies.
2. Grant me, O Lord, indulgence and patience in the face of the stubborn and annoying sick. Let me be moderate in everything, but may my love for science be insatiable. Remove from my heart the presumption that there is nothing I do not know. Grant me the strength, the will and the opportunities to increase my knowledge.

   Grant that in every moment I acknowledge the presence of things whose existence I did not even suspect, because our art is vast and the human spirit never ceases to travel the path of knowledge.
3. Lord Jesus, Divine Doctor, who in your earthly life showed care for those who suffer, and have entrusted the ministry of healing to your disciples, make us always ready to alleviate the pains of our brothers. Let each of us, aware of the great mission entrusted to us, strive, in our daily service, to be always an instrument of your merciful love. Enlighten our minds, guide our hands, make our hearts attentive and compassionate. Grant that in every patient we see the features of Your divine Face.

   You who are the Way, grant us to know how to imitate you every day as doctors not only of the body but of the whole person, helping those who are sick to walk their earthly path with confidence, up to the moment of meeting you.

4. You who are the Truth, give us wisdom and science, to penetrate into the mystery of man and his transcendent destiny, while we seek to discover the causes of evil and to find the appropriate remedies.

   You who are Life, grant us to proclaim and bear witness to the "Gospel of life" in our profession, committing ourselves to always defend it, from its conception to its natural end, and to respect the dignity of every human being, especially the weakest and most needy.

   Make us, O Lord, good Samaritans, ready to welcome, care for and console those we meet in our work.

   Following the example of the medical saints who preceded us, help us to make our generous contributions to constantly renewing the tools for health care.

   Bless our study and our profession, enlighten our research and our teaching. Finally, grant us that, having constantly loved and served you through our suffering brothers, at the end of our earthly pilgrimage we can contemplate your glorious face and experience the joy of meeting you, in your kingdom of infinite joy and peace. Amen

Previously, Pope Pius XII, on May 10, 1957, had delivered another prayer, formerly known as the "Doctor's Prayer."

O Divine Physician of souls and bodies, Redeemer Jesus, who during your mortal life favored the sick, healing them with the touch of your almighty hand, we, called to the arduous mission of doctors, adore you and recognize our sublime in you—model and support. May our minds, hearts and hands always be guided by you so as to earn the praise and honor that the Holy Spirit ascribes to our office (cf. Ecclesiastes,. 38).

Increase in us the awareness of being your collaborators in some way in the defense and development of human creatures, and instruments of your mercy.

Enlighten our intelligences in the bitter test against the innumerable infirmities of the bodies, so that, by rightly availing ourselves of science and its progress, the causes of evils are not hidden from us, nor do their symptoms mislead us, but with sure judgment we can indicate the remedies offered by your Providence.

Expand our hearts with your love, so that, recognizing You Yourself in the sick, particularly in the most desperate, we respond with tireless solicitude to the trust they place in us.

Make us, imitating your example, paternal in compassion, sincere in advising, diligent in curing, alien to deceiving, gentle in heralding the mystery of pain and death; above all that we be firm in defending your holy law of respect for life, against all assaults of selfishness and perverse instincts.

As doctors who take pride in your name, we promise that our work will move constantly in observance of moral order and its laws. Finally, grant that we ourselves, for Christian conduct of life and the correct exercise of the profession, deserve one day to hear from your lips the beatifying sentence, promised to those who visited You, sick in brothers: "Come, you blessed of the Father mine, take possession of the kingdom prepared for you" (Matthew 25, 34). So be it!

Ethical Analysis and Conclusion

Codes, oaths, and prayers of medical ethics have come to light over the centuries from different sources, at different times, from disparate societies, organizations, and perspectives. An ethical analysis of the codes of Medical Ethics indicates that they were not really developed, and were only basic theories of medical ethics. Codes—at least modern ones—are the product of many discussions, debates, and revisions.

Codes, oaths, and prayers come from various contexts, representing different professional groups, public and private agencies, lay organizations such as churches and patient groups. Not surprisingly, radically different ethical conclusions have been reached, based on fundamentally different roots and various methods of ethical reasoning.[4] From the expressions used, like any other formulation or, more properly, "prayer," the ground shared with ethical provisions is evident and, having to do with medical activity, is described adequately as "Medical Ethics."

Several developments within the Catholic Church have affected the ecclesial mission of health care. These include significant changes in religious orders and congregations, in the growing involvement of lay people and women, a greater awareness of the social role of the Church in the world, and of developments in moral theology since Vatican Council II.[5]

One contemporary understanding of the Catholic health ministry has taken account of the new challenges presented by transitions both in the Church and in the societies involved. The dialogue between medical science and the Christian faith has, for its primary purpose, the common good of all humans. It assumes that science and faith do not contradict each other. Both are founded in respect for truth and freedom. As new knowledge and technologies expand, each person must build their correct conscience based on moral norms for proper health care.[6] There are constant changes in clinical practice due to technological advances. The health system is under discussion in relation to both institutional and social factors.

Over the centuries many new principles have emerged and express the medical and moral teachings of the Church. These principles, often referred to as "directives," may provide the correct rationale and the direction for the revision of ethical and religious guidelines. The purpose of these ethical and religious directives is twofold, first: to reaffirm ethical standards of behavior in health care, and second, to provide authoritative Catholic guidance in relation to certain moral issues relating to health today. They involve sponsors, trustees, administrators, chaplains, doctors, health personnel and patients or residents of these institutions and services. Since they express the moral teaching of the Church, these Directives will be useful to Catholic professionals engaged in health services in related areas. The Directives

[4] May (2000), p. 116.

[5] Vatican Council II comprised four sessions from 1962 to 1965, under the pontificates of St. John XXIII and Paul VI.

[6] Sritharan et al. (2001). USCCB States Conference of Catholic Bishops, Ethical and Religious Directives for Catholic Health Care Services, Fifth Edition: 1-43, Copyright © 2009.

have been refined through extensive consultation with bishops, theologians, sponsors, administrators, doctors, and other health professionals. Furthermore, they will be periodically reviewed, in order to deal with new knowledge from theological and medical research or the new needs of the Church's public policy.[6]

Religion and Medical Ethics

A few religions have shared the dictates of medicine and some prayers attest to this. The prayers used by the Roman Catholic religion, reported here, are not the only evidence. Perhaps some curious readers, familiar with other cultural and religious traditions, will be able to offer very valuable comments on this subject and enrich this information. At the time of writing we can provide the following information.[7]

Religious traditions of medical ethics tend to differ from more secular approaches by emphasizing limitations to autonomous decision-making, evaluating the experience of suffering more positively, and tapping into beliefs and values that go beyond empirical verification.[7] The impact of the world's great religious traditions seems related to four major issues: (1) religious conscience in dealing with medical treatments; (2) end-of life decisions, including euthanasia, physician-assisted suicide, and withholding life-sustaining treatments; (3) the definitions of moral personhood (defining life's beginning and end); and (4) human sexuality.

The reality is that there are also differences within the single religions, let alone among different ones. For example, the Islamic approach differs regarding the suspension of life support such as nutrition, artificial hydration or the interruption of life-sustaining treatments. In conclusion, within a single belief there are numerous approaches and individual interpretations.

Of fundamental importance is the morality of an intervention and the age-old principle of non-maleficence, that is, to cause no harm.

"*Doctors should listen to patients' religious views and opinions with an open mind and treat them with the utmost seriousness.*" Despite this, "*a doctor should not proceed with a treatment, the request for which is based on a profession of faith of the client, which harms or does not bring any benefit to the patient himself.*"

Religion may be profoundly important to some people but it cannot oblige doctors to violate their own fundamental ethical values. In the event of disagreement, a "spiritual care professional," such as a priest or an imam, with greater knowledge of the patient's faith, can help resolve any tensions and reduce the "spiritual distress."

Moreover, a Few Comments

The values of secular medicine and those of religion, two important factors relating to human suffering, are occasionally destined to intersect, with evident repercussions on medical ethics. The findings of such tensions can shape patient values and

[7] Green (2013), Sokol (2020), Virtual Mentor (2009) and Post (2009).

treatment decisions in ways that doctors may not fully grasp. Likewise, the beliefs of the "caregiver" can come into conflict with the obligations of the profession, as is sometimes seen in the exercise of conscientious objection and/or in particular medical services. Comparisons and clashes between religion and medicine suggest how health professionals can effectively respond.

> *Fields once closely tied to religion, such as government, philosophy, and education, have sought nonsectarian grounding that opens them to members of any religious community or even none at all. Medicine and medical ethics have likewise sought to separate themselves from confessional stances. At the same time, medical ethics has demanded a respect for patients' religious and spiritual beliefs.*[8]

Clinical decisions ideally bring together the physician's expertise and the patient's values to arrive at a treatment that maximally benefits the patient. Religion and spirituality often shape a patient's values in ways that sometimes may even run counter to what physicians might consider best in that case.

Today, this conflict frequently arises with regard to health care, for instance, contraception, abortion, and fertility therapies. In the current debate the issue is usually framed as a clash between an individual caregiver's right to refuse to provide services of this kind on religious grounds and the profession's larger secular commitment to make these services accessible to all.

From the dawn of civilization spirituality and religion have defined human experience. It is from religious worship, beliefs, rituals, and practices that cultures emerge and that the great majority of lives are still shaped in most parts of the world, especially in times of severe illness or catastrophe when people tend to pose deep questions about their lives. These big questions do not go away: is there a purpose to life? Is there hope for humanity? Do love and compassion go with or against the grain of the universe? Is there a higher power and can our lives be lived in accordance with it? Are we morally accountable to it?

> *Modern times are as defined by spirituality and religion as any other in history, perhaps more so insofar as technological innovations force us to ask questions about our growing capacities to modify the essential nature of humans and to bring our species to an end through massive violence and ecological perils. We all know that religions can bring out the very best in people and the very worst too, like corporations, politics, and even the profession of medicine itself.*[7]

[8] Shinall (2009).

References

Angelo P. Distinzione tra promessa fatta a Dio, voto e giuramento. (IT. Distinction between a promise made to God, a vow, and a sworn oath). Amici Domenicani, Pub; 12 May 2009.

Green RM. Religion and medical ethics. In: Handbook of clinical neurology, vol. 118. Elsevier; 2013. p. 79–89.

May WF. Code, covenant, contract or philanthropy. In: Veatch RM, editor. Cross cultural perspectives in medical ethics. 2nd ed. Boston/Toronto/London/Singapore: Jones and Bartlett Pub; 2000.

Monteleone M. Preghiere e formule religiose. La civiltà romana - Mito e religione. (IT. Prayers and religious formulas. The Roman civilization – myth and religion). Oilproject; 2004.

Post SG. The perennial collaboration of medicine and religion, www.virtualmentor.org. J Ethics. 2009;11:807–10.

Shinall MC Jr. The separation of Church and Medicine. Virtual Mentor. 2009;11(10):747–9.

Sokol D. Religion and spirituality in medicine: friend or foe? BMJ. 2020;368:m106.

Sritharan K, Russell G, et al. Medical oaths and declarations. BMJ. 2001;323(7327):1440–1.

Virtual Mentor. American Medical Association. Religion, patients, and medical ethics. J Ethics. 2009;11(10):745–828.

Ethics in the Twentieth and Twenty-First Centuries

15

This chapter deals with some statements and guidelines in the field of clinical research and medical ethics. In particular, the following:

(a) Belmont Report, 1979.
(b) Nuffield Council on Bioethics, 1991
(c) CIOMS, 1993
(d) Good Clinical Practice, 1997
(e) Italy

Belmont Report (U.S.A.)

Historical Notes

On 12 July 1974 the National Research Act was signed in the USA, establishing the National Commission for the Protection of Human Subjects of Biomedical and Behavioral Research. One of the Commission's main tasks was to identify the fundamental ethical principles of biomedical and behavioral research relating to human subjects and to develop guidelines to ensure that such research is conducted in accordance with those principles.

The Belmont report, drawn up by the United States Department of Health and Human Services, addressed this and summarized the fundamental ethical principles.[1] The Report concerns "ethical principles and guidelines for the protection of subjects in research." Dated 18 April 1979, it owes its name to the Belmont

[1] Office of the Secretary (1979), Department of Health, Education, and Welfare; National Commission for the Protection of Human Subjects of Biomedical and Behavioral Research (2014) and The Belmont Report; The National Commission for the Protection of Human Subjects of Biomedical and Behavioral Research (1979).

R. G. Russo, *Medical Ethics*, https://doi.org/10.1007/978-3-031-42444-1_15

Conference Center, formerly part of the Smithsonian Institution, in Elkridge, Maryland and now part of Howard Community College.

It is subtitled "Ethical Principles and Guidelines for the Protection of Human Subjects of Research" and was produced, in two volumes, by The National Commission for the Protection of Human Subjects of Biomedical and Behavioral Research, according to the conclusions set out in discussions in 1976, 1977, and 1978. The final report was drawn up in 1978, then published in the U.S. Federal Register. The report discussed ethical principles and guidelines for the protection of clinical research subjects.

The summary contains all major assumptions:

"In carrying out the above, the Commission was directed to consider:

1. the boundaries between biomedical and behavioral research and the accepted and routine practice of medicine,
2. the role of assessment of risk-benefit criteria in the determination of the appropriateness of research involving human subjects,
3. appropriate guidelines for the selection of human subjects for participation in such research,
4. the nature and definition of informed consent in various research settings".[1]

Moreover, the Belmont Report does not make specific recommendations for administrative action by the Secretary of Health, Education, and Welfare. Rather, the Commission recommended that the Belmont Report is considered part of the Department's policy.

The following are the **Basic Ethical Principles: Three basic principles among those generally accepted in our culture are particularly relevant.**

1. **Respect for Persons.** "Individuals must be treated as autonomous agents and anyone with diminished autonomy is entitled to protection." Research participants voluntarily agree to participate and obtain enough information to make that decision. Individuals who lack this ability, in whole or in part, are considered vulnerable because they may not have the maturity or the ability to make an informed decision.
2. **Beneficence.** "Do no harm" is a Hippocratic principle of medical ethics but it is not enough, even if its extension to research implies that "One must not injure a person regardless of the potential advantages that towards others." The Hippocratic Oath also requires that doctors benefit patients "according to their best judgment."
3. **Justice** (equal distribution of the benefits and burdens associated with research).[2] The current use of informed consent and many other clinical trial practices respect some of the ethical principles illustrated in the Belmont report.

[2] Lantos and Spertus (2014), Scialpi (2015) and Wood (2009).

Ethical Principles and Guidelines for Research Involving Human Subjects

The term "research" means any activity that aims to test a hypothesis, draw conclusions, and then develop or contribute to knowledge. The Report aims to minimize therapeutic misunderstandings, when the purpose of clinical research is dealing with rather than acquiring knowledge.

The purpose of "practice" is to provide diagnoses, treatments, and preventive strategies for particular individuals. Risks and benefits are related to the probability/possibility of harming the persons. The study must not be influenced by social, racial, sexual, and cultural prejudices and the consent process must stress three fundamental elements: Information, Understanding, and Voluntariness.

Applications

1. Informed consent

   Voluntary participants in research, to the extent that they are capable, must be given the opportunity to agree on what will or will not happen to them.

   The consent process must include three elements:
   - Information,
   - Understanding,
   - Voluntary agreement to participation.
2. Assessment of Risks and Benefits:

   The nature and extent of the risks and benefits must be systematically assessed.

   The term "risk" refers to the possibility of harm. There are many types of risk, such as psychological, physical, legal, social, and economic. The term "benefit" in the context of research refers to something positive relating to health or well-being. The risks and rewards affect not only individual participants but also their families and society at large.
3. Selection of participants:

   This must be done fairly, in terms of procedures and results.

   The principle of justice ensures that the benefits and risks of research are fairly distributed. Special classes of injustice arise when participants are drawn from vulnerable populations, such as institutionalized or incarcerated people, particular racial groups, economically disadvantaged or very ill minorities.

Nuffield Council on Bioethics (London)

> We support, enable, and encourage people to improve their health to help them make the most of life.

The Nuffield Foundation examines and explores ethical questions arising from recent scientific advances in medical and biological research. It was founded in 1943 by William Morris, Lord Nuffield, the founder of Morris Motors; by 1990–1991 it enjoyed an excellent international reputation as an independent consultancy body.[3]

Here are some notes from the general outline from the Nuffield Council on Bioethics Strategic Plan 2012–2016 to illustrate its vast and widely-divided structure. Since 1994 the Council has been fully funded by the Nuffield Foundation, the Medical Research Council, and the Wellcome Trust.

The Board selects the topics which will then be studied in depth. Its members meet four to six times a year to decide on the Foundation's fields of intervention, listed below in alphabetical order:

Abortion, Resource Allocation, Personalized Health Care, Autism, Relationship Autonomy, Children, Biofuels, Bioinformation, Biotechnology and their Globalization, Stem Cells, Genetically Modified Cell Cultures, Culture of Scientific Research, Neonatal Medicine, Beauty Care, Biological Data and Health, Dementia, Dignity, Mental Disorders, Mitochondrial DNA Disorders, Health Inequalities, DNA and Patents, Organ Donation, Ethics of Health Care in Developing Countries, Pharmacogenetics, End of Life and Euthanasia, Genetics and Behavior, Genome, Neurotechnology, Privacy, Clinical Research in Children, Research with Human Subjects, Research in Developing Countries, Research on Embryos, Assisted Reproduction and Therapeutic Cloning, Genetic Resources and Their Equal Sharing (Nagoya Protocol), Genetic Screening, Prenatal Screening, Solidarity, Suppression of the supernumerary chromosome in Down's syndrome, Technologies in health and social care, Innovative therapies, Genetic tests and screening, Use of animals in research, Use of human tissues, Xenografts.

Once the Board has identified the main ethical issues, an expert meeting is convened, consisting of an independent chairman and 7–14 members, designated by the Board, to review the issue and report. Their aims are as follows:

- to identify and define ethical issues arising from recent advances in biological and medical research to anticipate or respond to public concerns;
- to examine and report these issues in a way that promotes public understanding and discussion;
- to publish such data in an appropriate manner, according to the Board's opinion.

The Nuffield Foundation is aware that researchers, sponsors, and all those involved in health care research are faced with different and sometimes conflicting guidelines, and works to present an ethical framework that serves as an international indicator.

[3] Nuffield Foundation https://it.wikipedia.org/wiki/Nuffield_Foundation.
http://www.nuffieldfoundation.org, http://www.efc.be/organisation/thenuffieldfoundation// it.wikipedia.org/wiki/Council_forinternational_Organizations_of_Medical_Sciences.

Nuffield and Medical Ethics

In addition to exploring ethical issues in biology and medicine that can crop up especially in daily work, the Nuffield Council has investigated non-invasive prenatal tests, genomic tests, cosmetic procedures, and time limits for the maintenance of human embryos in ethical research, and is specifically active in evaluation of the use of animals for testing new medicines.

Activities for Ethical Issues in Medicine

The activities of the Nuffield Council for Bioethics give a good introduction to the use of animals in different types of research and to the three "Rs": Refinement, Reduction and Replacement.

The Ethics of Animals

Some experiments actually cause suffering. Is it ethically acceptable to use animals to test new drugs for safety and efficacy?

CIOMS (Switzerland)

Historical Notes

The Council for International Organizations of Medical Sciences (CIOMS) is an international non-governmental organization that has official relations with the World Health Organization (WHO). The CIOMS[4] was founded in 1949 and is based in Geneva. Its mandates include the maintenance of collaborative relationships with the United Nations and its specialized agencies. In 2013, CIOMS counted 49 international and other organizations, representing many biomedical disciplines, national academies of science and medical research councils.

The first version of the CIOMS guidelines (1982) focused on ethics in biomedical research. Since then the Council has been involved in drafting guidelines, setting out ethical principles, with detailed comments, and how to apply them.

The second version of the CIOMS guidelines (1993) saw the explosion of the HIV/AIDS pandemic and proposals for prevention and treatment. These developments raised new ethical questions never previously considered and spurred the preparation of international guidelines for ethical review of epidemiological studies and biomedical research related to human subjects.

The third version of the CIOMS guidelines was completed in 2002.

[4] CIOMS books https://www.thriftbooks.com/a/cioms/690670/.

In the fourth version, dated 2016, the working group decided to expand the 2002 guidelines from "biomedical research" to "health research." CIOMS answers a number of pressing questions in research ethics. The Council stresses the need for research of scientific and social value, providing specific guidelines for health even in low-income sectors, specifying the conditions and methods for involving vulnerable groups and describing under what conditions biological samples and data relating to health can be used for research.

In following versions, published almost yearly, CIOMS hopes to ensure that ethical guidelines remain as a self-renewing document to address the challenges of modern research. They are considered the reference point for the biomedical scientific community in the world.

Main Objectives

- To facilitate and promote international activities in the field of biomedical sciences
- To maintain collaborative relationships with the United Nations and its specialized agencies and serve the scientific interests of the biomedical community

To achieve its objectives, CIOMS has initiated and coordinates the following main long-term programs:

- Bioethics
- Ethics
- Health policy
- Drug development and use
- International Nomenclature of Diseases.

CIOMS also does a variety of work in the health and pharmaceutical sectors, including:

- Studies of the physiological, biochemical, and pathological processes in response to a specific intervention, in healthy or sick subjects;
- Diagnostic, preventive or therapeutic measures in the population, taking account of individual biological variability;
- Studies on human behavior in different circumstances and environments.

Since 1999 the "CIOMS Form 1" has been used all over the world for the exchange of information, mainly based on pharmacovigilance, between the authorities, ministries, and pharmaceutical companies. CIOMS texts are employed as operational guides in many sectors of biomedical research and drug safety.[5]

[5] GCP https://it.wikipedia.org/wiki/Buona_pratica_clinica. Guidelines For Good Clinical Practice, 10 June 1996.

Ethics in CIOMS

In Geneva, in 2016, the International Ethical Guidelines for Health-related Research Involving Humans was prepared by the Council for International Organizations of Medical Sciences (CIOMS) in collaboration with the World Health Organization (WHO).[5] The guidelines are protected by Copyright© 2016.

The fourth version of the CIOMS Guidelines (2016). During its annual meeting in 2009 the Executive Committee of CIOMS considered the desirability of a revision of the CIOMS Ethical Guidelines for Biomedical Research. Since 2002 several developments had taken place including: heightened emphasis on the importance of translational research, a need to clarify what counts as fair research in low-resource settings, more emphasis on community engagement in research, the awareness that exclusion of potentially vulnerable groups in many cases has resulted in a poor evidence base, and the increase of big data research.

Moreover, the Declaration of Helsinki of 2008 was revised again at that same time.

The Executive Committee therefore first explored the need for revision. The titles of the Guidelines are:

1. Scientific and social value and respect for rights
2. Research conducted in low-resource settings
3. Equitable distribution of benefits and burdens in the selection of individual and groups of participants in research
4. Potential individual benefits and risks of research
5. Selecting controls in clinical trials
6. Caring for participants' health needs
7. Community engagement
8. Collaborative partnership and capacity-building for research and research review
9. Individuals capable of giving informed consent
10. Modifications and waivers of informed consent
11. Collection, storage, and use of biological materials and related data
12. Collection, storage, and use of data in health-related research
13. Reimbursement and compensation for research participants
14. Treatment and compensation for research-related harms
15. Research involving vulnerable persons and groups
16. Research involving adults incapable of giving informed consent
17. Research involving children and adolescents
18. Women as participants
19. Pregnant and breastfeeding women as participants
20. Research disasters and disease outbreaks
21. Clusters of randomized trials
22. Use of data obtained from online environments and digital tools in health-related research
23. Requirements for establishing research ethics committees and for their review of protocols

24. Public accountability for health-related research
25. Conflicts of interest

    APPENDIX 1 Items to be included in a protocol (or associated documents) for health-related research involving humans

    APPENDIX 2 Obtaining informed consent: essential information for prospective research participants

    APPENDIX 3 CIOMS working group for revision of the 2002 international guidelines for biomedical research involving humans

Fundamental Ethical Principles

All research involving human subjects must be conducted in compliance with three fundamental ethical principles:

1. Respect for people: a) respect for personal autonomy; b) protection against harm or abuse of persons with reduced autonomy (vulnerable people).
2. Charity: moral obligation to maximize benefits and minimize harm, prohibiting intentional harm to people: this is equivalent to "non-maleficence" (do no harm).
3. Justice: moral obligation to treat every person in accordance with what is morally right; fair distribution of burdens and benefits.

Research involving human subjects includes:

- Studies of a physiological, biochemical or pathological process or the response to a specific physical, chemical or psychological intervention;
- Verifying diagnostic, preventive or therapeutic measures, taking account of individual biological variability;
- Studies to determine the consequences of specific preventive and therapeutic measures;
- Behavioral studies related to human health in different circumstances and environments.

Paragraph 32 of the Declaration of Helsinki reads: "For medical research using identifiable human material or data, such as research on material or data contained in biobanks or similar repositories, physicians must seek informed consent for its collection, storage and/or reuse. There may be exceptional situations where consent would be impossible or impracticable to obtain for such research. In such situations the research may be done only after consideration and approval by a research ethics committee."

A Few Extracts from the CIOMS Guidelines

Clinical Trials Must Be Preceded by Laboratory or Animal Testing

1. Ethical justification and scientific validity of biomedical research involving human beings; prospects for discovery of new ways to benefit people's health.

......

3. Ethical review of sponsored research. Ethical and scientific examination: there must be a guarantee of independence and the absence of conflict of interest.
4. Individual informed consent. For any biomedical research involving humans, the researcher must obtain voluntary informed consent in a language that suits the individual's level of understanding, or else the permission of a legal guardian. The consent requirement, in whole or in part, may be waived when the research project involves no more than a minimum risk.
5. Essential information for informed consent: The investigator must inform the subject as follows:
   (a) participation in the research/study is voluntary
   (b) the subject is free to refuse, with no penalty or loss of benefits;
   (c) an explanation must be given of how research differs from routine medical care;
   (d) for controlled clinical trials: example(s) of randomization, double-blinding;
   (e) at the end of the study information will be given on the results in general;
   (f) subjects have the right to access their data on request;
   (g) the foreseeable risks, pain or discomfort or other inconvenience to the individual associated with participation must be illustrated, including any risks to the health or well-being of the spouse or partner;

   ....

   (n) respect for the subjects' privacy and confidentiality of data;
   (o) possible consequences of breaches of confidentiality;
   (p) use of genetic test results and family genetic information:
   (q) study/trial sponsors, the institutional affiliation of investigators, the nature and sources of funding for the research;

   ....

   (z) details of the ethics committee that approved or authorized the protocol.
6. How to obtain informed consent: sponsors' and investigators' obligations.

....

8. Benefits and risks for participants in the study: the potential benefits and risks are sufficiently balanced and the risks are minimized. The well-being of the human subject must take precedence over the interests of science and society.

....

11. Choice of control in clinical trials. Placebo can be used:
    – when there is no effective established intervention;
    – when it is believed that the effective established intervention would expose the subjects to greater temporary discomfort or delay the relief of symptoms;

- when the use of an effective established intervention as a comparator would not produce scientifically reliable results and the use of placebo would not add any risk of serious or irreversible harm to the subjects.
- ....

16. Women as participants:

Investigators, sponsors, or ethics review committees should not exclude women of reproductive age from biomedical research. The risks to the pregnant woman and the fetus must always be taken into account for a clinical study. Women in most societies have been discriminated against in their involvement in research, especially in clinical trials of drugs, vaccines and medical devices that could pose undetermined risks to the fetus.

17. Pregnant women as participants: Pregnant women should be eligible for participation in biomedical research and should be adequately informed of the risks and benefits to themselves, their pregnancies, the fetus and subsequent offspring, and their subsequent fertility.
18. Protection of confidentiality. Patients have the right to expect their doctors and other healthcare professionals to keep all information concerning them strictly confidential. Data from genetic research are treated the same way.

......

21. Ethical obligation of external sponsors to provide health care. External sponsors are ethically obliged to ensure the availability of:
    - any health services essential for the safe conduct of research;
    - treatment for individuals suffering harm as a result of research. Individuals who suffer as a result of research interventions must receive free medical care, and compensation for death or disability resulting from any such injury;
    - services that are a necessary part of a sponsor's commitment to a charitable intervention or to develop a research study
    - test product(s) reasonably available to the population or an interested community.
    -

Appendix 1 Discusses

4. Investigators' views on ethical issues;

10. Names, addresses, institutional affiliations, qualifications and experience of the principal investigator and other investigators;

11. The aims of the study or trial, its hypotheses or research questions, and its variables;

13 The number of subjects needed to achieve the aims of the study;

14. The criteria for inclusion or exclusion of potential subjects;

20. Clinical and laboratory tests and other tests required;

24. The known or foreseeable risks of adverse reactions to any proposed intervention and for any drug, vaccine or procedure to be tested;

28. The potential benefits of the research to individuals and others.

Good Clinical Practice (GCP): EU, U.S.A., Japan, etc.

"Good Clinical Practice (GCP) is an international ethical and scientific quality standard for designing, conducting, recording, and reporting trials that involve the participation of human subjects. Compliance with this standard provides public assurance that the rights, safety, and well-being of trial subjects are protected, consistent with the principles that have their origin in the Declaration of Helsinki, and that the clinical trial data are credible".[6] The standards that the governments of individual countries can apply are defined by the International Conference for the Harmonization of Technical Requirements for the Registration of Medicinal Products for Human Use (ICH), an international body established in 1997 to which the European Union, United States of America, and Japan all belong.

The GCP guidelines define the protection of human rights as subjects of clinical trials and provide assurances about the reliability of the data produced by the trials. The guidelines specify how clinical trials must be conducted, define the roles and responsibilities of sponsors, investigators and monitors (sometimes called Clinical Research Associates (CRA) in the pharmaceutical industry).[7]

There are a few reasons to point to the responses to this: increased ethical awareness, improved clinical trials, less fraud, fewer accidents during data collection, and possibly others.

All clinical trials must be conducted according to ethical principles, scientific evidence, and clear protocols. The benefits must outweigh the risks; the rights, safety, and well-being of study participants are of paramount importance, along with correct informed consent and confidentiality. The data must be easily accessible and recoverable for correct reporting, verification, and interpretation. In conclusion: clinical research must be carried out according to Good Clinical Practice.

Human rights have been violated enough in recent times, and the Declaration of Helsinki and the Nuremberg Code remain the basic defense.[8] The protection of clinical trial subjects is consistent with the principles set out in the Declaration of Helsinki, the statement of ethical principles developed by the World Medical Association.

In Italy GCP guidelines were first adopted in national legislation with the Ministerial Decree of 15 July 1997 (Transposition of the European Union guidelines of good clinical practice for the execution of clinical trials of medicines); the latest EU directives on the subject were implemented with Legislative Decree 211/2003 (Implementation of Directive 2001/20/EC on the application of good clinical practice in the execution of clinical trials of medicinal products for clinical use) and 2000/2007 (Implementation of Directive 2005/28/EC laying down detailed principles and guidelines for good clinical practice relating to investigational

[6] EMeA, ICH Topic E 6 (R1) Guideline for Good Clinical Practice, Step 5, July 2002.

[7] Vijayananthan and Nawawi (2008).

[8] GCP https://it.wikipedia.org/wiki/Buona_pratica_clinica.
Guideline GCP. 1996. Op.cit. McCormick (2013).

medicinal products for human use, as well as requirements for authorization of the manufacture or import of such medicinal products).

The basic indications are summarized here. For details and further information, the original documents can be consulted in their entirety.

Background

Providing a common standard for the European Union, Japan, and the United States was the goal of the GCP currently adopted by the World Health Organization (WHO). GCP is an international standard of ethical and scientific quality for the design, conduct, performance, monitoring, audits, recording, analysis, and reporting of clinical studies.[9]

Human rights having been violated enough in recent times, the Declaration of Helsinki and the Nuremberg Code stand as the basic defense.[10]

There are several advantages of these conditions: increased ethical awareness, better clinical trials, less fraud, and fewer accidents during data collection—and possibly others. All clinical trials must be conducted according to ethical principles, scientific evidence, and clear protocols. The benefits must outweigh the risks; the rights, safety, and well-being of participants are of paramount importance, together with complete informed consent and confidentiality. The data must be easily accessible and recoverable for correct reporting, verification, and interpretation.[10]

Trials are primarily intended to be run at all stages of drug development, before and after product registration and marketing, but are also applicable, in whole or in part, to biomedical research in general. They are addressed to researchers, ethics review committees, pharmaceutical manufacturers and other sponsors of research, and drug regulatory authorities. They protect the rights and safety of individuals, including patients, with public health objectives.

All research relating to human subjects must be conducted in accordance with the ethical principles set out in the Declaration of Helsinki. Three fundamental ethical principles must be respected: justice, respect for people, and charity.

Italy: The National System of Guidelines (Fauci et al. 2021)

The Official Gazette no. 66 of 20 March 2018 published the ministerial decree of 27 February 2018 on the establishment of the National Guidelines System (SNLG), on the subject of professional responsibility and safety of care. A Strategic Committee at the Istituto Superiore della Salute is responsible for management of the SNLG.

---

[9] Berghammer (2014).
CIOMS https://cioms.ch/ https://it.wikipedia.org/wiki/Council_for_International_Organizations_of _Sciences.

[10] Gazzetta Ufficiale della Repubblica Italiana (It: Official Gazette of the Italian Republic) no. 66, p. 16–18, 3 March 2018.

Article 3 (Functions of the Strategic Committee)
The Strategic Committee has the following functions:

(a) defines the priorities of the SNLG, regarding clinical activity, public health and organizational issues, based on the following criteria:
   1. epidemiological impact of diseases on the Italian population;
   2. variability of professional practices not justified by the available evidence;
   3. inequalities of care processes and outcomes;
   4. potential benefits deriving from the production of guidelines;
   5. type and quality of available evidence;
   6. high clinical risk;
   7. social demands and needs perceived by the population.

(a) promoting the efficient production of national guidelines, avoiding duplication and overlap the System, the production times of the guidelines and any critical issues that emerged in their evaluation, the rate of dissemination, the implementation of the guidelines by the recipients, and the impact on results;
(b) annually monitoring the SNLG, the number of guidelines proposed for inclusion and subsequently inserted in
(c) annually submitting a report to the Ministry of Health on the work completed;

2. For the exercise of its functions, the Strategic Committee can use data that may be made available, in compliance with current laws, by the competent central and peripheral authorities, in the epidemiological and pharmacoeconomic fields, on health technologies, socio-health organization, and the state of health of the population.

References

Berghammer G. Good clinical practice (GCP): a universal call for ethics in biomedical research. Taylor & Francis online; 15 May 2014.

Department of Health, Education, and Welfare; National Commission for the Protection of Human Subjects of Biomedical and Behavioral Research. The Belmont Report. Ethical principles and guidelines for the protection of human subjects of research. J Am Coll Dent. 2014;81(3):4–13.

Fauci AJ, Coclite D, Napoletano A, D'Angelo D, et al. Italian National Institute of Health guideline working group on major trauma. Ann Ist Super Sanita. 2021;57(4):343–51.

Lantos JD, Spertus JA. The concept of risk in comparative-effectiveness research. Mary Beth Hamel, editor. NEJM. 2014;371(22):2129–30.

McCormick TR. Principles of bioethics, ©2013. University of Washington; 1 October 2013.

Office of the Secretary. The Belmont report: ethical principles and guidelines for the protection of human subjects of research; 18 April 1979.
Scialpi V. FareRicerca Clinica.com (It. Doing clinical research.com); 10 March 2015.
The Belmont Report; The National Commission for the Protection of Human Subjects of Biomedical and Behavioral Research. Ethical principles and guidelines for the protection of human subjects of research. Appendix Volume II. Washington, DC: U.S. Government Printing Office; 18 April 1979.
Vijayananthan A, Nawawi O. The importance of Good Clinical Practice guidelines and its role in clinical trials. Biomed Imaging Interv J. 2008;4(1):1–4, e5.
Wood AJJ. Progress and deficiencies in the registration of clinical trials. NEJM. 2009;360(8):824–30.

16 Medical Ethics and Bioethics in the Twentieth Century

> Firstly, physicians in the twentieth century have achieved the respectability and social authority that their nineteenth-century predecessors had desired.[1]

In the twentieth century there has been a foreseeable and intense renewal of the concept of medical ethics. This "revolution" had already been seen in the American Medical Association (AMA)[2] texts and in the flourishing specific medical literature.[3]

The American Revolution[2]

"The American Medical Ethics Revolution" whose subtitle already suggests "How the AMA (American Medical Association) Code of Ethics has transformed the physician's relationship with patients, professionals and society," collects historical, philosophical, and critical essays originally presented on the occasion of the 150th anniversary of the Code of Medical Ethics, as a national code of professional conduct. In fact it covers the professional history inside and outside medical activity. In addition, there are essays by experts from different fields of bioethics (medicine, law, philosophy, sociology) who investigate the legitimacy of professional self-regulation and wonder whether in fact the doctors themselves—or others—should debate and control the scope and nature of medical ethics.

Finally, a series of essays addresses contemporary issues of bioethics: bioethics and human rights, standards of medical ethics in the developing world, treatment in alternative medicine, the challenge of "population drugs," and the question of universal access to health care. The appendix contains the specific complete code dated

[1] Jonsen (2000), p. 96.

[2] Baker et al. (1999), Lederer (2004), Maehle (2002). Codice Etico Medico dell'Associazione Medica Americana (1847).

[3] Hospers (1980).

R. G. Russo, *Medical Ethics*, https://doi.org/10.1007/978-3-031-42444-1_16

1847 and some important supporting material, from subsequent versions up to the current one, dated 2016. This volume has dealt with the history of medical ethics and probably has discussed the fundamentals of present and future problems in professional ethics and healthcare. Table of Contents covers all the main recently debated topics:

I. Historical reflections
1. Setting: moral philosophy, Benjamin Rush and medical ethics in the United States before 1846;
2. The American Medical Ethics Revolution;
3. The rebellion of the 1880s against the AMA Code of Ethics: "Scientific democracy" and dissolution of orthodoxy;
4. The challenge of the specialty in 1900;
5. Medical and media ethics: oaths, codes and popular culture;

II. Professionalism and Professional Ethics
6. 150 years later: the moral state and relevance of the AMA code, in:
7. Professionalism and institutional ethics
8. Practice, positivism and its complications
9. Who should control the scope and nature of Medical ethics?
10. Medical ethics as *materia medica*
11. Professionalism and professionalism
12. Who needs the professional ethics of doctors?

III. Current Challenges to Medical Ethics
13. Visible and invisible codes: the fate of the 20th century since the 19th century
14. Alternative medicine and the AMA
15. The challenge of serving both the patient and the population
16. The challenge of universal access to health care with limited resources

IV. Future challenges to biomedical ethics
17. Future challenges to medical ethics and professional values
18. Can ethics help the future of biomedicine?
19. Bioethics in the developing world: national responsibilities and international collaboration
20. Medical ethics and human rights: reflections on the 50th anniversary of the Nuremberg Code

Appendices: AMA Codes and main principles of medical ethics, in medical profession, 1847–1997

A. Note to 1847
B. Introduction to the 1847 Code of Ethics
C. Code of Ethics (1847)
D. Principles of medical ethics (1903)
E. Principles of medical ethics (1912)
F. Principles of medical ethics (1957)
G. First Principles of medical ethics (1980)

H. Fundamental elements of the patient-doctor relationship (1990/1994)
I. Approved opinions and reports; reports on "Financial incentives and the practice of medicine" and "Sex trade union in the practice of medicine".

Preamble

The medical profession has long subscribed to ethical statements for the benefit of the patient. As a member of this profession a physician must first of all recognize responsibility towards the patient, as well as society, other health professionals and also themselves. The following principles adopted by the AMA are not laws, but standards of conduct that define the essential elements of honorable behavior for the physician.

AMA Principles of Medical Ethics

1. A physician shall be dedicated to providing competent medical care, with compassion and respect for human dignity and rights.
2. A physician shall uphold the standards of professionalism, be honest in all professional interactions, and strive to report physicians deficient in character or competence, or engaging in fraud or deception, to appropriate entities.
3. A physician shall respect the law and also recognize a responsibility to seek changes in those requirements which are contrary to the patient's best interests.
4. A physician shall respect the rights of patients, colleagues, and other health professionals, and shall safeguard patients' confidences and privacy within the constraints of the law.
5. A physician shall continue to study, apply, and advance scientific knowledge, maintain a commitment to medical education, make relevant information available to patients, colleagues, and the public, obtain consultation, and use the talents of other health professionals when indicated.
6. A physician shall, in the provision of appropriate patient care—except in emergencies—be free to choose whom to serve, with whom to associate, and the environment in which to provide medical care.
7. A physician shall recognize a responsibility to participate in activities contributing to the improvement of the community and the betterment of public health.
8. A physician shall, while caring for a patient, regard responsibility to the patient as paramount.
9. A physician shall support access to medical care for all people.

Medical Deontology

In defining this Code we have the advantage of inferring the rules from the conduct of many eminent doctors who have graced the profession. From the age of Hippocrates to the present, in the annals of every civilization there is abundant evidence of the devotion of doctors to relieving their patients from pain and disease, regardless of the privations and dangers encountered.

The Introduction to The American Medical Ethics Revolution (1999) (pages xiii–xiv) clarifies that: "The Code of Ethics of 1847 is the first national code of professional ethics, of medical ethics. It is the ancestor of all professional codes of ethics, medical or non-medical." At its time, the AMA code of ethics was really a revolutionary document, and professional oaths were considered descendants of the classic Hippocratic Oath. Since they are activated by the performative expression "I swear" and are drawn up in the first person singular, they appear intrinsically personal.

"Ethics" and "Medical Ethics"

Medical ethics is the most debated topic that has received new, in-depth attention in relation to:

1. the doctor–patient relationship,
2. experimentation with genetic material,
3. the outcome of brain surgery for psychological disorders,
4. population control.

Professional competence in the U.S.A. has resulted in the formulation of a new medical ethics by numerous authors who list the duties of the modern physician, usually in accordance with the Hippocratic Oath.

Multiple comments help doctors (Catholics, Protestants, and Jews) to understand the complex moral questions.[4]

During the 1950s and 1960s a series of revolutionary cognitive and therapeutic developments were seen in the biomedical sciences: the discoveries of molecular biology, advances in resuscitation techniques, advances in pharmacology and the advent of transplant medicine. This progress has sometimes been perceived by public opinion as potentially threatening to humanity and the dignity of people.

The claim of the biological sciences to know and manipulate the fundamental mechanisms of life and human behavior has been considered a risk for the freedom and dignity of man.[5] Since the twentieth century, some moral theologians and philosophers began to question the possibility that medical ethics, based on the moral

[4] Jonsen (2000), pp. 84–95.

[5] Babu (2015), Williams (2005, 2008).

principles of deontological codes, could ensure respect for people's individual rights. Also the rights of doctors were identified.

Several factors (philosophical, psychological, religious, social, political, etc.) have been examined. The term "medical ethics" expresses a well-defined concept, but is not universally described and accepted. Perhaps only the Hippocratic Oath, long beyond its time, with its hard to decipher terminologies, often inappropriate or inaccurate today, still embraces all doctors, all over the world, in a single ideal, largely superior to any understanding: that of Man who dedicates himself to Man.[6]

Causes of Problems in Medical Ethics

The doctors' power over life and death is great as is as their recognized potential for abuse or neglect. Medical ethics can be considered an investigation of the values formed in the relationship between doctors and patients. This implies that it must be clearly distinguished from medical jurisprudence or forensic medicine on the one hand, and medical etiquette or conventions on the other.

Below are three examples of the potential areas for change.

1. One of the main acknowledged reasons for the increasing ethical problems in healthcare is the advance of technology. Today doctors have many means of keeping people technically alive—for example, thanks to machines, but these are usually expensive and invasive. So who decides what to do and when to do it, and when to accept death, especially if family members disagree among themselves?
2. Doctors have the means to perform organ transplants (kidney, lung, heart). However, there is increasing demand for organs for transplantation, so what priorities can be established, and what criteria should be used to make the decision?
3. Another important source of ethical difficulties in medicine is the cost of health care and the consequent question of how the costs must be assigned and who should pay.

The World Medical Association (WMA)[7] has taken on the primary goal of establishing and promoting the highest standards of ethical behavior and care by physicians and has adopted global policy statements on a range of ethical issues relating to medical professionalism, patient care, human research, and public health. The WMA is backed by the "WMA International Code of Medical Ethics," which

[6]Association for Medical ethics, 2005. http://www.ethicaldoctor.org Gale (2000).

[7]Tra le principali Organizzazioni internazionali: (IT. Some of the main international organizations): Amnesty International, International Federation of Associations of Pharmaceutical Physicians (IFAPP), International Federation of Pharmaceutical Manufacturers & Associations (IFPMA), Physicians for Human Rights (PHR), International Society for Health and Human Rights (ISHHR).

Falkenheimer (2014) and Walters and Moraczewski (2003).

reached its third edition in 2015.[8] Since its official launch in January 2005, the Code has been distributed to medical journals and societies around the world. It has been translated into 23 languages, but not yet into Italian:

- English (WMA)
- French (WMA)
- Spanish (WMA)
- Macedonian (Macedonian Medical Association)
- Albanian (Macedonian Medical Association)
- Traditional Chinese (Taiwan Medical Association)
- Korean (Korean Medical Association)
- Indonesian (Muhammadiyah University of Yogyakarta)
- German (German Medical Association)
- Arabic (University of Tunis Faculty of Medicine)
- Turkish (Turkish Medical Association)
- Russian (Russian Medical Society)
- Bulgarian (Bulgarian Medical Association)
- Japanese (Japan Medical Association)
- Estonian (Estonian Medical Association)
- Georgian (Georgian Medical Association)
- Slovak (Slovak Medical Association)
- Lithuanian (Lithuanian Medical Association)
- Latvian (Latvian Medical Association)
- Persian (Urmia University of Medical Sciences)
- Ukrainian (Ukrainian Medical Association)
- Polish (Polish Chamber of Physicians and Dentists)
- Slovenian (Medical Faculty, University of Maribor)

Medical Ethics in the World

WMA

The World Medical Association (WMA)[7] is an international and independent confederation of free professional medical associations representing physicians worldwide. Today (2021) it counts 115 Constituent Members and 1467 Associate Members, with more than 10 million registered physicians. It was founded on September 18, 1947, and has Headquarters location: Ferney-Voltaire, France.

WMA provides formulated declarations and resolutions to help guide national medical associations, governments, and international organizations around the

[8] WMA International Code of Medical ethics. 19499, 1968, 1983, 2006. WMA Manual, 2005 WMA Medical ethics, 2017.

WMA Principles of Medical Ethics, 2001.

World Medical Association (1949).

world: it works with an international network of academic and non-academic centers that aim to promote research, education and consultation in the field of biomedical ethics, support for students, faculty and researchers, and the organization of annual conferences.

Since it was founded, a central objective of the WMA has been to establish and promote the highest possible standards of ethical behavior and care by physicians. In pursuit of this goal, the WMA has adopted global policy statements on a range of ethical issues related to medical professionalism, patient care, research on human subjects and public health. The WMA Council and its standing committees regularly review and update existing policies and continually develop new policy on emerging ethical issues.

The WMA serves as a clearinghouse of ethics information resources for its members. To achieve this goal, the WMA cooperates with academic institutions, global organizations, and individual experts in the field of medical ethics. The WMA has adopted numerous policies that are recognized internationally as the global ethical standard for the topics they address. The following selection represents some of the most important ethics policies of the WMA.

EACME

The European Association of Centers of Medical Ethics (EACME) was founded in the early 1980s by a small group of theologians, philosophers and medical doctors involved in the new discipline of medical ethics—*bioethics*.

These "founding fathers" set out to build a network of centers of medical ethics in Europe with the aim of reinforcing the teaching, research, communication, and debate on ethical issues in medical practice, health policy, and medical sciences. The EACME officially started work on December 2, 1986, in Lyon, France. The centers (including the Bulletin of Medical Ethics) were located in France (Lyon, Paris), Spain (Barcelona), Belgium (Brussels), the Netherlands (Maastricht), and the United Kingdom (London). The strong presence of clergymen on the original Board explains why the EACME has stressed from the outset its pluralist approach to bioethical issues.

The Association expanded in the 1990s, when bioethics centers in Europe were increasingly cooperating in research and teaching projects funded by the European Union. This was the background for the "professionalization" of the young association, strengthened by efficient organization and administration under the guidance of the EACME Board and Bureau. New centers joined, from all over the European continent, stimulating and strengthening the Association's pluralist character.

EACME aims to promote and strengthen the debate on moral values and ethical theory in relation to health practice, biomedical research and health systems, from the individual, social and legal points of view. It also strongly backs cooperation with other societies and associations in the field of bioethics, philosophy of medicine and social medicine, both nationally and internationally, in particular with regard to medical ethics. It focuses on Eastern and Southern Europe, with close attention to supporting and promoting young talents and young researchers.

Code of Medical Ethics of the Federal Council of Medicine of Brazil[9]

The codes of 11 countries were compared: Argentina, Chile, Canada, United States, Portugal, United Kingdom, South Africa, Egypt, China, India, and Australia. The Brazilian Federal Council of Medicine approved the current Code of Medical Ethics in January 1988.

The code "contains the standards that govern doctors; those who violate this code are subject to disciplinary action as established by law."

Features of the code include: (1) statements regarding occupational health and the natural environment, (2) the right of doctors to go on strike, and (3) the requirement for medical research protocols to be submitted to an independent committee for approval and monitoring.

Research Ethics Committee. South Africa Medical Association, 1992 (SAMAREC)

SAMAREC was established by the South African Medical Association (SAMA) to examine the ethics of research protocols for clinical trials in the private health sector, guaranteeing the protection and respect of the rights, safety and well-being of the participants, and providing the public guarantee of this protection and fully informed consent. SAMA comprised a variety of medical groups representing various interests. It is a voluntary membership association to serve the best interests and needs of its members in all health-related matters.

Vision: To be the leading and preferred membership organization advocating and supporting medical practitioners in South Africa.

Mission: Being the custodians of growing advocacy platform that will unite, guide, and support members for the health of the nation.

Seychelles Medical and Dental Council (SMDC), 1994

The SMDC Board decided to provide some training in medical ethics. The Practical Guide to Ethics and Medical Law explains the main principles and theories of medical ethics and medical legislation. It describes 25 cases based on real events and sets out the key facts, laws, and theories for finding solutions and making informed decisions.

[9] Federal Medical Council (1994).

SMDC PRINCIPLES:

1. SMDC seeks to implement good governance in all its actions (good governance refers to: efficiency, efficacy, accountability, transparency, responsiveness, equity, respect for the law and natural justice)
2. SMDC collaborates with other national and international regulators to protect the health and safety of the public
3. SMDC seeks to achieve excellence in everything it des and will continually improve its own performance

Medical and Dental Council of Nigeria, (MDCN), 1995

Nigerian doctors' knowledge of medical ethics is seriously inadequate. There is an urgent need to improve the teaching of the discipline both at undergraduate and postgraduate levels. Considering the scarcity of books on medical ethics in Nigeria, the WMA Code serves as an information booklet for medical students, medical teachers, and practitioners engaged in medical law as well as lay people and patients who may wish to seek information on these aspects of the medical and dental professions.

Vision: To be the foremost professional regulatory body in Nigeria.

Mission: To regulate the practice of Medicine, Dentistry and Alternative Medicine in the most efficient manner that safeguards best healthcare delivery for Nigerians.

India Ethics Committee: Notified, 6 April 2002 (Babu, India)

Chapter 1-1. Medical Code of Ethics: Following the formulation of the Code of Medical Ethics, as stated in the Indian medical regulation of 2002, ethics in the Indian context is closely linked to indigenous classical and folklore traditions. Emphasis is laid on Indian concepts of ethics and medicine in the Hindu tradition. The classic Ayurvedic texts including *Carakasamhita* and *Susrutasamhita* propose hypotheses on the body, the self and the *gune* (Sanskrit term meaning: "merit," "quality," "virtue"). Karma, the notion that every action has consequences, provides a basis for medical Morality. Research on COVID-19: in the need for credible technical information on COVID-19, the Training Division at the Public Health Foundation of India conducts a series of online seminars.

Association for Medical Ethics, 2008: Cambridge, Massachusetts, USA

The Association for Medical Ethics (AME) is made up of doctors of all medical specialties. The Association's purpose is to promote good patient care and evidence-based medicine. The issues tackled include the ethics of responsible patient care and the identification of the (often widespread) influence of industry on many healthcare providers and their patients. Research on COVID-19.

Patients are faced with so many questions as they navigate the healthcare system. To answer a number of questions about topics from Physician Owned Distributorships to the newest drugs or latest surgery options, we have compiled a number of articles to give some easy to understand answers. Moreover, there are many types of biases in research that have been categorized.

They fall mainly into three groups with subcategories in each. The Association for Medical Ethics (AME) consists of physicians from every specialty of medicine. The purpose of the Association is to promote patient care and good, evidence-based medicine.

Australian Medical Association (Aust MA)

Code of Medical ethics 2004, Revised 2006, 2016.

The four pillars of medical ethics are: charity (do well), non-maleficence (do no harm), autonomy (respect the patient's wishes), and justice (for the allocation of resources).

The updated Code of Ethics of the Australian MA lays stress on the importance of:

- close personal relationships;
- patients with impaired or limited decision-making capacity;
- patients' relatives, caregivers, and other important figures, including lawyers;
- work with colleagues, with attention to bullying and harassment;
- work with other healthcare professionals;
- supervision/tutoring for health regulations; quality and safety.

Most nations have agreed on the active application of medical ethics. Many of them have long-standing texts and others have more recent ones. The latter are often in developing countries.[10]

Twenty-First Century: U.S.A., Europe

After the close and fairly exhaustive definitions of ethics in the nineteenth century, the search for similar perspectives continued in the twentieth century and now in the twenty-first.[11] In the twentieth century and the early twenty-first the ethical implications of medicine were not the object of much attention outside the medical environment. Some theologians, mostly Catholics, have put forward guidelines on

[10] Olweny (1994) and Zumla and Costello (2002).

[11] Parker and Hope (2000).

controversial issues such as abortion, contraception, and eugenics. The twenty-first century brought new deontological theories, together with new rules relating to morality, thanks mainly to several factors:

Technological Advances

The rapid expansion of scientific knowledge, especially in the fields of electronics, computers, molecular biology, genetics, and immunology, and their applications to medicine.

Pluralism of Values

Values tend to fall into two main groups: one that seeks to incorporate a religious point of view, be it Catholic, or in any case Christian, but also Jewish or Muslim or of other beliefs, having Man as the primary standard.

Patients' Rights

Rising health care costs raise serious concerns for the public and governments; the public turns to the Internet for information on medical issues.

Concern for Faith

There is growing attention to the role of faith in daily life, especially for those involved in the charismatic renewal in various communities, with an active religious approach.

Other Important Topics

Many of the issues today are considered pertinent to bioethics—the patient's rights, the protection of experimental subjects, whether animal or human, euthanasia and assisted suicide, the right not to know, and confidentiality, acknowledgment of medical errors and inequalities in access to care. These had all been widely discussed even before the term "bioethics" was introduced in 1970.

In 1971, Dutch physician Andre Hellegers and his colleagues from the newly created Kennedy Institute of Ethics in Washington appropriated the term to refer to a discipline aimed at addressing the religious and ethical dimensions of concrete medical issues. Autonomy was further strengthened with the enormous progress made by medicine in the twentieth century. The American government's investment in bioethics continued up into the 1990s.

Issues relating to recombinant DNA techniques in particular, and genetic engineering in general, raised questions about the limits of human self-control and nature. The cloning of humans and the use of stem cells for research and therapy have posed major challenges.[11]

Medical ethics, however, appeared to be more than just an oath; the term referred to codes of conduct developed by physicians to encourage self-regulation and reflection on the issues posed by disease, treatment and the physician's role. The *National Endowment for the Humanities* (NEH)[12] encouraged the development of the discipline of bioethics by funding several academic departments. It funded the Society for Health and Human Values, which offered medical faculties expertise in humanities and ethics.

Bioethics has aroused international interest and investment. Similarly to the Americans, governments, and organizations in other nations have set up special committees responsible for defining guidelines in medicine and biology.

Bioethics developed as a separate discipline in the second half of the twentieth century. The World Health Organization (WHO) and the United Nations Educational, Scientific and Cultural Organization (UNESCO) appointed committees on mapping the human genome, political organization, and the philosophy and history of the various countries. The numerous bioethics committees have reached different conclusions regarding the rules of clinical trials and issues such as euthanasia and the use of genetically modified organisms.

During the 1950s and 1960s, the biomedical sciences saw a number of revolutionary cognitive and therapeutic developments: the genetic code, breakthroughs in molecular biology, advances in resuscitation techniques, advances in pharmacology, and the advent of transplant medicine (just to name a few). These made the prospect of the control of life, death and disease by scientific medicine seem reality.

However—as we said earlier—advances in knowledge and the application of biomedical sciences are increasingly perceived by public opinion as potentially threatening humanity and people's dignity. The biological sciences' claim to understand and manipulate the fundamental mechanisms of life and human behavior are often considered harmful to the freedom and dignity of Man.

In the following years the emergence of bioethics[13] has pushed aside traditional medical ethics and codes of ethics. The increase in the possibilities of medical intervention, with the decrease in risks, has given the impression that we have gained access to a new ethical branch.

This arose in America and then—though not without opposition and widespread discontent—spread throughout the world. Bioethics abandons medical paternalism

---

[12] Il NEH è un'agenzia federale indipendente creata nel 1965. È uno dei più grandi finanziatori di programmi umanistici negli U.S.A., trasmettendo le lezioni della storia a tutti gli americanil sussidi NEH si rivolgono a istituzioni culturali, come musei, archivi, biblioteche, università, università, televisione pubblica e stazioni radio e a singoli studiosi. [IT. The NEH is an independent federal agency set up in 1965. It is one of the largest financers of humanistic programs in the USA, transmitting history lessons to all Americans. NEH funds go to cultural institutions such as museums, archives, libraries, universities, public television and radio stations, and scholars.)

[13] Jonsen (2000). Op cit. From Medical Ethics to Bioethics, pp. 115–120.

and takes respect for people's independent decision-making as its moral principle. This, in medicine, is embodied in the practice of informed consent and the various strategies aimed at protecting individuals who are unable to make autonomous choices, while always with the intention of causing the patient the least possible harm. The new biomedical ethics started above all from the philosophical-legal assumptions about informed consent and the possibility that the patient has the right to refuse or withdraw from treatment.[14]

In 1985 the first Chair of Bioethics in Italy was established at the Faculty of Medicine and Surgery of the Catholic University of Rome; the Institute of Bioethics was set up in the same faculty in 1992.

Forecasts for the Twenty-First Century

The traditional Hippocratic medical ethics seems taken for granted, exhorting doctors to observe certain strategies that have become largely obsolete and inadequate nowadays, and bioethics is increasingly addressing current "needs" and may even answer them, thanks to advances in medical and surgical science. But many of the "old" issues remain, at least for a large part of the world population. A work with this perspective was published in 2000 by Parker and Hope.[11] They took on the burdensome (and hypothetical) commitment of trying to predict what the task of medical ethics might involve in the twenty-first century. Their forecast is that: "Medical ethics will likely have to increasingly address the ethical problems arising from discrepancies in health care in different countries. Increasing longevity will lead to problems in the allocation of resources that become increasingly problematic within medicine".[11]

In the future we can largely forecast the main directions medical ethics will take—probably similar to those seen at the beginning of the twentieth century. However, the key problems will be quite different and biological technology will affect several main areas:

1. a substantial increase in life expectancy among the wealthiest nations;
2. growing evidence of the biological determination of human behavior;
3. the responsibility of young people today;
4. improvements in biological methods.

In richer nations, the balance of knowledge between doctor and patient will change, and consequently the issues of informed consent and patient choice will be profoundly different. Perhaps medical ethics will contribute to increasing globalization as one of the key issues in the twenty-first century. They will concern poor countries and the interactions between rich and poor nations. The main ethical issue in medicine will be shortages of health care for most of the world's population.

[14] Corbellini (2010).

The other issues that have to be taken into account, overlapping some of those above:

- the effect of a substantial increase in longevity;
- improving the growth of children;
- the biological determination of behavior;
- therapeutic research.

Other Aspects

Globalization: In the twenty-first century many processes will inevitably relate to common or very similar economic and information issues. A substantial increase in longevity: medicine might add 10 years to our lives. Medical developments over the next few decades will have a substantial effect on lifespans, which might even reach 120 years.

This will imply, first of all, that a larger proportion of each nation's wealth will have to be spent on medicine, because screening, prophylaxis and treatments will be routine Another inevitable consequence will be an increase in job opportunities and the reassessment of the retirement age.

Improvement of children's growth: modern genetics now offers the possibility of targeted treatments for the main killer diseases. This is probably its greatest beneficial impact. Biological determination of behavior and criminal responsibility too, for example, will have to be reassessed: the treatment of "criminals" will become a matter involving medical ethics.

Therapeutic research and clinical practice: There will be much more work in therapeutic studies, guided in part by the ideals of evidence-based medicine and in part by information technology (IT), making it possible to process data and unify test methods in many more centers.

Other authors consider different forecasts for the years to come.[15] In particular, there are concerns about the use of resources, one of the main issues relating to medical ethics:

1. technological advances are likely to continue producing promising and costly new therapeutic and diagnostic interventions;
2. treatment will often be only partially positive, leaving some individuals with an unacceptable quality of life;
3. resources for health care will be limited;
4. the moral authority that will decide the extent to which people can use their resources will also remain limited.

The options can therefore be reduced to three.

[15] Engelhardt (1991) and Irving (1999, 2003).

1. We can continue our commitment to providing optimal care equally for all, to the best of our ability;
2. a limited package of medical assistance and practice for all will be defined;
3. there will be a one-size-fits-all package that can be boosted by purchasing specific diagnostic and therapeutic interventions not included.

The doctor's role: It will be essential to grasp the fact that life is in fact finite, and so are medical capabilities, and economic resources. Moral authority will have to be exercised to set limits to health policy and health care in the future.

Medical ethics for the next century should focus on beneficence and temperance (*sophrosyne*) in our human condition.[15]

In Conclusion

Biological technology will have an impact on medical ethics in at least three main areas:

- it will lead to notable increases in life expectancy among the wealthiest nations;
- it will provide increasing evidence for the biological determination of human behavior, for example in criminal liability;
- it will consider our responsibilities in the enhancement of skills and competence, using biological methods.

Physicians' awareness and professionalism will help in developing socially useful programs. The contribution to establishing what the model of care might look like will be adapted to the relationship between patient and healthcare professional. Medical ethics will address the ethical issues deriving from differences between countries, often finding itself tackling the different conclusions already reached by secular bioethics (the natural law, or what we can understand as "right" or "wrong" with the help of reason alone) and by the medical ethics of each current religion (for example that interpreted by the *Magisterium* of the Church).[16]

The fundamental principles for the new millennium (starting with the year 2000) might be laid out as:

1. the primacy of the patient's well-being,
2. patient autonomy
3. social justice.

All these above will change medical ethics, as we know it so far. As a result, medical professionals will have great responsibilities as regards commitments relating to:

[16] Project of the ABIM Foundation, ACP-ASIM Foundation and European Federation of Internal Medicine (2002).

- professional competence;
- honesty with patients;
- patient confidentiality;
- maintaining adequate relationships with patients;
- improvement of the quality of care;
- improving access to care;
- fair distribution of resources;
- increases in scientific knowledge;
- maintaining trust through management of conflicts of interest.

Moreover[16]

Bioethics will specifically evaluate the ethics of the following: contraception; abortions; prenatal diagnosis of defective babies; human embryos and human fetal research; human cloning; formation of human chimeras; high-risk experimental research with the mentally ill; euthanasia; assisted suicide—to name just what comes to mind immediately. As there is no ethical code for bioethicists, there are several misunderstandings about bioethics: it is not just moral consensus but more of an academic theory, and should not be equated with the entire field of ethics but only with one of its sub-sectors.

On Hold

What ethics will be practiced in the twenty-first century? Lay bioethics or moral law? Obviously everyone has a choice. Even small differences or small errors in the choice of ethics might give rise to multiple harms for individuals, as well as for our culture and society. Medical ethics may therefore need to be considerably revised or even regenerated altogether.

References

Babu KG. Importance of ethics in today's society: special emphasis on medical ethics. RRJMHS. 2015;4(3)

Baker RB, Caplan AL, Emanuel LL, Latham SR, editors. The American medical ethics revolution. Baltimore/London: The John Hopkins University Press; 1999. 396 p.

Codice Etico Medico dell'Associazione Medica Americana. originariamente adottato dalla riunione aggiornata della Convenzione medica nazionale a Filadelfia, maggio 1847. (IT. Originally adopted at the National Medical Convention in Philadelphia, May 1847). Chicago: American Medical Associated Press; 1847.

Corbellini G. Storia dell'Etica Medica, Dizionario di medicina. (IT. History of medical ethics, Dictionary of medicine). Enciclopedia Treccani; 2010

Engelhardt HT. Medical ethics for the 21st Century. JACC. 1991;18(1):303–7.

Falkenheimer S. Medical ethics education in the U.S. and around the world. Christian Doctor – Spring 2014.

Federal Medical Council. Federal Medical Council (CFM) of Brazil adopts resolutions on criteria for death and on medically assisted procreation. Int Dig Health Legis. 1994;45(1):100–2. PMID: 11660644

Gale T. Encyclopedia of science, technology, and ethics, 2000

Hospers J. Bibliographical essay: The literature of ethics in the twentieth century. Bibligraphical Essay in Literature Liberty. 1980;3(3)

Irving DD. Which medical ethics for the 21st century? Eighth Annual Rose Mass. Brunch, The Grand Hyatt Hotel, Washington, DC. CERC Catholic Education Resource Center; 14 March 1999.

Irving DR. Which medical ethics for the 21st century. Linaore Quart. 2003:46–59.

Jonsen AR. Medical history in India and China in a short history of medical ethics. Oxford/New York: Oxford University Press; 2000.

Lederer SE. La seconda rivoluzione scientifica: scienze biologiche e medicina. Dall'Etica Medica alla bioetica. (IT. The second scientific revolution: biological sciences and medicine, From medical ethics to bioethics). Enciclopedia Treccani. Storia della Scienza (IT. History of Science); 2004.

Maehle A-H. The American medical ethics revolution. Med Hist. 2002;46(1):107–9.

Olweny C. Bioethics in developing countries: ethics of scarcity and sacrifice. J Med Ethics. 1994;20:169–74.

Parker M, Hope T. Medical ethics in the 21st century. J Intern Med. 2000;248:1–6.

Project of the ABIM Foundation, ACP-ASIM Foundation and European Federation of Internal Medicine. Medical professionalism in the new millennium: a physician's charter. Ann Intern Med. 2002;136:243–6.

Walters L, Moraczewski AS. Medical ethics, twentieth-century Catholic analysis. New Catholic Encyclopedia. Encyclopedia.com. The Gale Group Inc. http://www.encyclopedia.com (2003).

Williams JR. Medical ethics in contemporary clinical practice. J Chin Med Assoc. 2005;68(11):495–9.

Williams JR. Ethics at the World Medical Association: from policy to practice. JMAJ. 2008;51(4):290–3.

World Medical Association. International code of medical ethics. World Med Assoc Bull. 1949;1(3):109–11.

Zumla A, Costello A. Ethics of healthcare research in developing countries. J R Soc Med. 2002;95(6):275–7.

17 Ethics Committees

Comment:

Even if this chapter deals with a specific topic for events in Italy, it illustrates how various countries have reacted in the face of this new situation.

Birth of Ethics Committees

The U.S. House Committee on Ethics was created in 1967. It included five members from each party. In Italy ethics committees acquired legal status in July 1997. The establishment and functioning were defined in a Ministerial Decree dated March 18 and 19, 1998.[1]

[1] D.M. March 18, 1998 relativo alle Linee guida di riferimento per l'istituzione e il funzionamento dei Comitati etici (IT. relating to the reference guidelines for the establishment and operation of ethics committees) Published on Italian official. G.U. n.122 del May 28, 1998.

R. G. Russo, *Medical Ethics*, https://doi.org/10.1007/978-3-031-42444-1_17

What Are They?[2, 3]

In Directive 2001/20/EC of the European Parliament,[4] the Ethics Committee is defined as:

> *An independent body, composed of health care and non-health care personnel, responsible for ensuring the protection of the rights, safety, and well-being of trial subjects and for providing public assurance of this protection by, for example, issuing opinions on the trial protocol, the suitability of the investigator(s), facilities, and the methods and documents to be used to inform trial subjects prior to obtaining informed consent.*

Summarized below, in chronological order from (1) to (5), with some clarifications or comments, are the main documents relating to Ethics Committees in Italy:

1. Filosa A.M. Legislation and Role of Ethics Committees. Approval of the ethical-scientific aspects by a competent body.Diritto.it, 1996.[3]
2. **DECREE March 18, 1998.** Procedures for exemption from investigations on medicines used in clinical trials. [GU, (Official Gazette) General Series no.122 of 28-05-1998][1]

   Ethics Committees are legally recognized in healthcare facilities in Italy, in accordance with Ministerial Decree (M.D.) of 27 April 1992 (Provisions on technical documentation to be submitted in support of applications for marketing authorization of medicinal products for human use, also in implementation of Directive no. 91/507/EEC. [GU no.139 of 15 June 1992—Ordinary Supplement no. 86).)
3. **MINISTERIAL CIRCULAR April 8, 1999, n. 6**

   Clarifications on the ministerial decrees of 18 and 19 March 1998 published in the Official Gazette no. 123 of 28 May 1998 (GU General Series no. 90 of 19 April 1999).[2] Directive 2001/20/EC of the European Parliament and of the Council of 4 April 2001, concerning the approximation of the laws, regulations and administrative provisions of the Member States relating to the application of good clinical practice in clinical trials of medicinal products for human use.[4]

---

[2] D.L. 12-05-2006. Requisiti minimi per l'istituzione, l'organizzazione e il funzionamento dei Comitati etici per le sperimentazioni cliniche dei medicinali. (IT. Minimum requirements for the establishment, organization and operation of ethics committees for clinical trials of medicines.) Published onItalian official GU DM_12_Maggio_2006_CE, n. 194, pp 4–8.

[3] Comitato Etico, Wikipedia.

Filosa (1996), Mosconi et al. (2006), Istituto di Ricerche Farmacologiche Mario Negri et al. (2007).

McLean (2007) and Presidenza del Consiglio dei Ministri: I comitati per l'etica nella linica (IT. Presidency of the Council of Ministers: The ethics committees in clinics Pp 1–23, March 31, 2017.

[4] Direttiva 2001/20/CE del Parlamento Europeo del Consigli (IT. Directive 2001/20/CE of the European Parliament of the Council 2001/20/CE del Parlamento Europeo del Consiglio April 4, 2001.

4. **DIRECTIVE 2001/20/CE** of the European Parliament and of the Council of April 4, 2001 on the approximation of the laws, regulations and administrative provisions of the Member States relating to the application of good clinical practice in the execution of clinical trials of medicinal products for human use.[4]
5. **LAW DECREE** (D.L.) n. 211 of June 24, 2003: Implementation of Directive 2001/20/EC on the application of good clinical practice in the conduct of clinical trials of medicinal products for clinical use. (Official Gazette General Series n.184 of Sept. 08, 2003—Ordinary Suppl. N. 130).[5] The topics of the ethics committee are reported in the following Articles:

   Art. 2—Definitions
   Art. 3—Protection of the subjects of clinical trials
   Art. 4—Experimentation minors clinic
   Art. 5—Clinical trial on adults unable to validly give their informed consent
   Art. 6—Ethics Committee[6]
   Art. 7—Single opinion
   Art. 8—How to submit the application for the opinion of the committee ethics
   Art. 9—Beginning of a clinical trial
   Art.10—Conducting a clinical trial
   Art. 11—Exchange of information
   Art. 12—Suspension of the trial or infringements
   Art. 15—Verification of compliance with the rules of good clinical practice and manufacturing of investigational drugs
   Art. 16—Notification of adverse events
   Art. 17—Notification of serious adverse reactions
   Art. 22—Sanctioning system

Article 6. Ethics Committee

1. The ethics committee must issue its opinion before the start of any clinical trial about which he was consulted.
2. The ethics committee formulates the opinion referred to in paragraph 1, taking into particular consideration:
   (a) the relevance and relevance of the clinical trial and study design;
   (b) whether the assessment of the foreseeable benefits and risks satisfies the provisions of Article 3, paragraph 1, letter a), whether the conclusions are justified;

[5] Decreto Legislativo June 24 2003, n. 211. "Attuazione della direttiva 2001/20/CE relativa all'applicazione della buona pratica clinica nell'esecuzione delle sperimentazioni cliniche di medicinali per uso clinico" (IT. Legislative Decree June 24 2003, n. 211. "Implementation of Directive 2001/20/EC relating to the application of good clinical practice in carrying out clinical trials of medicinal products for clinical use") Published on official GU n. 184 del August 9, 2003 - Supplemento Ordinario n. 130.

[6] Article 6 is reported in full, as it presents many useful clarifications.

(c) the protocol;
(d) the suitability of the investigator and his collaborators;
(e) the dossier for the investigator;
(f) the adequacy of the health facility;
(g) the adequacy and completeness of the written information to be communicated to the subject and the procedure to be followed to submit informed consent to the same, as well as the justification for research on persons who are unable to give their informed consent regarding the specific restrictions set out in Article 3;
(h) the provisions regarding compensation in the event of damage or death attributable to the clinical trial;
(i) the provisions on insurance relating to compensation for damages caused to subjects by the trial activity, to cover the civil liability of the investigator and the promoter of the trial;
(l) the amounts and any modalities of remuneration or remuneration or emoluments of any kind to be paid in favor of the investigators and any indemnity of the subjects included in the trial and the relevant elements of the contract between the promoter of the trial and the experimental center;
(m) the methods of recruiting the subjects and the information procedures to spread the knowledge of the trial in compliance with the provisions in this regard by the rules of good clinical practice and in compliance with the regulations in force.

3. The ethics committee in the case of monocentric trials, within 60 days from the date of receipt of the application submitted by the promoter of the trial in the prescribed form, communicates its reasoned opinion to the promoter, the Ministry of Health and the competent authority. In the case of multicenter trials, the provisions of Article 7 apply.
4. The ethics committee, during the examination period of the application referred to in paragraph 3, may ask once to acquire additional information to that already provided by the promoter of the trial; in this case, the term provided for in paragraph 3 is suspended until the above information is acquired.
5. No extension to the term referred to in paragraph 3 is allowed, except for trials that use products for gene therapy and somatic cell therapy, as well as all medicines that contain genetically modified organisms, for which an extension of 30 days. For these products, the term is extended by another 90 days pending the authorization issued by the Ministry of Health.

   For xenogenic cell therapy there is no time limit for the application assessment period.
6. The contract referred to in paragraph 2.1 must be stipulated between the legal manager of the trial center or person delegated by him and the promoter of the trial, within the time limits allowed by article 9 for

assessment of the applications to be submitted to the competent authority, it being understood that the entry into orce of this contract is subject to the favorable opinion referred to in paragraph 1, and to completion of the procedures referred to in Article 9.

7. Without prejudice to the provisions of Article 12-bis, paragraph 9, of Legislative Decree 30 December 1992, no.502, and subsequent amendments, with the decree of the Minister of Health, in agreement with the Minister of Economy and Finance, the minimum requirements for the establishment, organization and functioning of the ethics committees are updated, without variance in expenditure. for clinical trials of medicines.

This decree entered into force on January 1, 2004.

6. **DECREE of May 12, 2006** Minimum requirements for the establishment, organization and operation of the Ethics Committees for clinical trials of medicines.[7] Specific points are dealt with, after the Epigraph and the Introduction:
   - Ethics Committee,
   - Establishment and composition,
   - Independence of ethics committees,
   - Organization,
   - Functioning of the ethics committee,
   - Economic aspects,
   - Single opinion,
   - Subsequent activation of the experimental centers,
   - Suspension of the trial,
   - Communication of the establishment of the committees,
   - Reference requirements,
   - Repeals,
   - Entry into force
   - Financial invariance clause.
7. Mosconi P, Colombo C, Labianca R, Apolone G. Oncologists' opinions about research Ethics committees in Italy: an update, 2004. European J Cancer Prevention 15: 91–94, 2006.
8. MINISTERIAL DECREE of February 8, 2013[8] "Criteria for the composition and functioning of ethics committees": the need to avoid the coexistence of different ethics committees in a single unit is further emphasized by local health company and for each individual hospital. The internal composition of the

[7] DM 12 maggio 2006.

[8] D.M. 8 febbraio 2013, n.96. Criteri per la composizione e il funzionamento dei comitati etici.(IT: Criteria for the composition and functioning of ethics committees).

Ethics Committees must ensure the presence of the necessary experience to fully evaluate the ethical and scientific methodological aspects of the proposed studies. As these activities are often very complex, it is necessary that in the ethical committee, there are different components to be able to discuss scientific and non-scientific aspects, before authorizing and create a research protocol.

Specifically, the Ethics Committees must include, in accordance with the law:

(a) three clinicians;
(b) a local general practitioner;
(c) a pediatrician;
(d) a biostatistician;
(e) a pharmacologist;
(f) a pharmacist of the regional health service;
(g) in relation to studies carried out at its headquarters, the medical director or his permanent substitute and, (and if a "Scientific Hospitalization and Care Institute" (IRCCS) is involved, also the scientific director where the trial is located);
(h) an expert in legal and insurance matters or a medical examiner;
(i) a bioethics expert;
(j) a representative of the field(s) in which the health professionals involved in the trial practice;
(k) a representative of the voluntary service or patient protection associations;
(l) an expert on medical devices;
(m) a clinical engineer or other qualified professional figure in the medical-surgical field of the medical device under study;
(n) a nutrition expert in studies of food on humans;
(o) a clinical expert in the relevant sector in studies of new invasive and semi-invasive technical, diagnostic, and therapeutic procedures;
(p) an expert in genetics in studies on genetics.

It is also preferable that the chairmanship of the Committee be entrusted to a member who is not dependent on the institution itself.

9. In date **January 27, 2014** the article n. 1 of Ministerial Decree February 8, 2013 (Criteria for the composition and functioning of Ethics Committees), by AIFA (Italian Agency of Medicines) has reported the following instructions:

Ethics Committees are independent bodies that are responsible for ensuring the protection of the rights, safety and well-being of persons undergoing trials and for providing a public guarantee of such protection. Where not already assigned to specific bodies, the Ethics Committees can also carry out consultative functions in relation to ethical issues connected with scientific and welfare activities, in order to protect and promote the values of the person. Furthermore, the ethics committees can propose training initiatives for health professionals in relation to bioethical issues.

According to the reorganization of the Ethics Committees, it is also certified that "*the competence of each EC concerns, in addition to the clinical trials of drugs, any other issue on the use of medicines and medical devices, on the use of sur-gical and clinical procedures, on the study on man of food.*"

10. **The AIFA Statement no. 550,** dated May 10, 2017[9] states that:

> *The creation of a coordination center for Ethics Committees at AIFA, the rationalization and reduction of existing ones and the introduction of standard procedures, are elements of absolute innovation. With this legislation new weapons are made available to the public and private research system aimed to compete on an international level and produce research of ever higher quality, creating added value for patients and for the entire research chain.*

The aim is to be able to guarantee:

- the feasibility of a research project in terms of the ethical and scientific correctness of the experiment
- the protection of the rights of subjects taking part in the clinical trial
- the adequacy of the relationships between the center where the research is conducted and the sponsor of the study (the sponsor is the person, company, institution or body that takes responsibility for initiating, managing, and / or financing a clinical trial).
- The ethics committee for clinical trials of medicines has the task of evaluating and validating the adequacy of the applicability of the protocol (objectives, design, conduction, evaluation of the results), the competence and suitability of the researchers, and all ethical aspects, with particular reference to informed consent, data protection and confidentiality to safeguard the rights, safety, and well-being of the subjects in the trial.[10]

11. **AIFA press release, 2017**. "This is excellent news for the healthcare world and for clinical research." This is how the Director General of the Italian Medicines Agency (Mario Melazzini) commented the approval by the Chamber of Deputies. "The measure introduces fundamental innovations, awaited for years, which have the merit of aligning the country with the rest of Europe and with the most advanced realities in the world in the field of clinical trials." The press release repeated the statement that the creation of a coordination center for ethics committees at AIFA adds new weapons to public and private research systems to compete on an international level, producing research of ever higher quality.
12. **Law 1/11/2018, n. 3.** Delegation to the Government in matters of experimentation in clinical medicine as well as provisions for the reorganization of professions health and for the health management of the Ministry of Health. (GU General Series n.25 of Jan.31, 2018).[11] The law contained some provisions that had immediate effect, postponing the definition of many issues to a series of

[9] N17aaa DDL 25 ottobre 2017, Lorenzin.

[10] AIFA Comunicato Stampa n. 550.

[11] GU Serie Generale n.25 del 31-01-2018.

decrees (legislative or ministerial) still to be approved, including the organization and activity of ethics committees.

13. **Ministerial Decree April 19, 2018**: the Ministry of Health regulated the composition of the National Coordination Center of local ethics committees for clinical trials. The Center counts 15 members, including the presidents of the National Bioethics Committee, the National Committee for Biosafety, Biotechnology and Life Sciences and the National Institute of Health. The general manager of AIFA also participates in the meetings of the Coordination Center. The center carries out tasks of coordination, direction and monitoring of the evaluation of the ethical aspects relating to clinical trials on medicinal products for human use, delegated to local ethics committees. It still has the following functions:
    - support and advice, at the request of individual local ethics committees;
    - definition of general directives aimed at ensuring procedural uniformity and compliance with the terms for the assessment by the local ethics committees of clinical trials on medical devices and Phase I, II, III, and IV trials of medicinal products for human use;
    - monitoring the activities of local ethics committees and reporting to their coordinators any non-compliance with the deadlines set by the committees themselves;
    - proposal to the Ministry of Health to suppress a local ethics committee in case of inaction or failure to comply with a regulation;
    - ensure the homogeneity of the administrative, economic and insurance aspects;
    - express an opinion, at the request of AIFA, for clinical studies that need to be reviewed following the reporting of adverse events;
    - identifies the local ethics committee should the promoter fail to indicate it.[12] Up to 40 local ethics committees will be identified.
14. **AIFA press release, 2018.** Establishment of the national coordination center of territorial ethics committees for clinical trials on medicinal products for human use and medical devices.[13] (GU General Series n.107, May 10, 2018).
15. The national coordination center of local ethics committees for clinical trials concerning medicinal products for human use and medical devices, had been confirmed by The Decree of the Minister of Health dated May 27, 2021. The meetings are attended by **AIFA Director General,** who ensures the coordination of the Center's secretarial functions (June 1, 2021).

Ethics Committees and Biomedical Research

Biomedical research with human subjects requires compliance with precise regulations and well-developed ethical and scientific standards. The guidelines that contribute to this activity are known and held in the highest consideration at international

[12] D.M 19 aprile 2018.

[13] GU Serie Generale n.107 del 10-05-2018.

and local level (see Declaration of Helsinki, CIOMS, GCP, WHO, and ICH guidelines). This ensures that rights are safeguarded and guaranteed, together with the dignity, safety, and well-being of the participants. Research Ethics Committees review all of this and monitor the studies once they begin, follow them up, with surveillance after the study ends.

The Committees have the authority to approve, reject or interrupt studies or request deemed appropriate. The Research Ethics Committees' functions include the identification of risks and benefits and also the evaluation of materials and documents (including checking informed consent and data confidentiality) and any other matters that may affect the ethical acceptability of the research.

Additionally, hospital ethics committees help clinicians address ethical challenges that have been raised in clinical practice. A thorough literature review and other measures serve to convey adequate information. The results in different countries are used in health policies. [14]

Bioethics vs. Medical Ethics[15]

BIOETHICS explains the moral principles of all areas of biomedical science including biotechnology, medicine, politics, law, philosophy, etc.

MEDICAL ETHICS specifically explains moral principles relating to clinical medicine.

Moreover: other details:

Bioethics refers to the ethics of medical and biological research; *medical ethics* is about the ethics of clinical medicine. Medical ethics, however, is a branch of bioethics since it focuses primarily on the ethics of medicine. Bioethics is multidisciplinary as it combines philosophy, law, and history with medicine, health, and nursing. Many terms are used for bioethics, sometimes interchangeably, although there are subtleties of meaning that we tease out below. In general, bioethics has become the main heading under which the others are gathered.

Medical Ethics refers to the ethics of the physician–patient relationship or the provider–patient relationship, including all the provider's general duties to a patient, such as helping the person and avoiding harming him or her, as well as specific rules of conduct, such as maintaining confidentiality. Medical ethics is an old traditional concept with a pedigree dating back to ancient Greece.[12]

Health Care Ethics covers almost the same things as medical ethics but is the preferred term when one aims to be inclusive of other healthcare providers such as nurses and physician-assistants or other members of the health-care team, or

[14] Hajibabaee et al. (2016) and Paternoster (2004–2005).

[15] Wikipedia (2017a, b) and Guraya Salman (2014).

supporters of the healthcare organization who have duties to patients; these include healthcare administrators, chaplains, and others.

Medical Humanities was initially coined to cover philosophical, literary, and humanistic approaches to problems in medicine. As such, medical humanities was thought to include bioethics since ethics is often conceived as an area of study in philosophy and philosophy is in the humanities. However, the usage of the term medical humanities has become more specialized. Now it mainly refers to the use of literature, creative writing or journaling, poetry, and film to increase appreciation for the humanistic, interpersonal, or empathetic aspects of medicine.

What's New About Bioethics?

As we have mentioned, ethical issues in the delivery of medicine go back more than a couple of thousand years. However, as was first noted by the contemporary casuist, Al Jonsen, ancient medical ethics was not a matter debated in the public square. Contemporary bioethics is different in that it engages the public. Such ethical issues are matters of concern at the bedside, in the board room, in legislatures, and debated around the dinner table. The work of bioethicists contributes to these debates but ultimately, bioethics is an ongoing societal dialogue that strives for and often achieves, a pragmatic consensus. It is this institutional and public nature of bioethics that leads so many to seek advanced education concerning bioethics such as graduate degrees.

General Conclusions

The first responsibility of the doctor will always be the care of the patient. Patients need some sort of moral guidance during illness. What they need, besides the proximity of an authoritative professional (the doctor), is also a system that helps them manage an often problematic relationship. The "doctor–patient" relationship is depicted in these terms.

Medical ethics has fostered this concept, promoting the essential values for the good output of a communication that recognizes trust, responsibility, and mutual respect. Certain ethical standards, including informed consent, privacy protection and confidentiality, provide additional benefit. They help build support for the same medical care. People—especially when in need—want to be able to trust quality and integrity in exchanges regarding health promotion and clarifications.

The purpose of doctor–patient interviews is therefore to help the patient cope with illness, disability, and death, or anyway relieve suffering. In all cases the doctor will have to help maintain the dignity of his patients and respect their autonomy. Some aspects of medical ethics are fundamental and timeless—basic in order not to delude the patient's expectations and to ensure the probity of the doctor himself regarding the appropriate care.

Doctor-Patient Relationship

This singular relationship can be presented as the natural conclusion of the long historical journey that medicine and ethics have made together, sometimes chasing each other or pushing each other ahead in order to reach the same final decision. Briefly, these are the main moments:

From Hippocrates' time, and perhaps even before then, to the present day there has been frequent confrontation between doctors and their clients. Doctors were initially taught how they should behave towards their patients to maximize the beneficial effects of their care. They had to reduce the risks and dangers arising from worry, errors or carelessness, in acute and chronic diseases.

"The relationship between doctors and patients has received philosophical, sociological and literary attention from Hippocrates onwards, and is the subject of around 8000 articles, monographs, chapters and books in modern medical literature".[16] Among the main functions (of the relationship) were the collection and communication of information, the development and maintenance of a therapeutic relationship, and the exchange of data from clinical programs. Doctors can and must observe many principles to maintain professional standards and sustain public trust.

It is hard to back the idea—which has lasted for millennia—that patients always follow their doctor's advice or directives, so it is hardly surprising that this particular controversy between patients and doctors may have created misunderstanding, confusion, and even a certain acrimony over time. In duties, doctors must always be ready to provide professional assistance to anyone who needs or expressly requests it, regardless of personal advantage. The "sick person" has always been expected to trust his doctor almost without being allowed to ask questions.[17] However, the "barriers" in communication can be put up by both parties. *"The indications of the doctor in the diagnostic and therapeutic fields frequently require, on the part of the patient, significant and often unpleasant changes in behavior. It follows that the patient generally tends to resist or oppose the prescriptions, all the more when he clearly sees the unpleasant effects but the advantages are not so clear."*

Similar situations can arise in the most complex situations and inevitably lead not only to a change in the relationship but also to inefficient therapeutic strategy.

More than the deontological ethics of the doctor's oath, in ancient times the teleological ethics of the virtues of Platonic origin were strongly present. For the early centuries of the Christian era, during the Middle Ages and the Renaissance, the rules governing the healer–patient relationship were based on the Hippocratic Oath, which circulated in a variety of translations and a variety of formulations.

The Hippocratic Oath actually makes no mention of the obligation for doctors to converse with patients. Specific duties are indicated differently: "... according to my ability, my judgment I consider a (therapeutic) regimen for the benefit of one of my patients and I refrain from anything harmful and malevolent." In "Decorum," which is part of the "Corpus Hippocraticum," Hippocrates admonished doctors to

---

[16] Goold (1999).

[17] Bert (2006).

"... do their duty calmly and skillfully, withholding most of the information from the patient while he is being treated."

Doctor and their patients, as it has been taking shape in the Western world, followed a precise order: the doctor's duty is to do the patients' good and the patient's duty is to accept it. In this "paternalistic" relationship the doctor's moral responsibility lies in the certainty that he is working for the absolute good of the patient.[14]

Without wishing to go deeper into this difficult question and even less to offer any quick solution to what can now be considered an everyday problem, it is worth contemplating how the doctor's word might have been taken, since ancient times. It is certainly interesting, stimulating—or even depressing at times—to be aware of the widely differing situations and the most varied and perhaps unexpected countries that may have encountered this substantial problem of ethics or personal or general morals.

There are of course different types of doctor–patient relationship, including:

- a contractual model, as presented by Hugo Engelhardt (Texas, 1941), according to which the principle of autonomy is more important than the principle of charity, but always with an ethical orientation;
- a utilitarian model, according to which "a norm is good when it produces the best good";
- the paternalistic models of the USA authors Pellegrino (1920–2013), and Thomasma (1930) according to which the best model is centered on the therapeutic alliance: the doctor must not only do physical good for the patient, but also psychological, social, and spiritual good, as well as enhancing autonomy and rediscovering mutual trust;
- a model by Veatch, currently a professor of medical ethics, according to which there must be a contractual relationship between doctor and patient which, however, must be based on the five fundamental points (autonomy, justice, keep promises, tell the truth, and do not kill).

Why is this? Starting from the concepts of right or wrong behavior over the course of history, we get to the current code of ethics. As a result, it is not the succession of events that is the most important: it is medical ethics itself, implying how to manage and guarantee the moral problems relating to the care of patients.

As an academic discipline, medical ethics includes the application of moral values and judgments to medical practice, its history, its philosophy and sociology.

Further clarification can be gained from the four fundamental principles of health ethics (commented several times in the text): autonomy, justice, beneficence, and no-harm.

References to the doctor–patient relationship appear frequently in various texts, indicating that the topic has been very much present and debated throughout the history of medical ethics. They are found in the current text from the time of Hippocrates, then in Rome, in the Middle Ages, among Jews and Muslims, and very often from the times of Gregory and Percival, from the early nineteenth century to today. The doctor–patient situation has changed considerably in all this time and medicine has acquired at least three new fundamental scientific values:

1. Treatment: diagnostic, prevention, treatment, and health promotion practices;
2. The availability of [modern] medical-surgical and therapeutic preparations;
3. The patient's new attitude—no longer just submissive and fearful, but collaborative and determined to heal.

Over time, a further predominant feature, the ethical one, has been added to the unquestionable basic requirements.

A thoughtful, meticulous report has recently been published[18] and others can be cited which, although starting from ancient Egypt, also come down to present times, and in any case always draw attention to the priority of the "patient" as an individual who experiences rather than just being the object of some disease or condition.[19]

The doctor's word is certainly important but in the end—and informed consent contemplates it—trust must be earned through conversation with the patient.

Thus one can glimpse a double truth, that of the patient, with all his fears and uncertainties and that of the doctor, with all his knowledge and diagnostic confidence. Ultimately, patient-centered medicine is "medicine for two people," so "the doctor and the patient influence each other at all times and cannot be considered separately" [rif?].

Sometimes they match and sometimes they don't, as everyone knows, often from personal experience.

Doctors "do not (always) agree with the theological principles of physics," as Albert the Great recalled in his work Metaphysica around 1270. This is still true, perhaps with fewer symptomatic doubts, but for this very reason with greater risks in application.

This new "therapeutic alliance," between doctor and client is certainly centered on the latter and leads to "understanding the complaints offered by the patient, the symptoms and signs found by the doctor, not only in terms of illness, but also as an expression of the patient's singular individuality, his conflicts and his problems," as already proposed in 1964.[20] Other authors also reached similar conclusions,[16] confirming the foundations for today's medical ethics, likely to be dominant from the twenty-first century onward.

The priority of life, beyond the simple jokes of politicians, religious figures or "*maîtres à penser*" in the most widely differing areas of science or daily existence, is invariably the object of public relations, private confidences or other reasoned expressions of the human race. Inevitably, we come to talk about health and the more or less habitual relationships between doctor and health worker, between us and our own doctor. Already St. John Paul II, at the Congress of the Italian Society

---

[18] Spinsanti (2010) and Paternoster (2005).

[19] Kaba and Sooriakumaran (2007) and Szasz and Hollender (1956).

[20] Balint (1964, 1969).

of General Surgery, in October 1980, insisted that "The patient–doctor relationship must return to being based on a dialogue made up of listening, respect, and interest."

Only in this way do "trust" and "conscience" meet and bring benefits, which may be vital. Most of the time they are in fact heedless of the socio-economic or religious reality in which they arise.

References

Balint M. The doctor, his patient and the illness. London: Pittman Medical; 1964.

Balint E. The possibilities of patient-centered medicine. J R Coll Gen Pract. 1969;17(82):269–76.

Bert G. Difference between bioethics and medical ethics Ethics in medical research. Recenti Progressi in Medicina. 2006;97(10):548–55.

Filosa AM. Legislazione e Ruolo dei Comitati Etici. Approvazione degli aspetti etico-scientifici da parte di un organismo competente (IT. Role of Ethics Committees. Approval of the ethical-scientific aspects by a competent body) Diritto.it; 1996.

Goold SD. The doctor-patient relationship (Challenges, opportunities and strategies). J Gen Int Med. 1999;14(Supp.1):S26–33.

Guraya Salman NM. Differenza tra bioetica ed etica medica Etica nella ricerca medica (IT. Difference between bioethics and medical ethics Ethics in medical research). N.p.; September 2014.

Hajibabaee F, Joolaee S, Cheraghi MA, Salari P, Rodney P. Hospital/clinical ethics committees' notion: an overview. J Med Ethics Hist Med. 2016;9:17.

Istituto di Ricerche Farmacologiche Mario Negri, Mosconi P, Apolone G. I comitati etici: ruolo e funzionamento. (IT. The ethics committees: role and functioning). Milano; 2 Feb 2007.

Kaba R, Sooriakumaran P. The evolution of the doctor-patient relationship. Int J Surg. 2007;5(1):57–65.

Mosconi P, Colombo C, Labianca R, Apolone G. Oncologists' opinions about research ethics committees in Italy: an update, 2004. European J Cancer Prev. 2006;15:91–4.

McLean SAM. What and who are clinical ethics committees for? J Med Ethics. 2007;33:497–500.

Paternoster M. Analisi comparativa dell'attività dei comitati etici nei principali paesi europei (IT. Comparative analysis of the activity of ethics committees in the main European countries). Dottorato di Ricerca in Ambiente, Prevenzione e Medicina Pubblica, Università degli Studi di Napoli Federico II, Facoltà di Medicina e Chirurgia. A.A; 2004–2005.

Spinsanti S. Cambiamenti nella relazione tra Medico e Paziente (IT. Changes in the relationship between Doctor and Patient). Enciclopedia Treccani online; 2010.

Szasz TS, Hollender M. The basic models of the doctor-patient relationship. Arch Intern Med. 1956;97:585–92.

Wikipedia. Bioetica ed etica medica (IT. Bioethics and medical ethics). Riflessioni morali. N.p., 03 febbraio 2010. Web. 02 May 2017a.

Wikipedia. "Principi di bioetica". Strumenti bioetici: principi di bioetica (IT. "Principles of bioethics". Bioethical tools: principles of bioethics). N.p., n.d. Ragnatela. 02 May 2017b.

Update to Years 2020, 2021, and 2022, with Information on COVID-19

18

This part of the text was added to the first edition after its publication, in Italian, in 2019. Here a few information are summarized on Medical Ethics in the years 2020, 2021, and early 2022. Some significant details of COVID-19 are explained.

Introductory Notes

Monsignor A. Manto, aged 53 y.o., doctor and lecturer at the Pontifical Lateran University, reflected on what is happening during the COVID-19 pandemic and its implications for the protection of health. He also commented on the bioethical aspects of the pandemic, and its social and economic repercussions throughout the world.[1]

> *I think no one can say they are ready to take this challenge alone. The challenge of an epidemic caused by a new virus, for which there is a lack of antibodies in the population and of an effective medical treatment, cannot be faced in isolation. It is necessary to share knowledge in the scientific community and to coordinate public health interventions. Nor can we face the challenge of developing ethical principles and medical ethics only unilaterally if under the pressure of an emergency.*

These straightforward words set me off on a quick excursus in the field of epidemics and pandemics.

[1] Quotidianosanità.it, (IT. Online newspaper), March 16, 2020.

R. G. Russo, *Medical Ethics*, https://doi.org/10.1007/978-3-031-42444-1_18

Infectious Diseases

Infectious diseases, mainly caused by viruses, bacteria or protozoa, which can be classified as micro-parasites, have spread throughout human history. They almost always developed following a similar pattern: an initial outbreak that resulted in an epidemic, and sometimes a pandemic, with different durations.[2]

In recent years, three such events have occurred, casting useful light for studying and understanding these diseases:

1. Establishment and implementation of an international infectious disease surveillance network, focusing on old and new diseases, sporadic, endemic or pandemic;
2. Advances in molecular diagnostics and sequencing techniques that offer important new possibilities for the control of various infectious diseases, and related basic and advanced diagnostics, resistance monitoring, mutations, etc.;
3. Prevention and therapy with new vaccines and improvement of those already available, and development and use of further antiviral drugs.

Summarized below are some of the main terms used in the scientific literature and sometimes also in the media. These are just succinct explanations, before we look more closely into the current pathology (known as COVID-19) and the questions of medical ethics it raises.

Viruses[3]

Viruses may have existed since the evolution of the first living cells. Despite attempts with molecular techniques to identify DNA or RNA in ancient fossils, it is still considered impossible to date them precisely.

Viral genetic material can occasionally be transmitted in the germline of host organisms, their descendants having integrated the virus into their own genome. This provides valuable information for virologists to trace the ancient viruses that existed freely up to millions of years ago. Some may have evolved from plasmids, or from transposons and retrotransposons, or as degradation products of the DNA of a cell, or even during the RNA phase of the world—that is, before the origin of life as we know it (see Footnote 3).

We have recently witnessed, as was to be expected, the intense production of texts and publications dealing with viruses and their characteristics. One of the first to be released on the market—and which became very popular in Italy—is

---

[2]Atti della Accademia Lancisiana: Anno Accademico 2018-2019, Seduta Inaugurale, (IT. Proceedings of the Lancisiana Academy: Academic Year 2018-2019, Inaugural Session), November 6, 2018, Vol. 63, no 1, January–March, 2019.
Weston et al. (2018).

[3]Anderson and May (1991).
Wikipedia: Virus.

mentioned.[4] As early as 1892, however, an article by Dmitri Ivanovsky described a non-bacterial pathogen capable of infecting tobacco plants; since then, some 5000 viruses have been described in detail, though there are probably millions. Viruses are found in almost all ecosystems on Earth and constitute the most abundant biological entity of all; they can exist as independent and inactive particles. Diseases attributable to viruses are defined acute (when the necessary treatments and investigations require hospitalization of the infected patient and/or when death occurs); recurrent (when there are repeated waves of more or less intensity in the population); non-appearing (when there are dormant infections without the virus being traceable); and sub-clinical (when there are no symptoms even though the virus is traceable).

A human being's immune response (natural and acquired) is either humoral or cellular. The most important humoral mechanism is complement activation and the acquired response gives rise to antibodies. The most important cell mechanism in the natural response is the activation of macrophages and natural killer (NK) cells, while in acquired immunity CD4+ and CD8+ lymphocytes are activated. Cytokines play a major role in both responses. The immune response can apparently range from non-existence to persistence throughout life in the patient, or it can cause what is known as chronic immune pathology, when a disease is induced directly by the immune response.[5,6,7,8,9,10,11,12,13]

Influenza viruses can be spread through coughing, sneezing, and droplets of saliva. Noroviruses and rotaviruses—common causes of viral gastroenteritis—are transmitted by the fecal-oral route, but can also pass from person to person through direct contact with food and drink. In infected cells viruses lose their structural individuality, which consists of nucleic acids, and their derivatives take over part of the cell's biosynthesis work, and produce new virions (single viral particles).

---

[4] Lodish et al. (2000). Section 6.3, Viruses: Structure, Function, and Uses. New York: W. H. Freeman, 2000.
Burioni (2020).

[5] Shors (2008).

[6] Barry (2004), Osterholm (2005), and Browne (2006).

[7] OMS, World Health Organization (2019).

[8] Selgelid (2005) and Selgelid et al. (2011).

[9] McIvor (2016).

[10] Upshur (2008).

[11] DuVal et al. (2005).

[12] Grady et al. (2001).

[13] Quarantena, Wikipedia.
Quarantena. Vocabolario Treccani *on line, Istituto dell'Enciclopedia Italiana,* Institute of the Italian Encyclopedia.

RNA Viruses

RNA viruses can be classified in to four different groups based on how they replicate. A first inspection establishes whether the genetic material is single or double stranded. All RNA viruses use their own enzymes and replicate to make copies of their genomes. Lacking the tools necessary to produce proteins and metabolize sugars, viruses need a host cell to proliferate. The number of genes in the RNA chain varies from 3 to 250, fewer even than those of a simple bacterium.

Some of the best-known viral diseases are measles, mumps, respiratory syncytial infection, influenza, rabies, hepatitis A, common cold (caused by over 200 different types), poliomyelitis, rubella, HIV/AIDS, severe acute respiratory syndrome (SARS), West Nile/encephalitis, and Ebola/hemorrhagic fever.

Effects on the Host Cell

Viruses have a wide range of structural and biochemical effects on the host cell, called cytopathic effects. Most viral infections eventually cause the death of the host cell due to lysis, changes in the cell's surface membrane, and apoptosis—a form of programmed cell death. Some viruses cause no apparent changes to the infected cell.

Epidemiology

Viral epidemiology is a branch of medical science that studies the transmission and control of infections in humans. They can be transmitted at home between relatives of the same family, or passed from one person to another; the latter appears to be the most common route of diffusion. The virus can be transmitted, as already mentioned, by inhalation or in exhaled airborne droplets of saliva. The rate or speed of transmission of viral infections depends on various factors including population density, the number of non-immune individuals, the quality of health care, and the continuing infectious capacity of the virus.

Once identified, the chain of transmission can sometimes be interrupted by a vaccine; when this is not available, adequate measures of hygiene, disinfection and isolation of infected people ("quarantine"—*see below*) are recommended (see Footnote 5).

Outbreaks

Infectious disease outbreaks often involve scientific uncertainty, social and institutional perturbation, and a general climate of fear and mistrust. It is essential, first of all, to identify the virus and its source(s). Public health professionals, on the orders of policy makers, are required to assess and prioritize ethical values dictated by the time available and the economic and scientific resources to draw on.

We speak of an epidemic when an infectious disease increases the number of cases in a community or a well-defined area. To identify the origin, an epidemiological investigation of the infection is needed and, ideally, the movements of those affected should be mapped.

Epidemic

This term refers to the frequent and localized manifestation, limited in time, of an infectious disease, with widespread transmission of the causal virus. An epidemic occurs when a sick person infects more than one person and the number of cases rises steeply.

The World Health Organization (WHO) recommends that states prepare themselves, in compliance with International Health Regulations (IHR), to be able to ensure maximum protection against the spread of diseases from one country to another. WHO recommends proceeding gradually with deciding on the means to be prepared and the measures to be adopted, to take account of the level of risk.

WHO constantly monitors the circulation of viruses to detect potential pandemic risks: 153 institutions in 114 countries are involved in global surveillance and responses. The Organization calls on the collaboration of proven scientific personnel to formulate the correct diagnosis, identify vaccines and specific antiviral treatments.

Pandemic

This is the spread of a disease in several continents or in any case in large areas of the world. The WHO distinguishes five phases: Interpandemic—Alert—Pandemic—Transition—Final. In the last century, new epidemics have appeared, often causing pandemics. Several influenza waves (1918, 1957, 1968, and 2009) and the spread of AIDS (starting from 1983) have shown their transmissibility. The SARS coronavirus spread between 2002 and 2004, followed by avian flu in 2005/2006. In spring 2009, the H1N1 flu virus also spread, causing fever, cough, cold, sore throat, chills, headache, muscle and joint pain, exhaustion, and lack of appetite. In 2013 Ebola plagued the population of West Africa. The whole world is currently facing a pandemic which started in 2019 (COVID-19, Corona Virus Disease).

In a pandemic, firm decisions must be made to contain the spread of the disease, regarding the allocation of resources, antivirus treatments or vaccines, the need for restrictive measures and isolation of infected people (quarantine), the level of risk for health workers, and restriction of people's movements.

In less well-informed times, in broad terms and with different degrees of scientific approximation, this situation was already tackled in some fairly old publications (see Footnote 6).

1. In 1918 a new flu virus was identified, which came to be known as the cause of Spanish flu. Experts now think that pandemic may have led to at least 40 million deaths but it has been speculatively suggested that the death toll might have reached 100 million. Even taking the lowest estimate and without adjusting for population growth (up 250%), that virus caused more people to die in 24 weeks than AIDS has in 24 years.

   Most of the viruses responsible for pandemics have originated in Asia, but every nation must be involved in the development and production of vaccines, providing the producers with the necessary guarantees and subsidies. Antiviral drugs can limit the severity of an attack and in some cases even prevent disease; the prophylactic effects last as long as they are taken. Legal and ethical issues affecting public health need to be resolved promptly (Barry 2004 (see Footnote 6)).
2. The production of a vaccine takes at least 6 months, once the circulating strain has been isolated. An international action plan must be agreed for the use of antiviral drugs, to encourage the production of masks to protect the respiratory tract, antibiotics for the treatment of secondary bacterial infections, and detailed burial plans to manage the enormous number of corpses (Osterholm 2005 (see Footnote 6)).
3. Early on in the pandemic it was said that by 2020 it would become common practice to wear surgical masks (or those indicated FFP2) and perhaps rubber gloves in public, to prevent the epidemic developing its most serious form—a disease similar to pneumonia—which can affect both lungs and the bronchi and tends to be refractory to traditional treatments.
4. COVID will be particularly disconcerting because, after having caused a winter of absolute panic, it will seem to disappear completely for another 10 years, making it even more difficult to discover its cause and develop a cure (Browne 2006 (see Footnote 6)).

Ethics in Infectious Diseases

Five main ethical problems arise from the need to control infectious diseases:

1. support for infected people: adequate and recurrent care;
2. vaccines—when available they can be made mandatory from the epidemic phase;
3. isolation—infected individuals are asked to isolate themselves for a certain time while receiving the necessary medical care;
4. quarantine—an adequate period of isolation recommended for infected individuals, but also as a precaution for healthy potential carriers;
5. travel and movement restrictions, in order to prevent the spread of the disease.

A few reports illustrate the topic.

1. **WHO** (see Footnote 7)

Already on 20 January 2019, this international organization recalled the need to protect the health of the whole of humanity from epidemics of known diseases that can be prevented with vaccines (examples are measles and diphtheria), from an increase in drug-resistant pathogens, from rising rates of obesity due to physical inactivity, environmental pollution, climate change, and multiple humanitarian crises.

It was also hypothesized that new potential pandemics could arise that would seriously affect a large part of the world population. To address these and other threats, a 5-year strategic plan was laid out in 2019, implemented by WHO for the period 2019–2023.

2. **M.J. Selgelid** (see Footnote 8) argued that infectious disease should be recognized as a topic of primary importance for bioethics, but it has received relatively little attention compared to abortion, euthanasia, genetics, cloning, and stem cell research. The main ethical issues associated with pandemic planning are the following:
   (a) The consequences of the infection
   (b) Ethical issues—extremely hard to address
   (c) Justice and fairness as a central concern of ethics (especially in developing countries).

      Besides the dominant threat to global health, there may be tangible differences between different ethnicities or races. Individuals with infectious diseases such as AIDS or tuberculosis in particular are often stigmatized.

      A true understanding of the impact of an infectious disease on individuals and the community requires the integration of microbiology, immunology, clinical medicine, epidemiology, psychology, geography, anthropology, zoology, and many other disciplines. Unfortunately, only very few people have the competence necessary to achieve this.

3. **McIvor J**. (see Footnote 9)

   Ethical conclusions can be drawn about various infectious diseases through their similarities with or differences from other similar diseases. On the basis of their taxonomy (classification), the causes of the diseases themselves can be identified, as well as their control and important ethical considerations in a quick, organized and reasonable way. The result is a "ranking of infectious diseases" based on the ethically most important biological characteristics. The main questions related to their control, might be:
   (a) When is it appropriate to use an experimental treatment?
   (b) When is quarantine or isolation ethically justified?
   (c) What are the key ethical principles to be applied?
   (d) Do ethical principles differ between diseases? The ethical view can differ according to the physical differences between diseases.

4. **Upshur R.** (see Footnote 10)

   The surgeon general of the United States of America, William Stewart, said in 1967: "The time has come to close the book on infectious diseases. We [have] practically wiped out infection in the United States." This comment, however, was contradicted by later and even contemporary events. For example, from

1940 to 2004, especially in the 1970s and 1980s, several hundred new infectious diseases emerged, many of them zoonotic and bacterial. Infectious diseases are still an open book, as documented by historians.

A thematic issue of the Bioethics magazine in 2005 (see Footnote 11) is divided into 6 parts. Part I explores the relationship between bioethics and infectious diseases. Part II deals with ethics and their control; Part III deals with problems relating to the treatment of infected individuals; Part IV looks at ethical issues relating to mass vaccination programs; Part V devotes particular attention to developing countries and global health; Part VI addresses the bioethical conclusions of security, and "bioterrorism," This dossier will be particularly useful for public health or clinical ethics bodies.

5. **Grady C.** (see Footnote 12)

   In addition to the ethical issues already tackled by international organizations, these authors looked at some current ethical dilemmas: the treatment of participants in a clinical trial, informed consent, the obligations of researchers towards the study community, and the response to local health needs.

   The need for an ethical approach to serious communicable diseases was obvious during the outbreak of severe acute respiratory syndrome (SARS) in early 2003. Already then, the universal vulnerability of humans to communicable diseases and the need for coordinated and cooperative responses across national borders was evident. As the crisis deepened and restrictions were imposed, concerns remained about access to care, the allocation of medicines, the availability of safety equipment and the sharing of vital information. Specific information and conditions are constantly shifting and implementation decisions need to be made quickly.

Current Pandemic and Epidemic Risks Around the World

Chikungunya, cholera, Crimean-Congo hemorrhagic fever, Ebola virus disease, Hendra virus infection, influenza (pandemic, seasonal, zoonotic), Lassa fever, Marburg virus disease, meningitis, MERS-CoV, Monkeypox, Nipah virus infection, Plague, Rift Valley Fever, SARS, Smallpox, tularemia, yellow fever, Zika virus disease, Coronavirus (COVID-19).

Quarantine (See Footnote 13)

Quarantine, occasionally mentioned as *absentia*, is a period of isolation and observation for people who might be carriers of infectious germs. It is normally observed for *40 days*. The etymology of the word historically refers to the 40-day isolation imposed in the fourteenth century in Venice for ships and their crews coming from areas affected by the plague: in the Venetian language *quaranténa*. The earliest forms of quarantine are described for lepers in the Old Testament (Deut. 7:15; Lev. 5: 2,3; 13: 1–2; 14: 8,9; Num. 9:16) and in the writings of Hippocrates. The duration of 40 days was considered long enough for diagnosing chronic or acute diseases.

Venice was followed by Reggio Emilia in 1374 and Genoa in 1467. The first isolation hospital (Santa Maria di Nazareth) was founded in Venice in 1403 on a small island facing the lagoon. It was still used in 1799 for 225,000 slaves and immigrants, possible carriers of leprosy or plague.

In America, the first quarantine regulations were drawn up only in 1643 by the Massachusetts Bay Colony, against ships coming from Europe, then later from the United Kingdom, which in 1663 made it compulsory for plague sufferers. France followed in 1681; then Boston, New York and Philadelphia to combat yellow fever and smallpox epidemics in 1797.

Quarantine was reported to have returned in the early 1980s, with AIDS, and after the catastrophic attack of 11 September 2001, when the fear of biological weapons spread in the United States. Quarantine was also imposed for the SARS epidemic and later for Ebola (2014). In 2019, around 60 million people were quarantined in the Chinese province of Hubei (the Wuhan region) as a containment measure related to the COVID-19 epidemic.

Since 25 March 2020 around three billion people have been banned from leaving home, to prevent the spread of the virus.[14] An Ordinance of the Italian Ministry of Health (Official Gazette 22 February 2020) set the duration of the quarantine at 14 days.

The Ethical Issues of Quarantine[15]

The relationship between individual rights and the need to safeguard collective health will be one of the open themes and knots that humanity will have to unravel. It is neither easy nor painless to expect all the inhabitants of one or more cities to observe quarantine even though since the Middle Ages isolation of the sick has been used to protect the rest of society. With the discovery of antibiotics and vaccines, humanity seemed to have overcome forever the need to resort to drastic measures to combat and contain epidemics, but it was not to be.

Recent events have raised serious ethical questions about the solutions. The quarantine imposed to stem the pandemic spread of the virus involved measures that also limited individual rights to some extent. Tracking and recognition systems have been adopted as well, but they too are not respectful of citizens' privacy, and easily lend themselves to abuses that affect people's freedom.

[14] Popular Mechanics, New York, N.Y., U.S.A. March 6, 2020.
Post Editor, Milano, March 25, 2020, Time, London, May 18, 2020.

[15] Willis (2020).

Coronavirus[16]

It is estimated that the common ancestor of all existing coronaviruses has already existed for millions of years. Coronaviruses, a group of RNA viruses, are carriers of diseases in mammals and birds. These are "obligate" intracellular micro-parasites and can only multiply inside a living "host" cell. They were first discovered in the 1930s, in domestic poultry, when it was shown that an acute respiratory infection was caused by a bronchitis virus, which also caused gastrointestinal, liver, and neurological damage in the animals examined. Coronaviruses generally cause most of the colds that hit us throughout the year.

Identified in the 1960s, only seven coronaviruses are known to cause disease in humans. There is more than one type of coronavirus. Their genome size ranges from approximately 26 to 32 kb, which puts them among the largest RNA viruses. They are common in people and animals including bats, camels, cats, and cattle. SARS-CoV-2, the virus that causes COVID-19 originated in bats, similarly to MERS and SARS. Four coronaviruses frequently cause the symptoms of the common cold (serotypes 229E, OC43, NL63, and HUK1). Three others cause much more serious, sometimes fatal, respiratory infections (SARS-CoV in 2003, MERS-CoV in 2012, and SARS-CoV-2 in 2019 were identified). SARS-CoV-2 is the virus responsible for the disease called COVID-19. Among the human coronaviruses that have their origin in bats the ancestors of SARS-CoV initially infected those of the genus Hipposideridae, Rhinolophidae, then Asian palm civets and finally humans.[17]

Since SARS-CoV-2 only recently emerged as a human pathogen, and researchers are still not certain about its origins, it is often referred to as "a new coronavirus" and there is still great uncertainty about its transmission in different parts of the world. It can be transmitted between people through direct or indirect contact, just like other respiratory viruses that have been circulating in the human population for decades.[18]

There are some clear definitions so far:

A Confirmed Positive Case is a subject with the new coronavirus that has been tested and confirmed by the Centers for Disease Control and Prevention or the Ministry of Health.

An Alleged Positive Case subject with the new coronavirus that has been tested by a local or commercial laboratory, but has not been confirmed.

Isolation—The Ministry of Health can impose isolation for people affected by COVID-19; it can oblige patients to remain in their homes, or in the hospital ward where they have been admitted.

---

[16] Masters (2006).
Wikipedia. Coronavirus.

[17] Quammen (2012).

[18] Moriyama et al. (2020).

Transmission of the Coronavirus

The coronavirus mainly spreads from person to person, most often by coughing or sneezing. Droplets can be sprayed at a distance up to almost 2 m. When you breathe them in, the viruses can enter your body. Some individuals remain asymptomatic, but they can still spread the virus.

If the virus reaches a surface or an object it can live for several hours, and then later can infect a person's mouth, nose or possibly the eyes. For example, SARS-CoV-2 can persist on various surfaces for specified times. On copper for 4 h; on cardboard for up to 24 h; on plastic or stainless steel for 2–3 days. It is therefore important to disinfect surfaces.

Some dogs and cats have tested positive for the virus, but there is no evidence that they can transmit the virus to humans.

Incubation Period

This refers to the time between exposure to a virus and the first manifestation of symptoms. The incubation period for the new coronavirus can be from 2 to14 days.

Death Rate

Scientists and public health officials have estimated that the new coronavirus has a death rate of around 1%. The precise figure is not yet known, as asymptomatic patients typically do not seek treatment and are therefore not counted as survivors in the fatal accident pool.

Asymptomatic: a patient infected but showing no symptoms of COVID-19. Scientists believe the new coronavirus can spread in asymptomatic people.

High risk: this is generally related to age and/or underlying health risks, including people whose immune systems are compromised.

Ventilator: a device that introduces oxygenated air into the lungs of a person who is unable to breathe independently.

ARDS—"Acute respiratory distress syndrome." This serious complication can affect 1% of people infected with the virus, and many need ventilators for several whole weeks. The ARDS causes deaths in 30–40% of patients.

Vaccines/Therapy—Testing vaccines started in March 2020 and WHO announced that as of 23 April 2020, 83 potential COVID-19 vaccines were being evaluated[19] six have now been approved for human testing in clinical trials.

At present, there is no specific drug treatment for COVID-19. People who have a mild infection need treatment to relieve their symptoms, such as rest, fluids, and fever control.

[19] ISS Bioethics COVID-19 Working Group (2021).

Cycle of Disease with the Coronavirus

The viral pathogenesis comprises five main events:

1. The virus enters the host.
2. The virus replicates at the site of entry.
3. It diffuses from the implantation site.
4. It disseminates to target organs.
5. The virus is eliminated from the body and the infection is resolved.

Risk Factors

People over the age of 65 are more likely to have serious illness, as are those living in nursing homes or long-term care facilities, with weakened immune systems, or with mildly debilitating conditions, such as hypertension, heart disease, lung disease, asthma, kidney disease requiring dialysis, obesity, diabetes, cancer treatment (chemotherapy), liver disease, cigarette smoking (see Footnote 18).

Ethical Questions[20]

Of paramount importance is the necessity to protect the most vulnerable people.

A frequent problem is the allocation of medical resources. Serious situations have required important and burdensome decisions about who should receive the proper medical care and the protection afforded to all health care workers. Some regulations and guidelines have been prepared in this regard. A paper by the American bio-law expert Lawrence Gostin (see Footnote 20) in 2003 argued, following the spread of acute respiratory syndrome (SARS):

> a few coercive measures have been implemented, which, although violating individual rights, were found to be acceptable.

COVID-19

Symptoms

The first cases of COVID-19 relate to a live animal market in Wuhan, capital of the Hubei province in China, with a population of 19 million; Hubei province has a population of 58 million. These cases suggested that the virus was initially transmitted from animals to humans.[21]

[20] CBHD Staff (2020) and Gostin et al. (2003).

[21] Ren et al. (2020).

The outbreak in December 2019 indicated the main symptoms of the new disease (96%): fever, cough, shortness of breath, trouble breathing, fatigue, chills (sometimes with agitation), muscle aches, headache, sore throat, anosmia or ageusia (loss of sense of taste or smell), nausea, diarrhea. A striking feature of this virus is the rapid progression of respiratory failure soon after the onset of dyspnea and hypoxemia.

Patients with severe COVID-19 may also experience: acute onset of bilateral infiltrates, severe hypoxemia, pulmonary edema, heart failure (see ARDS), lymphopenia, central or peripheral nervous system disorders, heart, kidney, acute liver injury, cardiac arrhythmias, rhabdomyolysis, coagulopathy.

Worldwide, the WHO Stated on 11 March 2020 That the Disease Is a Pandemic[22]

A concomitant finding is a cytokine release syndrome, manifested by high fever, thrombocytopenia, and steep increases in inflammatory markers. This can lead to interstitial pneumonia, causing respiratory failure, septic shock, and death. Many complications can be caused by the various organs sharing the infection. People over the age of 65 are more likely to contract serious illness, especially those in nursing homes or in long-term care facilities, with a weakened immune system or with hypertension, heart disease, lung disease, asthma, kidney disease requiring dialysis, obesity, diabetes, cancer treatment (chemotherapy), liver disease, cigarette smoking.

SARS-CoV-2 recognizes interpersonal spread, but asymptomatic people can also spread the virus. In this regard, WHO and European authorities continue to encourage people to take care of their health and protect others:

- wash your hands frequently with soap and water or using a hand sanitizer product;
- maintain social distances (keep an interpersonal distance of at least 1 m);
- avoid touching your eyes, nose, and mouth;
- follow respiratory hygiene (covering your mouth and nose with a mask or behind an elbow when necessary);
- seek medical attention early if you have a fever, cough and breathing difficulties; And
- keep informed and follow the advice provided by health professionals.

[22] WHO Europe: COVID-19 outbreak a pandemic, 12-03-2020.
Lauer et al. (2020), Crist (2020a), Leung et al. (2020), Cubeta et al. (2020), Chow et al. (2020), and Smith (2020a, b).
Cochrane: COVID-19 Study Register, Special collection. 2020.
NEJM collection, Vol. 382 No. 25, June 18, 2020.
Fauci et al. (2020) and Rubin et al. (2020).

Other symptoms may also be present, but are less frequent: chills, aches, headaches, fatigue, and digestive system problems such as nausea, abdominal pain, vomiting or diarrhea. Conditions that may put a person at greater risk for severe COVID-19 are: asthma, dementia, cerebrovascular diseases (e.g., stroke), cystic fibrosis, hypertension, reduced immune defenses, pregnancy, liver disease, pulmonary fibrosis, cigarette smoking, type 1 diabetes, thalassemia.

Intensity and Severity

Scientists do not define the virus as a living being. Viruses have no metabolism and cannot grow or respond when stimulated. To reproduce, as we already explained, they need a host organism. When SARS-CoV-2 enters a host cell, a series of complex chemical reactions take place that enable it to reproduce. Our body responds with a fever, as our immune system activates itself to attack the virus.

SARS-CoV-2, which probably entered in France in the late 2019,[23] is one of the three types of coronaviruses that can cause serious illness[24] along with Middle East Respiratory Syndrome (MERS) and Sudden Acute Respiratory Syndrome (SARS). It spreads the same way as other coronaviruses. The virus can also infect people at low risk of consequences; in these cases the complications are generally mild or moderate,[25] especially in children and young adults. The precautions specified by the Ministry of Health must also be observed, in order to reduce the possibility of contagion.

A Necessary Choice in the Absence of Adequate Health Resources

Faced with the major problems that have involved the medical and nursing classes in the recent pandemic, a few completely unprecedented decisions have to be taken: which infected patients have priority in treatments, for medical care and for final or fatal measures?

Medical and political experts predicted that the numbers of coronavirus cases would drastically exceed the reception capacities of hospitals in many parts of the world. Doctors and nurses have also to face the prospect of selecting which patients should have priority for treatment. These decisions are contrary to everything that medical professionals stand for and are exceedingly painful. Deciding who to treat is an ethical dilemma raising far-reaching moral questions. This issue has been discussed in various publications.

---

[23] Deslandes et al. (2020).

[24] Berlin et al. (2020).

[25] Gandhi et al. (2020).

Serafini E.[26] asked: "Who does one save during a pandemic if not everyone can be cured, according to medical ethics?"

The Hippocratic Oath is brought to mind… and fortunately! Serafini concludes: "The emergency must not lead to the loss of the right, even if ruthless, clarity of ethical principles, waiting for the political class to question how to avoid, in the future, having to respond to the dilemma of choosing between the life and death of a citizen."

Romeo N. (see Footnote 26) "In Italy, infections rose rapidly to such an extent that doctors are responsible for assessing the appropriate treatments and interventions depending on the facilities available." Deciding who to treat therefore poses a heavy ethical dilemma.

According to the director of the Stanford Center for Biomedical Ethics, there are theories on how to make ethical "triage" decisions: egalitarianism, utilitarianism and prioritization. "Triage is terrible, it's traumatizing and doctors who have dedicated their careers to helping people now have to push people away. It's terrible."

Welch D. (see Footnote 26) The Australian government, noting increasing numbers of cases of contagion, has provided no guidelines for doctors working on the front line, who may be obliged to make difficult decisions regarding patients in critical conditions.

Minnelli C. (see Footnote 26) "Italy is one of the most affected European countries. In the northern regions, where a worrying number of infections have been found, the ever-increasing demand for care and attention has exceeded and undermined the hospital resources available at the time." Professionals had to assign priority to those patients who were most likely to survive. Together with the need to allocate the necessary financial resources, the analysis insists on the importance of an ethical perspective that did not leave the burden of these difficult choices solely to doctors.

Predictions for the Next Treatment[27,28]

A large part of society has responded positively to the more stringent impositions of the health authorities and has accepted the difficulties deriving from home isolation, quarantine, the use of masks, social allocation, temporary restrictions on movement or "leisure." There is now substantial debate about a vaccine, and a valid

[26] Serafini (2020), Romeo (2020), Welch (2020), and Mannelli (2020).

[27] Biskup and Prewitt (2020), Young (2020), Delbert (2020), Grein et al. (2020), Sahly et al. (2020), Gandhi (2020), Baden and Rubin (2020), Crist (2020b), Hussey and Budwick (2020), Preidt (2020a), Caddy (2020), Sax (2020), and Reinberg (2020).

[28] Astore et al. (2021).

pharmaceutical remedy still needs to be confirmed. A variety of guidelines and indications have been suggested anyhow.[29,30]

One strategy involves the use of plasma from infected and subsequently healed individuals. Together with the corpuscular portion, their plasma also contains the antibodies formed in response to exposure to the virus. These antibodies, injected into infected people, can antagonize the virus itself and block its spread and replication. Pharmacological possibilities are also being investigated, and the best results were initially obtained with the drug Remdesivir. Alternative therapies are discussed below.

A Few Further Notes

In addition to the general information, however, summary and constantly evolving, regarding the situation of cases and deaths, the distribution of the effects of COVID-19 in the world population is regularly reported, and some particularities of the current pandemic and conclusions relating to the medical ethics of the pandemic are briefly commented here, although obviously purely preliminary.

The information related to COVID-19 at the time of writing cannot be offered as a definitive analysis of the information that will surely be forthcoming in the next few years.

Forecasts: COVID-19: Certain and Uncertain Aspects of the Pandemic[31]

Two years after its discovery, SARS-COV-2 has been extensively studied, but its progenitor which allowed the spillover to humans, is still not known.[32]

How SARS-CoV-2 evolves over the coming months and years will determine the course of this global crisis, we do not know for sure whether the virus will turn into

[29] Circolare del Ministero della salute (IT: Circular from the Ministry of Health) March 9, 2020.

COVID-19. Aggiornamento della definizione di caso. (IT. Case definition updated) 0007922-09/03/2020-DGPR.

Circolare del Ministero della salute (IT: Circular from the Ministry of Health) Feb. 29, 2020. Linee di indirizzo assistenziali del paziente critico affetto da COVID-19. (IT. Guidelines for the care of the critically ill patient affected by COVID-19) 0002619-29/02/2020-GAB-GAB-P, Circolare del Ministero della salute (IT. Circular from the Ministry of Health) Feb 22, 2020.

COVID-2019. Nuove indicazioni e chiarimenti. (IT: COVID-2019. New indications and clarifications) 0005443-22/02/2020-DGPRE-DGPRE-P.

WHO announces COVID-19 outbreak a pandemic. March 12, 2020.

Collins (2020), Fagiuoli et al. (2020), and Wikipedia (2020).

Wikipedia, COVID-19 pandemic in Italy.

Rosenbaum (2020).

[30] Qui Finanza (2020a, b).

[31] Spriano (2022).

[32] May (2021).

something more threatening, almost eight billion vaccine doses have been delivered worldwide, and are changing the evolutionary landscape of the virus, but we have no way to predict the outcome.[33]

Vaccination Strategies: Serious Disease and Equity

So far, most COVID-19 vaccines have effectively prevented severe forms for all previous variants, including hospitalization and death, as this efficacy may depend mainly on T cell immune responses,[34] So far all the vaccines against COVID-119 are proving extremely safe and it is therefore hoped that, in the short term, everyone should be vaccinated.

Since it first appeared SARS-CoV-2 continues to surprise the scientific world, leaving many questions open for the 2022 research agenda:

In which populations will new variants arise?
What is the susceptibility to infection of vaccinated people compared to that of unvaccinated people?
Are breakthrough infections less transmissible and what are their phenotypic characteristics?
Can infections arise for different specific immune profiles and -specific viral strains?
How long does natural and vaccine immunity last, in terms of clinical protection and infection?[35]

New Variants

Some variants of the virus initially described have followed and others are still being further identified. The best-known variants identified to date are:[36]

- Alpha, considered by the WHO as a variant of concern (VOC), was first identified in Kent in the UK in September 2020 and triggered the UK's second wave of pandemic;
- Beta: First identified in South Africa in May 2020, Beta is also considered a VOC by the WHO;
- Gamma was first identified in Manaus, Brazil in November 2020 and is another WHO VOC. For the time being it is still the dominant variant in South America.
- Delta, the now dominant VOC in Europe and the United States continues to cause sharp rises in cases across much of Asia, including Bangladesh, Iran, Iraq,

[33] Callaway (2021).

[34] Karim et al. (2021).

[35] McIntyre et al. (2022).

[36] www.bmj.com; www.ecdc.europa.eu.

Japan, Kazakhstan, Malaysia, Myanmar, Pakistan, South Korea, Thailand, Vietnam, and India, where it was identified in October 2020;
- Delta plus: the Delta variant is also emerging with a mutation of the spike protein K417N, which was reported on 23 July 2020 in England (45 cases);
- Eta: Cases have been found in 72 countries including the UK and Nigeria, where it was first detected in December 2020;
- Iota: First identified in New York, USA, in November 2020, it has now been reported in 53 countries;
- Kappa: First detected in India in October 2020, it has now been reported in 55 countries;
- Lambda: First identified in Peru in December 2020, Lambda became the dominant variant within 3 months, accounting for 80% of all cases, It has been detected in 41 countries;
- Omicron: This variant was first isolated in samples collected on 11 November 2021 in Botswana and on November 14 in South Africa; by 22 December 2021 it had been isolated in 110 countries.

Epidemiological data supported the hypothesis that Omicron's rise was largely due to its ability to infect people immune to Delta through vaccination or previous infection. Certainly how SARS-CoV-2 evolves in response to immunity will have strong implications for its transition to the viral endemic.

COVID Vaccines

How Many and What COVID Vaccines Are There Around the World?

Vaccination is perhaps the only strategy to put an end to the COVID-19 pandemic. The only real hope for the current year lies entirely in the efficacy of the vaccines developed in such a short time against SARS-CoV-2. Unfortunately, this hope has been weakened in recent months by a new emergency: the circulation of multiple variants of the new coronavirus (see above) which probably leaves people less susceptible to the disease.

In Italy today there are four vaccines against COVID-19: Pfizer, Moderna, Vaxzevria (Astrazeneca), and Janssen (J&J). The American Food and Drug Administration (FDA) and the European Medicines Agency (EMA), however, are also examining the other vaccines against the new coronavirus. COVID-19, in fact, has caused an emergency that is slimming the bureaucracy required for obtaining authorization, All this was possible thanks to the identification of the best target of SARS-CoV-2, or the protein that constitutes the spike (S), to ensure an effective immune response against the pathogen.

The immune response obtained thanks to vaccines is characterized by:

- the production of neutralizing antibodies;

- a response mediated by T lymphocytes;
- the absence of diseases developing due to the antibodies produced by the vaccine (ADE).

These are the most widely licensed vaccines in various countries or in clinical trials:

- Sputnik V, whose technical name is Gam-COVID-Vac, was developed in Russia and is based on viral vectors such as that of J&J and AstraZeneca.
- CoronaVac, BBI-CorV, and WIBP: Sinovac and Sinopharm are two Chinese companies specialized in the production of vaccines based on inactivated viruses.
- NVX-CoV2373 or Nuvaxovid, produced by Novavax, a US company, is based on recombinant proteins.
- CVnCoV, developed by the German CureVac, is a messenger RNA vaccine, like those from Pfizer and Moderna.
- Vidprevtyn is produced by the French pharmaceutical company Sanofi Pasteur. This vaccine against COVID-19 is protein-based: it contains the recombinant Spike protein, grown in the laboratory, and an adjuvant.
- Convidicea: Ad5-nCoV, a vaccine against COvid-19 produced by the Chinese company CanSino Biologics, is based on a viral vector similar to that developed by AstraZeneca.
- Soberana and Abdala: these Cuban vaccines are still at various stages of independent research, politics and proved evidence of efficacy. Unofficial data show high efficacy rates and low costs; nevertheless WHO denies approval due to low production standards.

Medical Resources[37]

The new forms of pandemic have raised important ethical concerns as it causes serious damage to a significant number of people and can potentially overwhelm routine clinical services. In addition to age, doctors and health personnel have been advised to take into account the general health status of patients, particularly comorbidities, This is partly because early studies of the virus suggested that patients with pre-existing serious health conditions were significantly more likely to die.

The complex ethical situation associated with the allocation of scarce healthcare resources has involved all state and local structures. The advantages and disadvantages of the various health aims envisaged have been carefully debated. The results are based on data from 149 countries and regions. These findings can be used to support policy decisions as countries prepare to impose or revoke physical distancing measures in current or future epidemic waves.

[37] Emanuel et al. (2020), Ranney et al. (2020), and Rosenbaum (2020).

COVID-19 and Medical Ethics

Health officials need to consider taking steps to increase supplies and their allocation. Some brief but significant documents have been published.[38]

WHO Working Group on Ethics and COVID-19.

WHO has established an international Working Group on Ethics and COVID-19 in order to develop advice on key ethical questions that Member States need to address. Since its formation in February 2020, the group has been engaged in the following activities:

Advice on ethical considerations in COVID-19 research

Practical guidance on the application of ethical values central to COVID-19 research published in the journal "Public Health Ethics"

A policy on resource allocation and priority setting in COVID-19 care

Ethics input into the WHO's Clinical Management Guidelines and training

Feedback provided on the Solidarity Trial protocol Development of emergency standard operating procedures for human research committees to facilitate a review of protocols during the COVID-19 pandemic. Advice on the criteria that must be satisfied for SARS-CoV-2 challenge studies to be ethically acceptable

In Conclusion: Ethical Priorities

Blockade measures have helped reduce the number of COVID-19 cases in countries around the world, together with previously envisaged and imposed restrictions, such as school closures and the now well-known practices of limiting mass gatherings and the need for personal hygiene. Their combination has played a significant role in reducing cases of contamination and death. However, these rules, due to their incomplete acceptance and the difficulties of control, have not always gained the public's trust and therefore have not proved truly effective for a response to the pandemic.[39]

New medical and ethical issues will emerge that will shift the existing urgencies.

Many ethics experts have asked physicians to contribute to these guidelines and research on these topics. There is widespread conviction that ethics has a role in evaluating the issues involved in maximizing benefits during a public health emergency, and in response to the question of which issues are the most pressing, which have been overlooked, and which are the most complex, a substantial ethical contribution was needed.

The ethical implications of resource allocation are at the heart of the current COVID-19 pandemic. Doctors may be obliged to choose which life to save by deciding who to admit to intensive care. In this scenario healthcare decisions take on great ethical importance. In addition to the four general principles, often reported

[38] Agolia et al. (2022), Beigel et al. (2020), Crist (2020c, d), and Doheny (2020).

[39] Preidt (2020b).

and discussed (autonomy, non-maleficence, charity, and justice), there are many other, more specific ethical considerations, such as how to maximize benefits and what social and instrumental values to assign. Policy decisions must be established and implemented by public health officials. As a result, the appropriate facilities work with state and local health departments and hospitals to ensure consistent triage processes.

Actual needs will certainly broadly modify the care and assistance offered to patients in hospital or even at home.[40]

COVID-19 has raised many ethical issues since the start of the pandemic. Most of these have focused on issues relating to the treatment of large numbers of affected people in intensive care units. As the pandemic began, it quickly became apparent that, with the "lockdown" intensive care units could come under severe pressure. Doctors and ethics specialists soon began to develop guidelines and research to prioritize these emergency situations. Many routine medical practices have had to slow down, and some have actually stopped.

For example, in the light of the assault of COVID-19, some hospital patients had to be moved to intensive care from other wards, with substantial malaise and costs for patients not affected by the coronavirus. The excess death tolls among these other patients—whose necessary routine care had often to be postponed—may even have exceeded those of victims killed by the virus. For example, organ transplantation stalled, leading to increased mortality among those waiting for organs, and some cancer screening services also completely stopped. Hardly any documents have dealt with these important topics or with the increased risk of death among ethnic minorities, socio/economically disadvantaged.

Many ethics experts have asked physicians to contribute to these guidelines and research on these topics. There is widespread conviction that ethics has a role in evaluating the issues involved in maximizing benefits during a public health emergency, and in response to the question of which issues are the most pressing, which have been overlooked, and which are the most complex, a substantial ethical contribution was needed.

And finally, in the light of the most recent situation, I can only conclude by stating, on a personal basis:

> *Viruses know no defeats and, to counter the scientific remedies of the moment, they know how to change so as to replicate from individual to individual to gain unconscious supremacy without warlike warnings,*
>
> *The breadth of the shield embraced by man, in defense of the occasion, has contours and consistency dictated by scientific experience already gained, by the expertise and dedication of the health personnel involved, and by the need to observe the dictates that medical ethics of the past and present prescribe.*
>
> *It is not easy to conclude this chapter, which was mainly intended solely for information, as the pandemic is still ongoing and continues to claim victims and arouse continuous, and never disregarded, concerns and proposals for solution. It is not easy, as I said, and right now apparently impossible,*

[40] Shaw (2020).

Therefore, to conclude, we can only hope that the many problems existing in this sector will soon be relegated to an obsolete chapter in the history of medicine. The history of medicine, with all its meanings, is after all infinite.

References

Agolia J, Bayefsky M, Bharadwaj M, et al. Soled D, editor. Module 8: medical ethics in relation to COVID-19. 2022. https://www.ama-assn.org/topics/covid-19-ethics-guidance.

Anderson RM, May RM. Infectious diseases of humans. Dynamics and controls. Oxford: Oxford University Press; 1991.

Astore C, Zhou H, Jacob J, et al. Previsione di eventi avversi gravi, modalità di azione e trattamenti farmacologici per le complicanze di COVID-19. (IT. Prediction of serious adverse events, mode of action, and pharmacologic treatments for complications of COVID-19). Rappresentazione scientifica. 2021;11:20864.

Baden LR, Rubin EJ. COVID-19—the search for effective therapy. N Engl J Med. 2020;382:1851–2.

Barry JM. Viruses of mass destruction. FORTUNE Magazine, November 1, 2004.

Beigel JH, Tomashek KM, Dodd LE, et al. Remdesivir for the treatment of Covid-19, preliminary report. 2020. https://doi.org/10.1056/NEJMoa2007764.

Berlin DA, Gulick RM, Martinez FJ. Severe COVID-19. N Engl J Med. 2020;383(25):2451–60. https://doi.org/10.1056/NEJMcp2009575.

Biskup E, Prewitt E. NEJM Catalyst. 2020;1(3).

Browne S. Profezie. (IT. Prophecies). Milano: Ed. Oscar Mondadori; 2006. p. 220.

Burioni R. Virus. Milano: Ed. Rizzoli; 2020. p. 83–108.

Caddy S. Developing a vaccine for COVID-19. BMJ. 2020;369:m1790.

Callaway E. Beyond Omicron: what's next for COVID's viral evolution. Nature. 2021;600:204–7.

CBHD Staff. Coronavirus: explanations and ethical issues. Deerfield, IL: The Center for Bioethics Human Dignity, Trinity International University; 2020.

Chow N, et al. Preliminary estimates of the prevalence of selected underlying health conditions among patients with coronavirus disease, 2019—United States, February 12–March 28, 2020. Morb Mortal Wkly Rep. 2020;69(13):382–6.

Collins P. Claims of a weaker COVID-19 virus disputed. WebMD Health News, June 3, 2020.

Crist C. COVID-19 may have spread in China in August. WebMD News Brief, June 9, 2020a.

Crist C. COVID-19 treatment could get approval by September. WebMD Health News Brief, June 12, 2020b.

Crist C. COVID-19 shutdowns saved millions of lives. WebMD News Brief, June 9, 2020c.

Crist C. COVID-19 may have spread in China in August. WebMD News Brief, June 10, 2020d.

Cubeta RL, Shuster CE, Smith S. New models for a new disease: simulating the 2019 novel coronavirus. Alexandria: Institute for Defense Analyses; 2020.

Delbert C. How social distancing can defeat coronavirus. Popular Mechanics, March 13, 2020.

Deslandes A, Berti V, et al. SARS-CoV-2 was already spreading in France in late December 2019. Int J Antimicrob Agents. 2020;55(6):106006.

Doheny K. COVID-19 vaccine: latest updates. WebMD Health News, June 11, 2020.

DuVal G, Gensler G, Danis M. Ethical dilemmas encountered by clinical researchers. J Clin Ethics. 2005;16(3):267–76.

Emanuel EJ, Persad G, Upshur R, et al. Fair allocation of scarce medical resources in the time of COVID-19. N Engl J Med. 2020;382:2049–55.

Fagiuoli S, Lorini FL, Remuzzi G. Adaptations and lessons in the province of Bergamo. N Engl J Med. 2020;382:e71.

Fauci AS, Clifford Lane H, Redfield RR. COVID-19. Navigating the uncharted. N Engl J Med. 2020;382:1268–9.

Gandhi RT. Combination therapy for COVID-19. Lancet. 2020.

Gandhi RT, Lynch JB, del Rio C. Mild or moderate COVID-19. N Engl J Med. 2020;383(18):1757–66.
Gostin LO, Bayer R, Fairchild AL. Ethical and legal challenges posed by severe acute respiratory syndrome. JAMA. 2003;290(24):3229–37.
Grady C, Ramjee G, et al. Ethical and legal issues in infectious disease research and control. Emerg Infect Dis. 2001;7(7):534.
Grein J, Ohmagari N, et al. Compassionate use of remdesivir for patients with severe COVID-19. N Engl J Med. 2020;382:2327–36.
Hussey C, Budwick D. Moderna announces positive interim phase 1 data for its mRNA vaccine (mRNA-1273) against novel coronavirus, 2020.
ISS Bioethics COVID-19 Working Group. Ethical aspects of anti-COVID-19 vaccine trials. Version of February 18, 2021. Rome: Istituto Superiore di Sanità; 2021. (ISS COVID-19 Report No. 3/2021—Original in Italian).
Karim SSA, et al. Omicron SARS-CoV-2 variant: a new chapter in the COVID-19 pandemic. Lancet. 2021;398:2126–8. https://doi.org/10.1016/S0140-6736(21)02758-6.
Lauer SA, et al. The incubation period of coronavirus disease 2019 (COVID-19) from publicly reported confirmed cases: estimation and application. Ann Intern Med. 2020;172(9):577–82.
Leung GM, Bhutta ZA, Matzoso MP, et al. COVID-19: how a virus is turning the world upside down. BMJ. 2020;369:m1336.
Lodish H, Berk A, Zipursky SL, et al. Molecular cell biology. 4th ed. New York: W. H. Freeman; 2000.
Mannelli C. Whose life to save? Scarce resources allocation in the COVID-19 outbreak. J Med Ethics. 2020;46(6):364–6.
Masters PS. The molecular biology of coronaviruses. Adv Virus Res. 2006;66:193–292.
May M. Eight unanswered questions about the COVID-19 pandemic. Nat Med. 2021;27:2058–61. https://doi.org/10.1038/s41591-021-01598-x.
McIntyre PB, et al. COVID-19 vaccine strategies must focus on severe disease and global equity. Lancet. 2022;399(10322):406–10. https://doi.org/10.1016/S0140-6736(21)02835-X.
McIvor J. The ethics of infectious disease control: lessons from the Ebola outbreak and an ethical framework. Thesis, Victoria University of Wellington; 2016.
Moriyama M, Hugentobler WJ, Iwasaki A. Seasonality of respiratory viral infections. Annu Rev Virol. 2020;7:83–101.
OMS, World Health Organization. Ten threats to global health in 2019; 2019.
Osterholm MT. Preparing for the next pandemic. N Engl J Med. 2005;352:1839–42.
Preidt R. Face masks can help prevent viral spread. HealthDay News, May 22, 2020a.
Preidt R. Have lockdowns worked to control coronavirus? HealthDay News, July 16, 2020b.
Quammen D. Spillover. L'evoluzione delle pandemie. (IT. The evolution of pandemics). Milano: Adelphi Ed.; 2012.
Qui Finanza. Coronavirus, la situazione in Italia: la mappa dei nuovi focolai. (IT. Here finance. Coronavirus, the situation in Italy: the map of the new outbreaks), 2020a.
Qui Finanza. Coronavirus, scoperto il ceppo più diffuso in Italia: non è quello di Wuhan. (IT. Here finance. Coronavirus, the most widespread strain in Italy discovered: it is not that of Wuhan), 2020b.
Ranney ML, Griffeth V, Jha AK. Critical supply shortages—the need for ventilators and personal protective equipment during the COVID-19 pandemic. N Engl J Med. 2020;382:e41.
Reinberg S. COVID survivor blood transfusion a safe treatment. WebMD, Wesinghouse June 4, 2020.
Ren L-L, Wang Y-M, et al. Identification of a novel coronavirus causing severe pneumonia in human: a descriptive study. Chin Med J. 2020;133(9):1015–24.
Romeo N. The grim ethical dilemma of rationing medical care, explained, Vox.com, USA, Pub. March 31, 2020.
Rosenbaum L. Facing COVID-19 in Italy—ethics, logistics, and therapeutics on the epidemic's front line. N Engl J Med. 2020;382:1873–5.
Rubin EJ, Harrington DP, et al. The urgency of care during the COVID-19—pandemic learning as we go. N Engl J Med. 2020;82(25):2461–2.

Sahly HM, et al. Convalescent plasma has potential utility for managing COVID-19. JAMA Journal Watch, 2020.
Sax PE. Dexamethasone improves survival in COVID-19. NEJM Journal Watch, June 21, 2020.
Selgelid MJ. Ethics and infectious disease. Bioethics. 2005;19(3):272–89.
Selgelid MJ, McLean A, Arinaminpathy N, Savulescu J, editors. Infectious disease ethics—limiting liberty in contexts of contagion. Berlin: Springer; 2011.
Serafini E. Chi salvare durante una pandemia se non si possono curare tutti, secondo l'etica medica. (IT. Who to save during a pandemic if everyone cannot be cured, according to medical ethics). The Post Internazionale, March 27, 2020.
Shaw D. Triaging ethical issues during a pandemic: a rough guide. Basel: Institute for Biomedical Ethics; 2020.
Shors T. Understanding viruses. Sudbury: Jones and Bartlett Publishers; 2008.
Smith MW. WebMD Health News Reviewed, June 8, 2020a.
Smith MW. WebMD Health News Reviewed, coronavirus and COVID-19: what you should know, June 12, 2020b.
Spriano P. COVID-19: aspetti certi e incerti della pandemia. (IT: COVID-19: certain and uncertain aspects of the pandemic) Uniflash, 2022.
Upshur REG. Ethics and infectious disease. Bull World Health Org. 2008;86(8):654.
Welch D. Critical decisions about who will live or die during the coronavirus peak may be left to frontline doctors. ABC Investigations (Australia), Pub. April 5, 2020.
Weston D, Hauck K, Amlôt R. Infection prevention behaviour and infectious disease modeling: a review of the literature and recommendations for the future. BMC Public Health. 2018;18:336.
Wikipedia. Coronavirus pandemic in Italy; 2020.
Willis E. A cure worse than disease. Hist Today. 2020;70(3):22–4.
Young K. COVID-19: social distancing through 2022?/Infection in healthcare workers. NEJM Journal Watch, April 14, 2020.